ONCOLOGY NURSING REVIEW

ONCOLOGY NURSING REVIEW

SECOND EDITION

Connie Henke Yarbro, RN, MS, FAAN

Clinical Associate Professor
Division of Hematology/Oncology
Adjunct Clinical Assistant Professor
Sinclair School of Nursing
Editor, *Seminars in Oncology Nursing*
University of Missouri–Columbia
Columbia, Missouri

Margaret Hansen Frogge, RN, MS

Vice President, Strategic Development
and System Integration
Riverside Health Care
Kankakee, Illinois

Assistant Professor of Nursing
Rush University College of Nursing
Rush-Presbyterian-St. Luke's Medical Center
Chicago, Illinois

Michelle Goodman, RN, MS

Oncology Clinical Nurse Specialist
Rush Cancer Institute
Assistant Professor of Nursing
Rush University College of Nursing
Rush-Presbyterian-St. Luke's Medical Center
Chicago, Illinois

Jones and Bartlett Publishers

Sudbury, Massachusetts
BOSTON • TORONTO • LONDON • SINGAPORE

World Headquarters
Jones and Bartlett Publishers
40 Tall Pine Drive
Sudbury, MA 01776
978-443-5000
info@jbpub.com
www.jbpub.com

Jones and Bartlett Publishers Canada
2406 Nikanna Road
Mississauga, ON L5C 2W6
CANADA

Jones and Bartlett Publishers International
Barb House, Barb Mews
London W6 7PA
UK

Production Credits
Acquisitions Editor: Penny Glynn
Editor: John Danielowich
Production Editor: Linda DeBruyn
Vice President of Manufacturing and Inventory: Therese Bräuer
Editorial and Production Service: Innovation Publication Services
Cover Design: Dick Hannus
Text Design: Connie Leavitt, Bookwrights
Printing and Binding: Courier

Library of Congress Cataloging-in-Publication Data
Yarbro, Connie Henke.
  Oncology nursing review / Connie Henke Yarbro, Margaret Hanson Frogge, Michelle Goodman.—2nd ed.
    p. ; cm.—(Jones and Bartlett series in oncology)
  ISBN 0-7637-1635-9 (pbk.)
    1. Cancer—Nursing—Outlines, syllabi, etc. I. Frogge, Margaret Hansen. II. Goodman, Michelle. III. Title. IV. Series.
  [DNLM: 1. Neoplasms—nursing—Esamination Questions. 2. Neoplasms—nursing—Outlines.   WY 18.2 Y26o 2000]
  RC266.0565 2000
    610.73'698—dc21   00-062735

Cover illustration: Dick Hannus

Printed in the United States of America
04 03 02 01 00   10 9 8 7 6 5 4 3 2 1

CONTENTS

v

INTRODUCTION

Oncology Nursing Review is a comprehensive book and CD-ROM learning package that will help you review content related to oncology nursing and cancer care. From the authors of the authoritative *Cancer Nursing Principles and Practice* (5th ed.), this text contains 1,000 multiple-choice questions as well as five practice tests on the companion web site. Each question has an accompanying answer.

Organization

The book is organized into eight chapters corresponding to the areas tested on the Oncology Nursing Certification examination. The chapters include:

1. Quality of Life
2. Protective Mechanisms
3. Gastrointestinal and Urinary Function
4. Cardiopulmonary Function
5. Oncologic Emergencies
6. Scientific Basis for Practice
7. Health Promotion
8. Professional Performance

Each chapter represents an important content area in oncology nursing. The chapters are further divided into subsections to facilitate study of major topics within these areas.

How to Use the Book

There are two approaches to using *Oncology Nursing Review.* If you are just beginning to review the subject matter, you will probably want to spend more time with the book questions before you attempt the practice tests. If you are further along in your study, the practice tests and accompanying self-assessment can help you identify areas that need further review.

If you are just beginning to review, we recommend that you work through a small section at a time, reading the question and recording the answer. Then consult the correct answers and the explanations. Read the explanations both for the answers that you got correct and for those that you missed. You may find additional information presented that will augment your knowledge base and clarify points that you may have overlooked or misunderstood. If you answer a question incorrectly, consult *Cancer Nursing Principles and Practice* (5th ed.) and *Cancer Symptom Management* (2nd ed.) for more information.

About the Accompanying Web Site

The companion web site that accompanies this book is a useful learning tool that contains five practice exams. To access the web site, please to to http://onr.jbpub.com/ and follow the instructions on the screen.

When prompted for your pass code, enter 2A68X8HT.

Each practice exam, containing 200 questions, allows you to time yourself in preparation for the actual test. Allow three and a half hours to complete the test and check your answers. Your performance will give you a good idea of your knowledge of key content areas and your ability to function under time pressure.

Finding Out About Certification Requirements

If you want to obtain the Oncology Nursing Certification, it is important for you to contact the certifying organization, the Oncology Nursing Certification Corporation (ONCC). The ONCC publishes a *Test Bulletin,* which we suggest that you acquire. This bulletin provides important information about certification including test dates, application deadlines, test center locations, eligibility criteria, and information about the test itself, as well as sample questions.

You can contact the ONCC through its web site, www.oncc.org; via E-mail at oncc@ons.org; by telephone at (412) 921-8597; by fax at (412) 928-0926; or by mail at 501 Holiday Drive, Pittsburgh, Pa. 15220-2749.

QUALITY OF LIFE

COMFORT

Pain

1.1   Which of the following processes associated with the occurrence of pain is considered vague and subjective in that it encompasses complex behavioral, psychological, and emotional factors?
a.   transduction
b.   transmission
c.   modulation
d.   perception

1.2   The transdermal route of narcotic administration was first used with which opioid?
a.   methadone
b.   fentanyl
c.   morphine
d.   levorphanol

1.3   An example of counterirritant cutaneous stimulation is:
a.   subcutaneous administration of morphine
b.   minor surgery
c.   massage
d.   imagery

1.4   Directing one's attention away from the sensations and emotional reactions produced by pain is known as:
a.   distraction
b.   biofeedback
c.   autogenic relaxation
d.   hypnosis

1.5   The dimension of pain that encompasses the meaning that the pain experience has for a person is the:
   a.   behavioral dimension
   b.   affective dimension
   c.   sensory dimension
   d.   cognitive dimension

1.6   Of the following, which population is statistically likely to have the highest prevalence of pain?
   a.   patients in a hospice setting
   b.   patients in the general ward
   c.   patients in the early stages of illness
   d.   pediatric patients

1.7   Which of the following is *not* a common obstacle to successful pain management?
   a.   inaccurate knowledge about pharmacological principles
   b.   a lack of basic assessment skills
   c.   a lack of available knowledge in the field
   d.   legal impediments

1.8   Assessment of behavioral parameters in cancer pain includes an evaluation of:
   a.   the quality of the pain
   b.   associated psychologic problems
   c.   the effect of pain on activities of daily living
   d.   the duration of the pain

1.9   During a return visit to a man with metastatic prostate cancer to the ribs, the home health nurse notes that he is in pain and has not been receiving the morphine at the increased frequency prescribed 48 hours earlier. The wife is visibly upset at his discomfort, yet is concerned about his increased lethargy when the drug interval was first changed. The nurse's interventions at this point would be directed at:
   a.   explaining to the wife that increasing the frequency of the drug is what probably gave him some pain relief and his sleep was a sign that he was comfortable
   b.   empathizing with the wife over her concerns that the decreased drug interval was a sign that her husband was becoming addicted
   c.   congratulating the wife for being astute enough to recognize that the drug was building up in his system
   d.   changing the pain regimen to include a different narcotic

Fatigue

1.10   Which of the following is considered to be the most common side effect of cancer treatment?
   a.   nausea
   b.   vomiting
   c.   fatigue
   d.   pain

1.11   Subjectively defined fatigue has a/an _____ component, which differentiates it from weakness.
   a.   involuntary
   b.   voluntary
   c.   initiation
   d.   duration

1.12 Why are the possible cumulative effects of multiple surgical procedures important to those studying cancer-related fatigue?
    a. Fatigue is a consistent finding in patients who are recovering from surgery.
    b. It is not unusual for patients to undergo several surgical procedures for diagnosis and treatment of cancer.
    c. Both a and b are true.
    d. Neither a nor b is true.

1.13 Based on modality of treatment, which of your patients would you expect to have the most severe fatigue?
    a. Joe, who is being treated with biologic response modifiers
    b. Karen, who is undergoing chemotherapy
    c. Martha, who has just had surgery
    d. Thomas, who is undergoing radiation treatment

1.14 Which statement is true of individuals who have suffered from cancer-related fatigue once they have completed treatment?
    a. Fatigue will disappear almost immediately upon the conclusion of treatment.
    b. Fatigue may gradually fade after the treatment is finished.
    c. Fatigue absolutely should improve upon the completion of treatment.
    d. The use of assistive devices and systematic planning of activities should be unnecessary upon completion of treatment.

1.15 Mary says that she has been feeling tired for several weeks now. She finds it difficult to concentrate, and she does not have the energy to perform simple chores around the house. She still walks her dog and swims twice a week at the YWCA, but she feels very drained afterward. She's tried getting more sleep, but that does not seem to be helping. Mary is probably experiencing:
    a. acute fatigue
    b. chronic fatigue
    c. weakness
    d. depression

1.16 You see a colleague assessing his patient, Mark, for fatigue. He asks Mark about the activities he usually performs, and he gives him several tests for concentration. When you ask your colleague about it later, he says that he is trying to gather a thorough assessment of Mark's fatigue. You suggest:
    a. an exercise endurance test
    b. asking Mark's family for more information
    c. asking Mark to describe his fatigue
    d. choosing an objective indicator

1.17 You have a patient, Karen, who is experiencing some symptoms of anemia and chronic cancer-related fatigue. You ask your colleague, who has studied a great deal of outside information on the topic, what is likely to happen. He tells you to expect that her anemic symptoms will be treated:
    a. with similar expected results for both the anemia and the fatigue
    b. with better expected results for both the anemia and the fatigue
    c. with worse expected results for both the anemia and the fatigue
    d. with only marginal results expected

Pruritus

1.18 Mr. Allen has extensive pancreatic carcinoma with obstructive liver disease, for which he has recently completed radiation therapy. He takes oral morphine for pain. He has just begun to complain about pruritus. What is the *most likely* cause of his itching?
   a. oral morphine
   b. dry desquamation due to radiation
   c. liver disease
   d. all of the above

1.19 Pruritus frequently accompanies jaundice in patients with obstructive biliary disease. Which of the following best describes the mechanism of pruritus under these circumstances?
   a. Itching is primarily due to dry, flaky skin.
   b. Itching is caused by irritation of the cutaneous sensory nerve fibers by accumulated bile salts.
   c. Itching is due to poor body hygiene and the use of deodorant soaps.
   d. Itching is due to the accumulation of cholestyramine.

1.20 Which of the following is *not* effective treatment for pruritus?
   a. meticulous skin hygiene
   b. oil-based lotions and antihistamines
   c. cholestyramine
   d. vitamins A, C, D, and B complex

1.21 Nursing care of the individual with liver cancer involves:
   a. meticulous skin care for pruritus
   b. providing a low-protein, high-fat diet
   c. continuous administration of anticoagulants
   d. assistance with an abdominal binder

1.22 Mr. Marks has Hodgkin's disease. He has recently completed radiation therapy and chemotherapy. His chief complaints include pain, for which he is receiving morphine, and a generalized itching of unknown etiology. The itching is *most likely* due to which of the following?
   a. a systemic symptom related to Hodgkin's disease
   b. a side effect from opiate therapy
   c. dry skin due to radiation therapy
   d. all of the above

1.23 Mr. Elliot presented to the outpatient ambulatory care center with a complaint of recent-onset generalized itching. This itching, or pruritus, could be related to which of the following?
   a. CNS malignancies
   b. Hodgkin's disease
   c. occult metastases
   d. a and b
   e. b and c

1.24 Pruritus occurs in approximately 40% of patients with Hodgkin's disease and is most often associated with advanced disease.
   a. true
   b. false

1.25   Mr. Ely has recently been told he will be starting interleukin-2 (IL-2) therapy as part of a research protocol. Which of the following is *not* considered a side effect of IL-2 therapy?
   a.   moderate hair loss
   b.   moderate to severe itching
   c.   rapid weight gain
   d.   nausea, vomiting, and diarrhea

1.26   Which of the following measures is *not* therapeutic in the management of pruritus?
   a.   maintaining a warm and humid environment
   b.   cimetidine and diphenhydramine
   c.   moisturizing agents such as aquaphor, oil, and oatmeal baths
   d.   oral morphine as needed

Sleep Disorders

1.27   Research into the side effects of chemotherapy indicates that sleeping difficulty is reported by approximately what percentage of individuals?
   a.   50%
   b.   40%
   c.   30%
   d.   20%

1.28   Your patient has been receiving chemotherapy for some time and states that she has no energy to perform even the basic activities of daily living. Your advice to her is to do which of the following?
   a.   She needs to rest more because she needs to save her energy to resist infection.
   b.   Because it is possible that too much rest can exacerbate fatigue, she needs to be encouraged to establish an exercise program that is a balance between rest and activity.
   c.   She should be encouraged to take a sleep aid whenever she is unable to sleep.
   d.   a and c

1.29   According to research, which of the following nonpharmacological measures is *most effective* in relieving fatigue?
   a.   frequent napping
   b.   going to bed earlier
   c.   increasing the number of hours resting or sleeping
   d.   exercise

1.30   Your patient is receiving paclitaxel on a weekly basis. She commonly experiences nausea and is prescribed the antiemetic granisetron to take if she needs it. She complains that she is having trouble sleeping and often feels agitated at night. Which of the following is a logical explanation for her symptoms?
   a.   Her difficulty in sleeping is likely due to the decadron she takes to prevent hypersensitivity reactions to the paclitaxel.
   b.   She is probably feeling agitated due to the granisetron.
   c.   Adverse neurologic effects, including sleep disruption, are common in patients taking paclitaxel.
   d.   Insomnia and restlessness are common in anyone undergoing treatment for cancer.

1.31   Your patient experiences intense nausea and vomiting from chemotherapy and is given a prescription for lorazepam to take with her antiemetics at night. She wants to know why she is being given an antianxiety agent when she does not feel anxious. Your explanation would include which of the following?

    a.   The lorazepam is given to increase the effectiveness of the antinausea pills.

    b.   She probably does not realize how anxious she really is and that it is important to suppress that anxiety before it contributes to her problem.

    c.   The lorazepam is given to induce sleep, which is an important strategy for preventing nausea and vomiting with chemotherapy.

    d.   all the above

1.32   The role of sleep as it relates to the immune system has been studied extensively in recent years. Which of the following statements regarding sleep and its relationship to the immune system is false?

    a.   Sleep functions as an immunorestorative mechanism.

    b.   Growth hormone and prolactin are elevated during sleep.

    c.   Steroid levels, which are immunosuppressive, are reduced during sleep.

    d.   Growth hormone is immunosuppressive.

1.33   Early morning awakening, a form of insomnia, can be an important diagnostic indicator of depression.

    a.   true

    b.   false

1.34   Sleep aids are commonly prescribed to assist patients with insomnia to get to sleep and stay asleep. Which of the following statements regarding the newer nonbenzodiazepine sleep aids is false?

    a.   They suppress delta sleep similar to traditional benzodiazepine sleep aids.

    b.   They have a shorter half-life compared to traditional sleep aids.

    c.   They are likely to cause less feelings of sedation after awakening.

    d.   They are less effective in maintaining a sleep state.

Dyspnea

1.35   Ms. Howe has persistent productive coughing, which, she says, is exhausting. Which intervention should *not* be used?

    a.   Inspired air is warmed and humidified.

    b.   Cigarette smoking is discouraged.

    c.   Deep breathing and coughing techniques are taught and reinforced.

    d.   Narcotic medications are used for cough suppression.

1.36   Mr. Smith has laryngeal carcinoma with regional recurrence. During a routine physical exam you notice that he is experiencing stridor. This is most likely an indication of which of the following?

    a.   extrathoracic airway obstruction

    b.   intrathoracic airway obstruction

    c.   tumor

    d.   a and c

1.37   Mr. Allen has lung cancer and complains that he cannot catch his breath. He is scheduled to have a chest x-ray to determine the etiology of his shortness of breath and dyspnea. Which of the following statements would be accurate counsel for this patient?
   a.   His symptoms are probably due to the side effects of radiation and chemotherapy.
   b.   The chest x-ray will probably show that the tumor has grown, and he should think about palliative care.
   c.   Dyspnea in the person with lung cancer is often associated with pleural effusions, all of which are considered to be malignant.
   d.   If a pleural effusion is found, it is possible to manage the problem with a procedure called pleurodesis.

1.38   Which of the following sclerosing agents are used to manage recurrent pleural effusions?
   a.   bleomycin
   b.   doxorubicin
   c.   tetracycline
   d.   all of the above

1.39   Janis frequently experiences dyspnea due to recurrent pleural effusions. Her doctor has suggested that she have a more permanent device placed into her pleural space to make it easier to drain the fluid from her lung. Which of the following is an accurate description of this device?
   a.   A pleuroperitoneal shunt can be inserted to divert fluid from the chest cavity to the abdomen.
   b.   A pleural port can be implanted underneath the skin just below the ribs, with the catheter resting in the pleural space. The port is accessed with a 19-gauge Huber point needle whenever she complains of difficulty breathing.
   c.   A small-bore catheter may be placed into the pleural space and allowed to drain through a one-way valve by gravity drainage.
   d.   all of the above

1.40   Your patient with advanced lung cancer is experiencing acute dyspnea. You understand that his difficulty breathing is most likely caused by *all but* which of the following?
   a.   destruction of lung tissue by radiation
   b.   pleural effusion
   c.   airway obstruction by tumor
   d.   increased mucus production

1.41   Chest x-ray reveals that Mr. Stanton has a large pleural effusion contributing to his dyspnea and difficulty breathing. Once the fluid is drained, the physician instills a sclerosing agent into the pleural space. In preparing your patient for the procedure, you would be certain to mention *all but* which of the following?
   a.   The purpose of injecting bleomycin into the pleural space is to kill any cancer cells that might be there.
   b.   The procedure is painful, and therefore the patient will be given adequate pain medication prior to the procedure.
   c.   If the fluid reaccumulates, it can be drained again.
   d.   The sclerosing agent is given to obliterate the pleural space.

1.42   Dyspnea is often considered an early sign of cardiac tamponade. Which of the following statements best describes the symptom of dyspnea in a patient experiencing cardiac tamponade?
   a.   Dyspnea is caused by an increased cardiac output.
   b.   Dyspnea is caused by a decrease in lung expansion.
   c.   Dyspnea occurs because of pulmonary congestion.
   d.   all of the above

Fever and Chills

1.43   Mr. Tim has recently received intravesical bacillus Calmette-Guerin (BCG). The evening of his treatment, he calls complaining of nausea and a fever of 101°F. The *most likely* cause of his symptoms is which of the following?
   a.   Fever and nausea are common with BCG treatments, and he should take diphenhydramine and acetaminophen to lessen these symptoms of systemic hypersensitivity.
   b.   His symptoms indicate a possible systemic BCG infection, and he should report to the emergency room as soon as possible.
   c.   Because the BCG is given locally into the bladder, there are no systemic symptoms. He probably has the flu and should take medications to manage the symptoms.
   d.   Bladder infections are common with BCG injections, and he should bring in a urine sample as soon as possible.

1.44   Which of the following signs and symptoms are associated with disseminated BCG infection?
   a.   rash, nausea, and a low-grade fever
   b.   flu-like syndrome and organ dysfunction
   c.   persistent high fever, chills, and diarrhea
   d.   hematuria and dysuria

1.45   Which of the following is considered to be the cardinal symptom of infection?
   a.   pus formation
   b.   inflammation
   c.   fever
   d.   elevated white blood cell count

1.46   Your patient received chemotherapy 6 days ago and has now called with a fever of 101°F and chills. She has a productive cough, and, except for not being able to get warm, feels fine. You send her for a complete blood count and learn that her absolute granulocyte count is 500 cells/mm^3. You instruct her to come to the hospital to be admitted. Your decision is based on which of the following?
   a.   She is at risk for bleeding and severe anemia.
   b.   She probably has pneumonia and needs to be observed.
   c.   When the neutrophil count is 500 or less, approximately 20% or more of febrile episodes have an associated bacteremia.
   d.   She is past her nadir, but cultures need to be done to determine the source of a possible infection.

1.47   Endotoxins are a critical element in shock. Which of the following is *not* a function of endotoxins?
   a.   Endotoxins release endogenous pyrogens.
   b.   Endotoxins cause formation of microthrombi.
   c.   Endotoxins cause increased vasoconstriction and decreased capillary permeability.
   d.   Endotoxins cause the febrile response and activation of the complement, coagulation, and fibrinolytic systems and the release of bradykinin.

1.48 Fever and chills are a common symptom associated with sepsis. What percentage of patients with severe sepsis present with fever and chills?
  a. 38%
  b. 55%
  c. 68%
  d. 95%

1.49 Noah is a patient with testicular cancer who has just begun his 3-day course of aggressive chemotherapy, including cisplatin, etoposide, and bleomycin. During the evening shift, you notice he has spiked a fever and is experiencing chills. The etiology of his fever and chills is likely due to which of the following?
  a. Aggressive chemotherapy is frequently associated with myelosuppression, which presents as fever and chills.
  b. He most likely has a fever related to his recent surgical procedure.
  c. The fever and chills are probably related to the side effects of chemotherapy.
  d. He most likely has a nosocomial infection.

1.50 Your patient has a platelet count of 33,000/mm^3 and has had frequent nose bleeds. He is currently receiving his second platelet transfusion and is complaining of shaking chills and has a fever of 102.4°F. The cause of his chills and fever is *most likely* which of the following?
  a. He has aspiration pneumonia from his nose bleeds.
  b. He is having a transfusion reaction because of contamination of the platelet pack.
  c. Unfiltered platelet concentrates accumulate high levels of cytokines.
  d. His fever is most likely related to his pancytopenia.

1.51 Management of a febrile nonhemolytic transfusion reaction presenting as fever, chills, headache, hypotension, tachypnea, and dyspnea includes *all but* which of the following?
  a. Stop the transfusion and maintain patent IV line with normal saline.
  b. Notify physician and administer acetaminophen for fever, meperidine for chills and rigors, and antihistamine for dyspnea.
  c. Place the patient in the Trendelenburg position and administer a fluid bolus.
  d. Continue the transfusion if symptoms are not severe.

1.52 Which of the following statements regarding tumor fever is *not* accurate?
  a. Tumor fever is considered a paraneoplastic syndrome primarily associated with lymphomas and some solid tumors.
  b. Tumor fever is produced by tumor secretion of one or more pyrogenic cytokines.
  c. Treatment for tumor fever includes antipyretics and broad-spectrum antibiotics.
  d. NSAIDs have been used to distinguish between fever from infection and that caused by tumor.

1.53 Mrs. Andrews has just begun her first dose of Herceptin. One-third of the way through the infusion, she complains of feeling cold. She is experiencing a shaking chill and has a temperature of 101.4°F. Your interventions include *all but* which of the following?
  a. Stop the infusion and notify the physician that the patient is having a reaction to the Herceptin therapy.
  b. Monitor vital signs and administer diphenhydramine and acetamenophen as directed.
  c. Inform the patient that people who react to the Herceptin the first time are more likely to react more intensely with each subsequent treatment.
  d. Resume the infusion at a slower rate when vital signs are stable.

COPING

Spiritual Distress

1.54 Spirituality refers to that dimension of being human that:
a. represents and expresses one's life principle
b. prompts individuals to make sense of their universe and to relate harmoniously with self, nature, and others
c. involves reflecting systematically about right conduct and how to live as a good person
d. all of the above

1.55 Regardless of one's beliefs about religion, some individualized form of _____ prayer is known to be directly correlated with spiritual well-being.
a. petitionary
b. ritualistic
c. conversational
d. none of the above

1.56 The work of reconstructing a worldview to include new, wiser assumptions in response to trauma involves a process of balancing:
a. clarification and summarization
b. approach versus avoidance
c. identifying and appreciating cognitive strategies
d. none of the above

1.57 Which of the following is *not* considered to be a central aspect of spirituality?
a. an integrating energy
b. religiosity
c. a life principle
d. an innate human quality

1.58 Research into spirituality and death reveals many aspects of the relationship between spiritual issues and preparation for death. Which of the following assumptions regarding spirituality and preparation for death is *not* based in research and is considered to be false?
a. There is a direct relationship between spirituality and imminence of death.
b. The closer an individual gets to death, the more she or he will become aware of personal spirituality.
c. Praying, having faith, and hoping are used as coping strategies equally among persons with advanced cancer and those with early-stage cancer.
d. Religious faith or prayer are top-ranked coping strategies among over 80% of cancer survivors.

1.59 Although it is true that oncology nurses hold diverse perspectives about controversial issues such as physician-assisted suicide and active euthanasia, nurses' attitudes regarding end-of-life decisions are most significantly influenced by which of the following?
a. professional integrity
b. sanctity of life
c. personal religiosity
d. patient autonomy

1.60 Mr. Allen is distressed over his wife's apparent anger and rejection of God due to the recent discovery that her breast cancer has recurred. Your efforts to counsel him are based on which of the following cognitive strategies?
   a. Individuals assume that traumatic events such as cancer strengthen one's belief that there is meaning and worth.
   b. Individuals whose world is shattered will work to reconstruct their worldview so that it includes a rationale for God's failings.
   c. Individuals use strategies such as making comparisons to another situation to make the event meaningful.
   d. The nurse helps to construct for the individual a possible meaning for this event.

1.61 Spirituality is best defined by which of the following components?
   a. meaning and motivation
   b. religious beliefs and dogma
   c. ethics and religiousity
   d. self-transcendence and beneficence

Financial Concerns

1.62 Individuals with low annual incomes:
   a. are three to seven times more likely to die of cancer than those with high annual incomes
   b. rarely experience a definable difference in survivorship or treatment outcome based solely on their economic status
   c. are twice as likely to experience recurrence, treatment failure, or death as those with higher annual incomes
   d. none of the above

1.63 The differences in incidence, mortality, and survival among various ethnic groups has been studied, and it has been determined that poverty, not race, accounts for the lower survival rate. Poverty lowers the survival rate among the many ethnic groups by:
   a. 5–10%
   b. 10–15%
   c. 15–20%
   d. 20–25%

1.64 A primary barrier to cancer care for many of the ethnic minority population is:
   a. inability to pay for services
   b. language barrier
   c. cultural differences
   d. access to care

1.65 The growth of managed care and capitation have contributed to:
   a. a dramatic drop in coverage of prevention-oriented services
   b. driving the coverage of preventive services
   c. reduced funding for immunologic studies
   d. fewer elder care provisions

1.66   Rebecca's health plan committee at work has reviewed complaints from employees about their lack of ability to access care outside the present plan if they require a treatment found only in one of their city's two research hospitals. In response, the company switches to a plan that allows members to access out-of-plan providers but imposes strict utilization strategies. This is *most likely* a:
    a. point of service (POS) plan
    b. health maintenance organization (HMO)
    c. physician-hospital organization (PHO)
    d. preferred provider organization (PPO)

1.67   Middle- and upper-class families with adequate health insurance and relatively secure jobs:
    a. can still be excessively burdened by out-of-pocket expenditures for deductibles and copayments
    b. now can expect no gaps in insurance coverage
    c. represent the only segment of the population with no serious concerns about health expenses
    d. b and c

1.68   Nurses may use all of the following to justify needed resources *except*:
    a. feasibility studies
    b. cost-benefit analysis
    c. standards of quality care
    d. cost-effectiveness analyses

1.69   The demand for charity care is steadily increasing at a time when many hospitals have negative operating margins. A significant reason for the increased need for charity care is:
    a. the dramatic growth in ambulatory, hospice, and home care
    b. the number of people who are employed but not covered by employer health insurance
    c. a trend toward reduced Medicare and Medicaid coverage for outpatient services
    d. changes in federal and state guidelines regarding reimbursement to physicians for charity cases

1.70   Along with the quantity and quality of care provided by alternative care settings, the other important factor that influences the selection of a care setting for the cancer patient is:
    a. its proximity to the acute-care hospital
    b. its cost and the patient's financial resources
    c. the professional training of its medical staff
    d. its policies relating to the multidisciplinary team approach

Emotional Distress

1.71   A patient who has just been diagnosed with lung cancer denies the diagnosis and refuses to hear about it. The patient's denial behavior is:
    a. adaptive
    b. maladaptive
    c. value neutral
    d. none of the above

1.72 Two patients have the same stage II lymphoma diagnosis. One is 26; the other is 58. Younger patients report:
   a. less confusion about prognosis and treatment options than their older counterparts
   b. fewer adjustment difficulties in comparison to their older counterparts
   c. greater adjustment difficulties in comparison to their older counterparts
   d. a and b

1.73 In a recent article, a colleague, Richard, writes about the emotional aspects of dealing with a unique patient he worked with last year. In describing the kinds of psychological boundaries he established with this patient, you notice that he has drawn a diagram in which his and the client's boundaries are touching. You realize that his boundaries with this patient were:
   a. rigid; the patient's boundary was not allowed to intersect, or overlap, with Richard's
   b. clear; he was accessible, but did not get mixed up with the patient's personal priorities or goals
   c. diffuse; Richard became enmeshed with the patient and overinvolved
   d. diffuse; his boundaries made a limited intersection with those of the patient, yet Richard managed to keep a "professional" distance

1.74 A 68-year-old woman recently diagnosed with metastatic cancer confesses that she has no one to talk to and feels extremely depressed. She has a history of depressive disorder, but is currently not taking any medication. Your nursing action is based on which of the following?
   a. History of a previous psychiatric diagnosis increases the risk of developing depression after a cancer diagnosis.
   b. Severity of disease is associated with poorer psychological adjustment.
   c. Social networks have been found to increase psychological adjustment.
   d. all of the above

1.75 Which of the following statements regarding decision making in reference to treatment decisions is correct?
   a. The majority of patients prefer to take an active role in making the final selection of treatment.
   b. The majority of patients prefer to take a passive role, allowing the physician to make the final decision about treatment.
   c. The majority of patients prefer to collaborate with the physician in making decisions regarding treatment.
   d. none of the above

1.76 Ten-year-old Liza is to be assessed for possible acute myelogenous leukemia (AML) and acute lymphocytic leukemia (ALL). This proves to be quite a challenge since the two have similar symptoms. Liza has ALL and begins treatment with a combination of vincristine, prednisone, and L-asparaginase. The physician begins to express strong hopes for a remission, but Liza's mother takes you aside and says, "My husband's aunt died of AML at age 40—and she was very robust and athletic! What hope does a mere 10-year-old have? Liza's not exactly robust to begin with, and she's so young." You answer that:
   a. The physician is aware that the prognosis is grimmer when ALL affects children but that psychosocial support for Liza can make a world of difference in survival rate.
   b. Age and athletic ability have been shown to make no difference in the demographics of remission and survival rates in ALL.
   c. Complete remission is achieved in 93% of children with ALL, as opposed to 70–75% in adults.
   d. Remission rates in patients with ALL depend on etiology and stage of disease and are not reflected by age or activity levels.

1.77   Cancer patients who are *most likely* to exhibit psychosocial distress include all of the following *except*:
    a.   those who have been unsuccessful in resolving past stress situations
    b.   those who are dealing with stressors simultaneously
    c.   those who perceive minimal social support in the situation
    d.   those who cope principally through adaptive defense mechanisms

1.78   An example of an emotion-focused nursing intervention that might be used to foster the coping response of a cancer patient would be:
    a.   giving information to the patient about the subjective, environmental, and temporal features of diagnostic and treatment processes
    b.   referring patients for more specialized or intensive therapy
    c.   using role-playing to help the patient understand the impact of personal responses on others
    d.   practicing anticipatory socialization to expected life stressors and processes, such as loss and grief

1.79   Which of the following statements about psychosocial aspects of cancer care is true?
    a.   Denial or minimization may be an effective coping strategy, allowing individuals to assimilate the impact of the illness in manageable increments.
    b.   Psychosocial responses to cancer can be clearly identified as either adaptive or maladaptive.
    c.   A perception of uncertainty in a situation results in an appraisal of danger.
    d.   Distancing behaviors of health professionals are helpful in preventing overinvolvement.

Social Dysfunction

1.80   One dimension that is not as frequently represented in QOL is _____ well-being.
    a.   psychological
    b.   functional
    c.   spiritual
    d.   social

1.81   The QOL dimension of social well-being includes:
    a.   family functioning and intimacy
    b.   religious practices
    c.   positive and negative moods
    d.   all of the above

1.82   Research demonstrates that when patients with low and high levels of information about their disease are compared, which of the following is true?
    a.   Patients who know less about their illness experience less anxiety.
    b.   Patients and their spouses who know little about the disease tend to make conclusions by conjecture.
    c.   Patients and their spouses who know little about the illness tend to experience more denial and isolation as a couple.
    d.   b and c

1.83   As an individual cancer patient faces imminent death, certain losses and changes are experienced. The individual's response to these losses and changes is usually to do which of the following?
    a.   search for immortality
    b.   search for meaning
    c.   search for acceptance
    d.   search for forgiveness

1.84   It is not uncommon for the spouse of a person with cancer to be unwilling to discuss his or her concerns with the person because of fears that it might be distressing to the patient. However this need to "protect" can result in which of the following outcomes?
  a. increased caregiver burden
  b. decreased caregiver burden
  c. increased denial, fear, and isolation
  d. a and c

1.85   The family assessment in home care is *least likely* to include which of the following questions?
  a. What is the pattern of authority at home?
  b. What is the functionality of the caregiver?
  c. How many fire exits are available?
  d. What other support systems are there?

1.86   On conducting a family assessment, the home health care nurse identifies conflict among the family members caring for the patient. Upon inquiry, the nurse learns that the conflict is "not new" and has existed "for years." Using this information, the home health care nurse establishes a plan of care that:
  a. attempts to change the behavior among the family members because the patient is upset by the conflict
  b. involves having psychological services counsel the "conflicting members"
  c. schedules family meetings about how the conflict is affecting the patient and what can be done to resolve it
  d. is sensitive to the feelings of the members in conflict but does not attempt to treat the causes of the conflict

1.87   The psychosocial dimension of cancer care focuses on both the unique needs of the individual at risk for or with cancer and the:
  a. unique needs of other individuals in society
  b. clinical training of health care professionals
  c. social groups affected by that individual
  d. role of specific therapies in cancer treatment

1.88   Which of the following is *not* a strategy for family care?
  a. family-level teaching with respect to the disease, treatment, rehabilitation, and/or prognosis
  b. anticipatory guidance
  c. mobilization of health care and/or community resources
  d. the provision of intensive family therapy to all families of cancer patients

Loss and Grief

1.89   Which of the following grief reactions of an elderly woman who has lost her husband of 40 years would prompt the hospice nurse to suggest counseling?
  a. She takes out 40 years' worth of photograph albums and wants to review her marriage and life with her deceased husband with the hospice nurse.
  b. She refuses to let her sister and brother-in-law into her home anymore, blaming them for buying her husband cigarettes "all those years."
  c. She plans her husband's funeral by herself, listens to all his favorite classical music pieces, and chooses passages from his Bible.
  d. She delegates all the responsibility for disposition of her husband's belongings to the children.

1.90   While describing her sadness about her husband's imminent death, the wife of your patient says, "I have never been able to accept the death of our son, and now my husband is going too." Which of the following is the most appropriate response?
a.   "Do you feel your husband is dying soon?"
b.   "What was it like for you and your husband when your son died?"
c.   "Losing your son and your husband must be so difficult for you."
d.   "At least your son and your husband will be together soon."

1.91   One year following the death of her husband, Mrs. Ely still cries and rarely goes out with friends. As part of bereavement counseling, you conclude which of the following?
a.   This is a normal grief reaction. She could benefit from being seen more often.
b.   This is an example of unresolved grief, which is associated with increased risk of suicide.
c.   Acute grief can last beyond a year, but Mrs. Ely could benefit from a support group.
d.   Grieving beyond a year is often associated with unresolved guilt about the death of a loved one.

1.92   Which of the following tasks is *not* considered crucial to the normal grief process?
a.   acceptance of the reality of the loss
b.   experience the pain of grief
c.   adjust to a new environment where the deceased has never been
d.   withdraw emotional energy and replace it in another relationship

1.93   Which of the following excludes a patient from meeting criteria for hospice care?
a.   The family prefers that the nurse not talk about dying around the patient.
b.   The patient explains that he wants to continue to receive the new monoclonal antibody because he is certain it will be curative.
c.   The doctor orders two units of blood to be given at home along with pamidronate.
d.   The patient explains they are not ready to look at funeral homes.

1.94   A typical reaction of an adolescent following the death of a parent is to:
a.   blame the remaining parent and/or other family members for the parent's death
b.   shield the remaining parent from discussing distressing feelings
c.   withdraw from family relationships during a protracted period of grieving
d.   openly share information and feelings with the remaining parent and other family members

1.95   A deterioration in the relationship between patient and child is *most likely* to occur when the:
a.   relationship is father-son rather than mother-daughter
b.   patient is well adjusted
c.   relationship is father-daughter rather than mother-daughter
d.   prognosis for the patient is poor

1.96   The process by which a grieving person begins to work through part of his or her grief before the patient dies is termed:
a.   final reconciliation
b.   grief premonition
c.   resolution of guilt
d.   anticipatory mourning

Anxiety

1.97 Mr. Jantzen quits smoking. He is very anxious about his risk and asks, "How much will my risk be affected?" You explain that the rate of decline in his risk of developing lung cancer is determined by the cumulative smoking exposure prior to cessation, the age when smoking began, and the:
   a. degree of inhalation
   b. amount of passive smoke previously exposed to
   c. brand of cigarettes smoked
   d. amount of time that has passed since quitting

1.98 Factors that influence health behaviors include knowledge and education level, socio-economic status, race, and:
   a. residential location
   b. marital status
   c. age
   d. employment status

1.99 Alexis, 27, brings her mother Margie, 48, in for a breast exam. Both women have avoided regular medical care because they fear the discovery of problems. During the course of the interview, you discover that neither is familiar with the rationale behind regular BSEs or mammography. As part of your patient education plan, you intend to tell them that:
   a. Alexis should have a breast exam every year but should perform BSE monthly; her mother should do both every 6 months.
   b. Alexis should begin getting mammograms annually. Her mother should get one every 2 years.
   c. Margie is the only one who should be getting BSEs at this time; Alexis will, too, at 30 years of age.
   d. Alexis should have a breast exam every 3 years; Margie, every year.

1.100 Anxiety is defined operationally as an increased level of arousal accociated with vague, unpleasant, and uneasy feelings that occurs in response to a perceived threat. What is the source of this perceived threat?
   a. a nonspecific external stimulus
   b. a specific external stimulus, often a physical threat
   c. a nonspecific internal or external stimulus
   d. a specific internal stimulus, usually pain or inflammation

1.101 Empirical data suggest that anxiety is associated with selected patient outcomes. In one study, for example, women with high anxiety related to breast biopsy were found to have:
   a. a higher than average mortality rate
   b. elevated diastolic blood pressure
   c. recurrent nausea
   d. positively correlated critical thinking ability

1.102 Among the nursing interventions shown to be effective with cancer patients experiencing anxiety are all of the following *except*:
   a. helping the patient learn new coping strategies through anxiety-reducing role-playing
   b. helping the patient focus on the perceived threat and appraise the stimuli in a different way, thus reducing anxiety
   c. helping the patient identify stimuli that have resulted in a loss of self-esteem
   d. exploring perceived patient concerns and helping patients evaluate these concerns

1.103   According to a study by Hays, which of the following cancer patients is *most likely* to require inpatient hospice services?
   a.   a patient who experiences more physical symptoms but fewer symptoms that are uncontrolled
   b.   a patient who assumes the role of protector in an attempt to shield family members from emotional reaction
   c.   a patient who experiences fewer physical symptoms but more symptoms that are uncontrolled
   d.   a patient whose family experiences increased anxiety and fatigue in response to uncontrolled symptoms

Altered Body Image

1.104   A woman wishing to minimize the effects of breast surgery on her sexuality would be *most likely* to elect:
   a.   lumpectomy
   b.   modified mastectomy
   c.   radical mastectomy
   d.   any of the above might be selected by a woman; it is the opportunity to have input into treatment selection that is significant

1.105   Following four courses of chemotherapy, Albert shows you that his fingernails are having a strange reaction. They have developed transverse white lines or grooves. You explain to Albert that this symptom:
   a.   is a response to doxorubicin because pigmentation has been deposited at the base of the nail
   b.   indicates a reduction or cessation of nail growth in response to cytotoxic therapy
   c.   reflects a cytotoxic reaction to cyclophosphamide
   d.   is a partial separation of the nail plate called onycholysis and is a reaction to 5-FU therapy

1.106   Because of the staging of her cancer, the size of the tumor, and a number of other factors, Marcia will undergo immediate breast reconstruction after her surgery. Her surgeon has explained that the procedure most likely to be used in her case is the TRAM flap. You explain to Marcia that this will involve removing tissue from her _____ and tunneling it to the mastectomy site.
   a.   abdominal muscle
   b.   latissimus dorsi muscle
   c.   lower abdomen
   d.   buttocks

1.107   Two basic approaches to nursing intervention for alterations in sexual health of cancer patients are:
   a.   education and counseling
   b.   screening and role-playing
   c.   affective therapy and role modeling
   d.   enhancing reality surveillance and reinforcing personal power

1.108   Sexuality in the cancer patient may be affected by several factors, including each of the following *except:*
   a.   psychosexual changes associated with mutagenicity
   b.   physiologic problems of fertility and sterility
   c.   psychologic issues such as loss of self-esteem and fears of abandonment
   d.   changes in body appearance resulting from therapy

1.109   Mrs. Archer has recently had a radical cystectomy with resection of nearly one-third of the anterior wall of the vagina. She is approaching discharge and requires teaching regarding any changes she can expect in terms of her sexuality. It would be appropriate to include which of the following in your discussion?
   a.   The diameter of the introitus and the vaginal barrel may be compromised due to the surgery.
   b.   Intercourse may be restricted, even painful.
   c.   The clitoris may be injured or have compromised function because of scarring and fibrosis after surgery.
   d.   all of the above

1.110   Radiation is commonly used in conjunction with surgery as treatment for vaginal cancer. Patient education prior to discharge would include which of the following?
   a.   Vaginal fibrosis and scarring can occur due to a loss of blood supply; therefore, vaginal intercourse is to be minimized.
   b.   Vaginal intercourse and the use of a vaginal dilator are encouraged to prevent narrowing of the vagina.
   c.   Water-soluble lubricants or prescribed estrogen cream are effective measures to minimize functional loss.
   d.   all of the above

1.111   Mrs. Parnell received a bone marrow transplant and total body irradiation as treatment for her leukemia. She is two years post-transplant and returns for a doctor visit complaining of vaginal dryness, dyspareunia, and loss of femininity. Your assessment and management of her complaints are based on which of the following?
   a.   These symptoms are common following treatment for leukemia and are likely due to the radiation.
   b.   Approximately 50% of women experience fatigue and lack of energy following transplant that is severe enough to interfere with sexual function.
   c.   Most women experience depression and anxiety regarding sexual function following transplant and she needs a referral to a psychologist.
   d.   a and b

1.112   An individual's body image is affected by several factors, including all of the following *except*:
   a.   feedback from significant others and significant events
   b.   what one perceives as an "ideal" body or image
   c.   how one's body actually looks and functions
   d.   the various elements that refer to psychologic self

Alopecia

1.113   The degree of hair loss varies depending on the area of the body exposed to radiation, the dose, and the radiosensitivity of the exposed structures. Which of the following describes the correct order of *decreasing* radiosensitivity?
   a.   scalp, beard, eyebrows, eyelashes, axillary, pubic, and fine body hair
   b.   fine body hair, eyebrows, eyelashes, pubic hair, scalp hair, beard
   c.   beard, eyebrows, scalp, pubic hair, fine body hair
   d.   All body hair is equally sensitive to radiation.

1.114   Albert is about to undergo chemotherapy that is known to cause significant hair loss. Which of the following will *not* be part of your patient education plan for Albert?
   a.   Chemotherapy-induced alopecia occurs slowly and may not occur for several months after the treatment.
   b.   Once chemotherapy is complete, regrowth is visible in 4–6 weeks.
   c.   Complete regrowth of hair may take 1–2 years.
   d.   In situations involving very high doses of alkylating agents, hair may not regrow.

1.115   Jeanne is 34 years old and has just been diagnosed with ER(+) stage I breast cancer with a 1.5 cm tumor. She is being treated with cyclophosphamide, methotrexate, and 5-fluorouracil. Understandably, she is distressed over many aspects of the treatment, and you are trying to help her adjust. During her first week of therapy, she describes vividly how one of her aunts, who also had breast cancer, lost all her hair during chemotherapy. She wants to know if this will happen to her as well. You tell her that:
   a.   she will not lose significant amounts of hair
   b.   she may experience gradual thinning
   c.   she may lose all of her hair in 2–3 weeks
   d.   her hair will not start growing back for 6 months following the end of therapy

1.116   Your patient asks whether there is anything he or she can do to prevent hair loss with chemotherapy. Which of the following would *not* be an appropriate response?
   a.   Minoxidil might be helpful to prevent hair loss.
   b.   Avoid washing or combing the hair for as long as possible.
   c.   High doses of vitamin E have been shown to help prevent hair loss with chemotherapy.
   d.   all of the above

1.117   Which of the following chemotherapeutic agents is *not* associated with significant hair loss?
   a.   bleomycin
   b.   vincristine
   c.   carboplatin
   d.   doxil

1.118   A patient being treated with radiation to an abdominal field is concerned about hair loss that she expects to experience following radiotherapy. You can best reassure her by telling her that:
   a.   hair follicles are relatively radioresistant due to their low rate of growth and mitotic activity
   b.   radiation response is seen mostly in tissues and organs that are within the treatment field
   c.   alopecia is permanent only when radiation is administered in low doses over an extended period of time
   d.   alopecia is more closely associated with brachytherapy than with teletherapy

1.119 Chemotherapy agents damage the hair most when it is in which phase of hair growth?
   a. anagen
   b. catagen
   c. telogen
   d. transitional

1.120 Which of the following chemotherapy agents is *least likely* to cause hair loss?
   a. cyclophosphamide
   b. docetaxel
   c. vinorelbine
   d. etoposide

Cultural Issues

1.121 Respect for cultures other than one's own and for people's specific beliefs and behaviors that emanate from their cultural background is known as:
   a. multiculturalism
   b. cultural sensitivity
   c. ethnoculturalism
   d. developing rapport

1.122 Strategies for designing effective culturally sensitive patient education programs include which of the following?
   a. consulting with key members of the cultural community in designing the program
   b. limiting involvement of members of the community in program development
   c. presenting the program to the community leaders for their support
   d. teaching educational programs in high school

1.123 The first line of treatment in Hispanic cultures is the use of:
   a. home remedies
   b. prayer
   c. conventional Western medicine
   d. holistic medicine

1.124 Among the high-risk behaviors in the Hispanic population are:
   a. obesity
   b. heavy over-the-counter and street drug use
   c. voodoo practices
   d. all of the above

1.125 In Native American cultures, the singers are those healers who:
   a. can transform themselves into other forms of life to maintain cultural integration at a time of great cultural stress
   b. diagnose the cause of disharmony and may indicate a cure; their primary interest is care for souls
   c. treat illnesses and disharmony by laying on of hands, massage, sweatbaths, and the use of herbs and roots
   d. all of the above

1.126 In a culture plagued by poverty, secondary prevention may be absent because of:
   a. a lack of insurance, inability to pay for service
   b. a present orientation where survival needs take precedence over screening and early detection
   c. limited care access
   d. all of the above

1.127 Helen is preparing to discuss options with a patient who speaks only Spanish. Helen speaks only English. If given a choice, Helen will probably want to choose the use of:
   a. a professional interpreter
   b. a family member as interpreter because the family is an integral part of treatment delivery and involvement in most Hispanic cultures
   c. a friend as interpreter because of the emotional support friends lend in a Hispanic, extended-family social structure and because a friend is more likely than family to relay the complete message
   d. any of the above, as long as the interpreter is fluent in both languages

1.128 The basic unit of society is the:
   a. family
   b. social structure
   c. religious structure
   d. relationship of ethnicity and culture to role assignment

Loss of Personal Control

1.129 The most common means of reducing uncertainty for the patient is:
   a. providing prepatory information and education
   b. referring him or her to a professional therapist
   c. protecting the individual from all negative information
   d. a and c

1.130 One of the principal appeals of most alternative methods of treatment to the cancer patient is their:
   a. perceived absence of risks and side effects
   b. ready availability and modest costs
   c. level of acceptability to family and friends
   d. high degree of efficacy and safety

1.131 Which of the following reasons is *least likely* to explain a decision by a cancer patient to explore an alternative method of treatment?
   a. a desire for greater control over the treatment process
   b. pressure from family and friends
   c. valid data on the efficacy of the method
   d. resentment toward an impersonal medical system

1.132 *All but* which of the following are considered to be significant advantages of dying at home?
   a. It promotes personal control.
   b. It helps children understand and facilitates their grief process.
   c. It helps to keep down the cost of health care.
   d. It minimizes the risk of emergency medical intervention.

1.133 The federal Patient Self-Determination Act, enacted in 1991, was intended to accomplish which of the following?
   a. provide all patients with information about patient's bill of rights
   b. enable health care agencies to provide patients with information about their right to accept or refuse treatment
   c. enable health care agencies to provide ways to execute advance directives
   d. b and c

1.134 Marion performs breast self-examination (BSE) on a regular basis; Ginny does not. Marion is more likely to have:
   a. an external locus of control
   b. a low perceived susceptibility
   c. a high perceived benefits
   d. an internal locus of control

1.135 Two coping styles for dealing with cancer include monitoring and blunting. Blunters are individuals who:
   a. give high levels of attention to threatening health information but their stress levels blunt their ability to respond to conventional patient education interventions
   b. seek excessive participation in treatment decisions, thereby blunting the health professional's greater effectiveness
   c. avoid information that presents threatening health information
   d. a and b

1.136 Which of the following is one of the key issues for adult children of cancer patients?
   a. disruption of current family relationships
   b. behavior problems
   c. lack of involvement in decision making regarding the parent's illness
   d. assuming the protector role and shielding parents from discussing feelings

Depression

1.137 One major reason that a diagnosis of depression among cancer patients is often complicated is that:
   a. some cancer patients had preexisting depressive symptoms before the diagnosis of cancer
   b. instruments have yet to be developed to measure depression among cancer patients
   c. symptoms of depression are often identical to those of anxiety
   d. the signs and symptoms of cancer are markedly different from those of depression

1.138 With depression, responses to a perceived loss of self-esteem may be affective, behavioral, or cognitive. Which of the following is an example of a *behavioral* response associated with depression?
   a. lack of energy
   b. guilt
   c. indecisiveness
   d. suicidal ideation

1.139   The primary criteria for assessment of depression include all of the following characteristics *except*:
    a.   characteristics that are a change from previous functioning
    b.   characteristics that are persistent
    c.   characteristics that were preexistent
    d.   characteristics that occur more days than not

1.140   A nursing intervention for the treatment of patients with depression that deals with the patient's *affective* responses is:
    a.   negotiating goals for increasing independence in self-care and decision making
    b.   giving permission for expression of feelings
    c.   contracting short-term goals of care that the patient can achieve
    d.   encouraging physical mobility

1.141   Unlike anxiety and depression, which of the following statements is true of hopelessness as a response of patients to the cancer experience?
    a.   It involves a combination of affective, behavioral, and cognitive responses.
    b.   It has not been implicated in the development of cancer or in the quantity and quality of life after diagnosis of cancer.
    c.   It can be clearly distinguished from other, similar concepts using the accepted defining characteristics.
    d.   It appears to wax and wane with perceived changes in the patient's life.

1.142   Which of the following statements most accurately describes the relationship between family responses to a diagnosis of cancer and the responses of patients themselves?
    a.   Family responses are similar to patient responses.
    b.   Responses of anxiety and depression are less common among family members than among patients.
    c.   Responses of hopelessness and altered sexual health are less common among family members than among patients.
    d.   Family responses generally are not similar to patient responses.

1.143   Fatigue may produce anxiety or depression in some individuals with cancer. The best explanation for this effect is that:
    a.   fatigue-induced electrolyte imbalances often trigger feelings of anxiety or depression
    b.   fatigue, anxiety, and depression have the same etiology
    c.   treatment-induced fatigue may force the individual to give up usual social roles
    d.   anxiety or depression frequently forces individuals with cancer to expend too much energy

1.144   The majority of empirical studies dealing with the relationship of cancer to self-concept have focused on:
    a.   the total self-appraisal of cancer patients, both men and women
    b.   the effects of various treatments on relationships of cancer patients with significant others
    c.   women with gynecologic or breast cancer or males with testicular or prostate cancer
    d.   the interaction of variables such as age, depression, and activity status on the psychosocial aspects of sexual health

Survivorship Issues

1.145 Which of the following statements about employment among cancer survivors is correct?
   a. Approximately 40% of cancer patients return to work after being diagnosed.
   b. The work performance of cancer survivors differs little from others hired at the same age for similar assignments.
   c. "Job-lock" refers to the situation in which cancer survivors are reluctant to accept new jobs that might involve increased responsibilities.
   d. Most federal and state laws specifically include cancer survivors among the "handicapped or disabled."

1.146 Your new position in a cancer clinic gives you the opportunity to counsel cancer survivors. You are aware that the adult cancer survivor's ability to achieve optimal physical, social, and psychological function can be most significantly affected by:
   a. socioeconomic considerations
   b. disease trajectory considerations
   c. physical function and cosmesis
   d. all of the above

1.147 The most powerful predictor of cancer survival is _____ at diagnosis:
   a. advanced disease
   b. changes in appearance or body function
   c. comorbid physical or mental conditions
   d. a and b

1.148 Which of the following "directions" provides patients who are at risk for loss of decision-making ability the best chance of having their health care wishes carried out?
   a. power of attorney for health care
   b. verbal instructions to the attending physician
   c. a living will
   d. a do-not-intubate/ventilate order on admission

1.149 Survival analysis is defined as:
   a. the probability that an individual will live with or without cancer for a specified period of time
   b. a time interval without evidence of recurrence of disease
   c. an observation of individuals with cancer and a calculation of their probability of dying over time
   d. the length of time an individual with cancer survives with evidence of disease

1.150 According to research, the ability to conceive or father a child after BMT is *most likely* to be related to which of the following?
   a. age (older patients were less likely to reverse gonadal dysfunction)
   b. whether or not TBI is used
   c. the use of colony-stimulating factors
   d. a and b

1.151   Your patient Melissa is beginning her treatment for osteogenic sarcoma and is concerned that the chemotherapy and radiation therapy might cause congenital abnormalities in her future offspring. An appropriate response would include which of the following?
   a.   Explain that what she should be thinking about is her own situation instead of dwelling on what might never be.
   b.   Explain that this is a legitimate concern and reassure her that research has found no higher incidence of congenital malformation in the children born of women who have had treatment for cancer than in the general population.
   c.   Explain that it is difficult to answer her question because there is a much higher incidence of miscarriage in women who have been treated for cancer.
   d.   Explain that you understand how she feels and refer her for genetic counseling.

1.152   The late effects of cancer treatment on the endocrine system result from damage to the hypothalamus pituitary axis and/or to:
   a.   target organs (e.g., the thyroid, ovaries, testis)
   b.   the cortical areas of the brain
   c.   the chemical structure of key hormones (e.g., insulin)
   d.   epithelial tissue (e.g., blood vessel linings)

1.153   Growth impairment as a late effect of treatment for cancer occurs as the result of:
   a.   overproduction of thyroxine by the thyroid gland
   b.   deficient growth hormone release by the hypothalamus
   c.   primary hypothyroidism
   d.   a disruption in pituitary control of several target organs

SEXUALITY

Reproductive Issues

1.154   Both chemotherapy and radiation therapy are known to have teratogenetic effects on the fetus, causing spontaneous abortion, fetal malformation, or fetal death. These complications are *most likely* to happen during which trimester?
   a.   first
   b.   second
   c.   third
   d.   The risk to the fetus is equal among the three trimesters.

1.155   Janie is 7 months pregnant and has recently had a lumpectomy for breast cancer. She is scheduled to begin chemotherapy followed by radiation. She is debating whether to start her chemotherapy or delay it until after she has her baby. She is concerned about the effect of the chemotherapy on her baby. Your comments and counsel are based on which of the following true statements regarding the effect of chemotherapy on a developing fetus?
   a.   Chemotherapy during the second and third trimesters may cause premature birth or low birth weights.
   b.   Chemotherapy during the second and third trimesters is not associated with a higher incidence of congenital abnormality compared to the normal pregnancy incidence.
   c.   Alkylating agents and antimetabolites are most often associated with fetal malformations during the first trimester.
   d.   all of the above

1.156   The fertility of which of the following patients is most likely to be affected by chemotherapy?
  a.   7-year-old Kevin
  b.   60-year-old Dan
  c.   Elaine, who is over 30
  d.   Pamela, who is 15

1.157   It has been suggested that after cancer therapy an individual should wait a minimum of 2 years before attempting conception. One reason for this is to allow for the recovery of spermatogenesis or ovarian function. Another important reason is that:
  a.   residues from chemotherapy typically remain in the body for at least 18 months
  b.   the psychologic effects of cancer therapy may be felt for a prolonged period of time
  c.   germinal epithelium may have been damaged by chemotherapy and/or radiation therapy
  d.   recurrence is most likely within the first 2 years after cancer therapy

1.158   Which of the following statements about pregnancy and cancer is false?
  a.   Most cancers do not adversely affect a pregnancy.
  b.   In general, pregnancy does not adversely affect the outcome of a cancer.
  c.   Therapeutic abortion has been shown to be of benefit in altering disease progression.
  d.   Treatment options should be evaluated as though the patient were not pregnant, and therapy should be instituted when appropriate.

1.159   Invasion of a cervical carcinoma into underlying tissue is found in a woman during the third trimester of her pregnancy. Which of the following treatments is *most likely* to be followed?
  a.   Fetal viability is awaited and appropriate therapy is given after delivery of the baby by cesarean section.
  b.   Surgery or radiation therapy, without therapeutic abortion, is undertaken immediately.
  c.   A radical hysterectomy and pelvic node dissection are performed and combined with radiation therapy.
  d.   Therapeutic abortion is performed immediately and followed by standard treatment for advanced disease.

1.160   Evaluation of the placenta for evidence of metastasis to the fetus is *most likely* to be carried out under which of the following situations?
  a.   when the mother has received combination chemotherapy during the third trimester of pregnancy
  b.   when the mother has received low doses of radiation during the first trimester of pregnancy
  c.   when the mother has breast cancer or invasive cervical cancer
  d.   when the mother has a melanoma or lymphoma

1.161   Which of the following is *most likely* to involve risk to the fetus whose mother is being treated for cancer?
  a.   pelvic surgery on the mother during the second trimester of pregnancy
  b.   low doses of radiation associated with diagnostic x-rays
  c.   chemotherapy during the first trimester of pregnancy
  d.   the use of anesthetic agents during surgery on the mother during the second trimester of pregnancy

1.162   In a support group you are conducting for expectant mothers with breast cancer, the question is raised: "How likely is cancer to spread from the mother to the fetus?" You explain that only a few cancers spread from the mother to the fetus. Among the following cancers mentioned by the group, the cancer *least likely* to spread from the mother to the fetus is:
a. melanoma
b. NHL
c. leukemia
d. breast cancer

Sexual Dysfunction

1.163   Mr. Crane is about to undergo a radical prostatectomy. He is concerned about his ability to be sexually active following his surgery. Your preoperative teaching of this patient is based on which of the following factors that promote sexual function following prostatectomy?
a. age less than 50
b. stage of disease
c. preservation of neurovascular bundles
d. all of the above

1.164   For patients who undergo surgery for gastrointestinal cancer, possible organic sexual dysfunction is most closely associated with:
a. placement of a colostomy
b. removal of rectal tissue
c. changes in body image
d. responses by family and friends

1.165   Treatments for prostate cancer have the potential to alter sexual function, even though prostate cancer occurs mostly in older men. Permanent damage to erectile function with loss of emission and ejaculation is *most likely* to occur with:
a. radical prostatectomy
b. transurethral resection
c. bilateral orchiectomy
d. transabdominal resection

1.166   Which of the following statements about the relationship between gynecologic malignancies and sexual dysfunction is correct?
a. Pelvic exenteration results in relatively few problems with sexual dysfunction.
b. The procedures commonly used to treat carcinoma in situ are not likely to affect fertility or childbearing.
c. Menopausal symptoms are closely associated with radical hysterectomy.
d. The majority of gynecologic cancers result in some abnormality of the vagina.

1.167   Which of the following side effects is *least likely* to occur as a result of radiation therapy?
a. alterations in organ function (e.g., decreased vaginal lubrication)
b. enhanced hormonal activity (e.g., overstimulation of the hypothalamus or pituitary)
c. general or psychologic side effects of therapy that can alter sexual function (e.g., diarrhea, loss of sexual desire)
d. primary organ failure (e.g., ovarian failure)

1.168 A patient is about to receive radiation for prostate cancer. He is concerned about sexual dysfunction as a result. As part of your patient education plan, you tell him that radiation therapy can cause sexual and reproductive dysfunction through:
   a. primary organ failure
   b. alterations in organ function
   c. temporary or permanent effects of the therapy itself
   d. all of the above

1.169 Which of the following has been implicated in sexual dysfunction in both men and women receiving chemotherapy?
   a. depletion of the germinal epithelium
   b. treatment with estrogens
   c. combination chemotherapy with MOPP
   d. treatment with androgens

1.170 Marcia, a patient of yours, will be commencing chemotherapy in 2 weeks. She asks you to explain to her the risks and side effects of chemotherapy. You tell her all of the following *except:*
   a. Chemotherapy can cause ovarian failure.
   b. Irregular menses are a common side effect.
   c. Sexual dysfunction is normal.
   d. Hot flashes and night sweats are to be expected.

1.171 The traditional bilateral retroperitoneal lymph node dissection (RPLND) results in:
   a. the loss of antegrade ejaculation
   b. infertility from retrograde ejaculation
   c. impaired ability to experience a normal orgasm
   d. a and b

SYMPTOM MANAGEMENT

Dying and Death

1.172 You are working with Mr. Gunther and his family, who have just discovered not only that his lung cancer has recurred, but also that it is terminal this time. Which is *not* likely to be true regarding Mr. Gunther's psychosocial needs?
   a. When coping with a difficult disease like lung cancer, it is the discovery of meaning in the disease that gives one a sense of mastery.
   b. The recurrence of lung cancer can be a greater crisis than the initial diagnosis.
   c. Often the fear of dying is not as profound as the fear of suffering in the process.
   d. Patients who are allowed to indulge excessively in expressing their fears, concerns, and wishes regarding death are more prone to morbid depression.

1.173 Active euthanasia refers to:
   a. the intentional taking of one's own life
   b. direct intervention causing death
   c. letting a sufferer die by withdrawing life-sustaining care
   d. all of the above

1.174   The most frequently addressed factors contributing to cancer-related suicide or euthanasia are:
 a. pain and other symptom distress
 b. advanced illness and poor prognosis
 c. family history of suicide or personal suicide history
 d. hopelessness and loss of self-esteem or control

1.175   The basic medical and nursing approach toward patients in a hospice program is:
 a. acute care
 b. curative care
 c. palliative care
 d. euthanasia care

1.176   Which is preferable, the durable power of attorney or the living will, and why?
 a. The living will is preferable because it prevents more suffering.
 b. The durable power of attorney is preferable because it covers only terminal situations.
 c. The durable power of attorney covers not only decisions in a terminal situation, but also any treatment decisions and therefore is preferable.
 d. The living will is better because health care providers are concerned about the ethical issues in active, direct euthanasia.

1.177   The Patient Self-Determination Act (PSDA), passed by the United States Congress in 1990, provides for which of the following?
 a. The patient has a right to request euthanasia, provided it is in writing.
 b. The physician must by law inform patients of their right to determine the manner in which they will die.
 c. On admission to the hospital, all health care institutions receiving Medicare or Medicaid reimbursement must ask patients whether they have an advance directive.
 d. No patient admitted to a hospital that receives Medicare or Medicaid reimbursement may be denied terminal care at that institution.

1.178   The husband of a woman with end-stage breast cancer is concerned that his wife is sleeping more and is not even waking to eat or drink. The hospice nurse would explain to the husband that:
 a. these are signs of approaching death
 b. the pain medication has reached a high blood level and needs to be reduced
 c. there is no reason to be concerned
 d. her oncologist should be called to obtain some direction for her care

1.179   In our current health care environment, the *greatest* danger regarding euthanasia is that:
 a. it will be used as a simple method of eliminating persons whose care costs are too high or who are considered a burden to society
 b. caregivers will be tempted to regard certain individuals' lives as not worthwhile
 c. it will discourage caregivers from proposing aggressive treatment for the seriously ill older person
 d. it is inconsistent with the position of nonmaleficence

Local, State, and National Resources

1.180 Effective cancer control is influenced *most* by which of the following?
   a. government policy
   b. routine chest x-rays
   c. hygiene
   d. a low-fat diet

1.181 The hospice nurse may decide in the initial interview that patient criteria for hospice care will *not* be met because:
   a. the patient's spouse expresses his wish to be involved in his wife's care
   b. the patient has entered a clinical trial through the National Cancer Institute
   c. the patient's home is 5 minutes from the hospice offices
   d. the patient does not wish to be resuscitated if she stops breathing at home

1.182 The goals of the Cancer Patient Education Network (CPEN) include which of the following?
   a. to increase cancer patient educators' access to the materials, services, and technical expertise of NCI's Patient Education Section (PES)
   b. to encourage networking and sharing of information among cancer patient educators
   c. to provide the patient educator with a direct link to the issues and concerns of cancer patients
   d. all of the above

1.183 Which of the following most accurately describes the philosophy of the National Hospice Organization?
   a. Patients can be made comfortable with alternative and complementary care.
   b. Euthanasia is an integral aspect of care if the patient requests it.
   c. Palliative management is centered around providing relief from suffering.
   d. Hospice is specialized care for the dying that is nonphysician-based care.

1.184 Which of the following is *not* a characteristic of the American Cancer Society?
   a. It is part of the National Cancer Institute with branches in nearly every state.
   b. It is a voluntary health agency.
   c. It sponsors several publications.
   d. It promotes advanced nursing education.

1.185 Which of the following does the federal government insist on before a drug can be marketed?
   a. the safety of the drug only
   b. the efficacy of the drug only
   c. the safety and the efficacy of the drug only
   d. the safety, efficacy, and long-term value of the drug

1.186 Guidelines for the handling of antineoplastic agents in the home are in accordance with those established by:
   a. the Food and Drug Administration
   b. the Occupational Safety and Health Administration
   c. the American Nurse's Association
   d. the Health Care Financing Administration

1.187 Which of the following does COBRA, a federal law passed in 1986, do?
    a. It offers continued medical coverage to those who leave jobs.
    b. It provides low-cost insurance to cancer survivors and other high-risk individuals.
    c. It provides free group health insurance to individuals not otherwise covered by medical plans.
    d. It prohibits employment discrimination against cancer survivors.

1.188 The primary function of the Cancer Information Service (CIS), sponsored by the National Cancer Insitutute (NCI), is to:
    a. perform diagnostic screening on large numbers of high-risk individuals
    b. investigate suspected carcinogens in the workplace and home
    c. set standards for potentially hazardous products
    d. answer inquiries from the general public concerning cancer-related issues

Blood Products

1.189 Under which of the following circumstances is administration of platelet concentrate from a single donor or HLA-matched donor preferable to that of a random donor platelet concentrate?
    a. when the patient is severely immunosuppressed
    b. when cost is a major factor
    c. when a patient's red blood cell antigens (ABO) are not known
    d. when time is a major factor

1.190 Mrs. Ryan has metastatic cancer and develops fever, increased pulse rate, and flushing during her transfusion. As you are checking her vital signs, she experiences anaphylaxis. Mrs. Ryan's reaction is *most likely* due to:
    a. ABO incompatibility
    b. recipient antibodies against immunoglobulin in the plasma
    c. antileukocyte antibodies directed against the donor blood
    d. development of alloantibodies to transfused blood

1.191 Therapy for disseminated intravascular coagulation (DIC) often involves the administration of several substances. Which of the following is *not* a common treatment for DIC?
    a. heparin
    b. epsilon-amino caproic acid (ACA or Amicar)
    c. vitamin K
    d. platelet replacement

1.192 A patient is to receive a blood transfusion of two units of packed red blood cells that have been irradiated. The rationale for irradiating the blood is which of the following?
    a. to kill any possible cancer cells in the blood
    b. to prevent the spread of the AIDS virus
    c. to prevent graft versus host disease
    d. to sterilize the blood

1.193 Providing leukocyte-depleted blood products to patients is intended to accomplish which of the following?
    a. prevent febrile nonhemolytic reactions
    b. prevent transmission of viral infections such as CMV infection
    c. prevent alloimmunization to blood products
    d. all of the above

1.194 Mr. Svensen, who is scheduled for surgery, expresses an interest in autologous blood dona-
tion. Which of the following parameters must be met to qualify:
   a. He must be nonanemic.
   b. He can donate no more than 6 units of blood before surgery.
   c. The blood can be donated from 42 days to 72 hours prior to surgery.
   d. all of the above

1.195 Ms. Daniels, who had an allogencie BMT, is about to receive a blood product. You must
ensure that the blood has been specially treated to prevent GVHD. This means you will check
to be sure that the blood product has been:
   a. exposed to alloimmunization and platelet refractoriness
   b. infiltrated with saline solution
   c. treated via plasmapheresis
   d. irradiated

1.196 Which of the following is *least likely* to be a cause of anemia in the cancer patient?
   a. decreased red cell production
   b. iron deficiency
   c. the primary disease process
   d. radiation therapy

1.197 Stanley has lung cancer and is receiving chemotherapy every 3 weeks and erythropoietin
subcutaneously on a weekly basis. He has been doing well, but lately has begun to complain
of headaches and occasional dizziness. These symptoms are *most likely* the result of which of
the following?
   a. metastatic disease in the brain
   b. severe anemia
   c. hypertension due to erythropoietin
   d. all of the above

1.198 Myelophthisis is caused by *all but* which of the following?
   a. cancer that originates in the bone marrow
   b. cancer that metastasizes to the bone marrow
   c. toxic metabolic end products
   d. radiation therapy to the bone

Enteral and Parenteral Nutrition

1.199 The most important role of the nurse in home parenteral nutrition (HPN) is to:
   a. keep records of times of infusion, intake, and output
   b. deliver all supplies, equipment, and medicines to the patient
   c. evaluate the patient, the home environment, and the family's ability to manage HPN
   d. perform all infusion regimens at home

1.200 Total parenteral nutrition for prolonged periods or at home is indicated in *all but* which of
the following situations?
   a. as a treatment for cancer cachexia
   b. where enteral feedings are not feasible
   c. for patients with enterocutaneous fistulas
   d. for patients with acute radiation enteritis

1.201   Which of the following is considered to be one of the major advantages of enteral nutrition compared to parenteral nutrition?
   a.   Enteral nutrition is associated with less diarrhea.
   b.   Metabolic abnormalities are more common with parenteral nutrition.
   c.   With enteral nutrition, normal enzymatic and mucosal activity is maintained in the gut.
   d.   Enteral nutrition is less expensive.

1.202   Which of the following is considered to be a potential hazard of a macrobiotic diet?
   a.   protein deficiency
   b.   vitamin D and vitamin B_{12} deficiency
   c.   calorie and iron deficiency
   d.   all of the above

1.203   Mr. Smith, who seems healthy, is scheduled for surgical resection of an esophageal lesion. Which route of administration of nutritional support do you predict is *most likely* to be appropriate for Mr. Svensen immediately following surgery?
   a.   enteral nutrition
   b.   TPN for 7–10 days
   c.   home TPN
   d.   none of the above

1.204   Which of the following patients would generally *not* be candidates for home parenteral nutrition?
   a.   those who are terminally ill and unable to drink fluids
   b.   those with severe enteritis due to radiation
   c.   head and neck cancer patients who have an upper airway obstruction
   d.   those patients with significant gastrointestinal malfunction

1.205   Mr. Cruz is receiving enteral nutrition every 4 hours and complains of diarrhea and cramping. The *least likely* cause of his discomfort is which of the following?
   a.   The formula is probably too concentrated.
   b.   The formula is probably too cold.
   c.   The formula is probably infused too rapidly.
   d.   The formula probably has too little fiber.

1.206   Your patient with esophageal cancer is undergoing surgery for placement of a feeding tube. The most logical explanation for using this procedure instead of parenteral nutrition is which of the following?
   a.   Enteral feedings are more economical.
   b.   Parenteral nutrition is associated with more metabolic complications.
   c.   Enteral feedings maintain the normal stimulation of enzymatic and mucosal activity in the gut.
   d.   Parenteral nutrition is indicated when the patient needs long-term nutritional support.

Rehabilitation

1.207   Mrs. Howe is undergoing adjuvant therapy for breast cancer and asks you if it is a good idea for her to exercise while she is taking chemotherapy. Which would be the *most appropriate* response?
   a.   Exercise can intensify her feelings of nausea and she should avoid exercise for 3–4 days following her treatment.
   b.   Research shows that exercise following meals relieves heartburn and is a good idea.
   c.   Aerobic exercise is especially effective in relieving fatigue and is highly recommended for women undergoing adjuvant chemotherapy for breast cancer.
   d.   Exercise can lead to dizziness and she should consult with her doctor before engaging in any form of exercise.

1.208   All of the following are considered to be indications for limb-salvage surgery *except:*
   a.   a locally aggressive chondrosarcoma
   b.   the absence of soft-tissue invasion
   c.   a tumor that typically metastasizes late
   d.   a child younger than 10 years of age

1.209   Which of the following is considered an accepted means of communication for the person who has undergone a laryngectomy?
   a.   artificial larynx
   b.   esophageal voice
   c.   tracheosophageal puncture (TP)
   d.   all of the above

1.210   Six months after his surgery, Mr. Fox, after participating in extensive speech rehabilitation, learns to speak by diverting exhaled pulmonary air through a surgically constructed fistula tract directly into the esophagus. This method of speech is produced through:
   a.   an artificial larynx made available immediately after surgery
   b.   esophageal voice therapy
   c.   surgical voice restoration or tracheoesophageal (TE) puncture
   d.   none of the above

1.211   After surgery, part of Ms. Eliot's rehabilitation process involves restoring the swallowing function, because aspiration during swallowing is one of the major complications following supraglottic laryngectomy. Initially, _____ will be the most difficult thing for Ms. Eliot to swallow without aspirating.
   a.   soft, mashed foods
   b.   dry, crunchy foods
   c.   liquids
   d.   hard, bulky food boluses (especially meats)

1.212   After laryngectomy, heavy lifting is restricted because of the:
   a.   lack of thoracic fixation
   b.   risk of aspiration
   c.   risk of hiatal hernia
   d.   reduction in cough effectiveness

1.213 The overall goal of general home care is:
   a. to provide complete and holistic care for the patient
   b. to assist the patient in a peaceful death with dignity
   c. to provide palliative care
   d. for patients and families to assume responsibility for the care

1.214 A program that regards rehabilitation in cancer care as a dynamic rather than a passive process is *most likely* to emphasize both ongoing reassessment and:
   a. customary convalescence
   b. a hospital or community base
   c. redefinition of goals
   d. frequent nursing referrals

1.215 The overall goal of rehabilitation for the person with cancer is to:
   a. return to baseline performance before the cancer
   b. anticipate and prepare physically for future debilitating effects of cancer
   c. achieve optimal functioning within the limits of cancer
   d. maintain an active, busy life

1.216 Which of the following factors have been found to be *most closely* related to rehabilitation needs of the cancer patient?
   a. medical and family history
   b. type of treatment and side effects experienced
   c. cancer site and stage of disease
   d. severity or duration of disease

Vascular Access Devices

1.217 A major advantage of the peripherally inserted central catheter (PICC) is that:
   a. it does not require frequent flushing because of the one-way valve
   b. dressing changes are simpler and more cost-effective
   c. it can be inserted at home by a certified nurse
   d. it has a separate designated port for blood withdrawal

1.218 The cause of extravasation in implanted ports is generally which of the following?
   a. the caustic nature of the drugs
   b. misplaced or displaced needle
   c. retrograde or subcutaneous leakage from percutaneously inserted catheters obstructed by a fibrin sheath
   d. b and c

1.219 Mr. Good has had his implanted port for 4 months and has always had a blood return. Following needle placement, you notice that the port flushes briskly with no evidence of resistance or patient discomfort; however, you are unable to obtain a blood return. Following numerous attempts to reposition the catheter, you are unable to achieve a blood return and conclude which of the following?
   a. Never infuse any medication into a port that does not produce a blood return.
   b. Because the patient has no discomfort and there is no resistance, it is safe to use.
   c. The catheter probably has a fibrin sheath and instilling urokinase may restore a blood return.
   d. b and c

1.220 An Ommaya reservoir is generally placed underneath the skin of the scalp overlying the cranium with the catheter extending to the ventricle of the brain. The purpose of this catheter placement is which of the following?
   a. measurement of intracerebral pressure
   b. sampling of cerebral spinal fluid for tumor cells
   c. a portal for injection of chemotherapeutic agents
   d. b and c

1.221 Which of the following statements concerning peripherally inserted central catheters (PICCs) is *not* correct?
   a. PICCs are excellent for long-term, intermittent infusional therapy.
   b. They can be inserted at the bedside by specially trained nurses.
   c. They require sterile external site care and routine flushing.
   d. PICC lines are used for intravenous administration of antibiotics, chemotherapy, and TPN as well as for blood drawing.

1.222 Which of the following statements regarding use of the epidural implanted port is *not* correct?
   a. Epidural ports are used to administer intrathecal or epidural medications, including chemotherapy and analgesics.
   b. Only preservative-free medication is instilled or infused into the port.
   c. The port is flushed with preservative-free heparin after each use.
   d. A 24-gauge noncoring needle and meticulous sterile technique are used to access epidural ports.

1.223 Mr. Archer has had an implanted port for 4 weeks and recently complained of pain in his right neck and shoulder, just above the catheter insertion site. On examination, you notice slight swelling over the neck, face, shoulder, and arm. He also complains that his arm is cold at times and there is some tingling in his arm and shoulder. What is the *most appropriate* action to take?
   a. These symptoms are normal following port placement and should resolve in 2–3 weeks. Have him return to the clinic in a week if he is not better.
   b. Flush the line with heparin to make sure it is not clotted.
   c. Notify the physician to examine the patient. A venogram will probably demonstrate a venous thrombosis.
   d. Notify the physician to obtain an order for urokinase. The patient probably has a fibrin sheath formation around the tip of the catheter.

1.224 Ms. Charles needs a peripheral IV injection of doxorubicin, a known vesicant. When giving a vesicant:
   a. it is always better to have a blood return throughout the injection
   b. a smaller-gauge needle is preferable
   c. to patients with small veins, choose an angiocath that is thin-walled with an over-the-needle cannula
   d. a and c

1.225   Which of the following factors should influence the choice of catheter used in the BCT process for a patient?
    a.   The patient undergoing BCT requires a catheter that is stiffer than the traditional CVC used for ABMT.
    b.   The stiff catheters used in ABMT are not necessary in BCT pheresis because there is a less rapid withdrawal of blood in BCT.
    c.   High volume and pressure are needed during pheresis.
    d.   a and c

PHARMACOLOGIC INTERVENTIONS

Antimicrobials

1.226   After a long period of time, Ms. Daniels, who had an allogeneic BMT, develops recurrent varicella zoster virus (VZV). What is the *most likely* treatment approach?
    a.   cyclosporine
    b.   methotrexate
    c.   acyclovir
    d.   cyclosporine and methotrexate in combination

1.227   Ms. Linhorst is diagnosed with an early proliferation of MALT lymphoma, apparently due to her exposure to *H. pylori*. The *most likely* course of treatment for Ms. Linhorst is:
    a.   a course of antibiotics
    b.   a course of radiation and antiviral agents
    c.   antiviral agents alone
    d.   conventional anticancer therapy

1.228   Which of the following activities or facts is the home health care nurse most likely *not* to teach the patient and/or family in order to ensure safe antibiotic administration in the home?
    a.   at what temperature to store the medication
    b.   what signs/symptoms of drug side effects to report
    c.   how to withdraw heparin from a vial
    d.   how to prepare and mix the antibiotic

1.229   Which of the following measures has been found to be most consistently effective in preventing infection in the bone marrow transplant environment?
    a.   meticulous hand washing
    b.   scrupulous hygiene
    c.   protective isolation
    d.   all of the above

1.230   Which of the following agents is used to prevent GVHD in bone marrow transplant?
    a.   medroxyprogesterone acetate
    b.   cyclosporine
    c.   cyclophosphamide
    d.   dexamethasone

1.231   Risk factors for veno-occlusive disease of the liver in BMT include *all but* which of the following?
    a.   patients with hepatitis
    b.   antimicrobial therapy with acyclovir, amphotericin, or vancomycin
    c.   cytomegalovirus and fungi
    d.   chemotherapy and radiation therapy before transplant

1.232   Trimethoprim-sulfamethoxazole is generally the treatment of choice for pneumocystis carinii. Which of the following is *not* usually a side effect of this drug?
    a.   nausea and vomiting
    b.   hemolytic anemia
    c.   hepatotoxicity
    d.   myelosuppression

1.233   A patient diagnosed with candida esophagitis is about to receive her first dose of amphotericin B. Which of the following is *not* a side effect of this drug?
    a.   fever and chills
    b.   nausea and vomiting
    c.   hypertension
    d.   bronchospasm

1.234   Prevention of acute side effects of amphotericin B includes *all but* which of the following?
    a.   Pepcid 20 mg IV
    b.   IV meperidine
    c.   hydrocortisone sodium succinate
    d.   acetaminophen

Anti-inflammatory Agents

1.235   Elise develops GVHD after undergoing allogeneic BMT. Which of the following will probably *not* be part of Elise's treatment plan?
    a.   systemic immunosuppressive therapy
    b.   topical steroids
    c.   NSAIDs
    d.   fluoride therapy

1.236   James has recently received chemotherapy as treatment for his bladder cancer. He asks what he should take if he gets a headache. Which among the following would be an appropriate response?
    a.   Aspirin is discouraged because it can cause increased risk of bleeding.
    b.   If his platelet count is below 130,000, he should avoid taking nonsteroidal anti-inflammatory drugs.
    c.   Acetaminophen does not interfere with clotting and is safe to use.
    d.   all of the above

1.237   Nonsteroidal anti-inflammatory drugs (NSAIDs) are *most useful* for which of the following?
    a.   phantom limb pain
    b.   nonobstructive visceral pain
    c.   postoperative pain
    d.   pain due to leukemic infiltrates

1.238   Which of the following drugs is *most commonly* associated with platelet dysfunction?
a.   cimetidine
b.   heparin
c.   aspirin
d.   estrogen

1.239   Which of the following best describes the effect that NSAIDs have on platelets?
a.   NSAIDS enhance the platelet secretory process.
b.   NSAIDs increase epinephrine-induced aggregation.
c.   NSAIDs inhibit platelet function.
d.   all of the above

1.240   Nonsteroidal anti-inflammatory drugs (NSAIDs) have been purported to prevent which of the following?
a.   bladder cancer
b.   breast cancer
c.   colorectal cancer
d.   prostate cancer

1.241   NSAIDs are known to cause gastrointestinal (GI) side effects. The etiology of these GI effects is best explained by which of the following?
a.   NSAIDs cause GI side effects only in the presence of preexisting mucosal irritation, as would occur with chemotherapy.
b.   The increased release of prostaglandin increases GI side effects.
c.   The drugs directly irritate the gastrointestinal mucosa, which is why they should be taken with an antacid.
d.   The loss of the cytoprotective effect of prostaglandin causes increased GI side effects.

Antiemetics

1.242   The primary mechanism of action of granisetron and ondansetron as antiemetics is which of the following?
a.   dopamine antagonist
b.   serotonin antagonist
c.   sedation
d.   suppression of autonomic pathways

1.243   The primary mechanism of action of dexamethasone as an antiemetic is:
a.   anti-inflammatory
b.   inhibit prostaglandin synthesis
c.   dopamine antagonist
c.   histamine receptor antagonist

1.244   Delayed nausea and vomiting occurs more commonly with which of the following agents?
a.   carboplatin
b.   mechlorethamine
c.   cisplatin
d.   vincristine

1.245   Dexamethasone is usually administered along with granisetron or ondansetron. The purpose of the dexamethasone is to do which of the following?
   a.   to treat delayed nausea
   b.   to prevent side effects of granisetron or ondansetron
   c.   to potentiate the antiemetic effect of the granisetron or ondansetron
   d.   to produce euphoria

1.246   Which of the following is *not* a side effect of the serotonin antagonists?
   a.   dizziness
   b.   constipation
   c.   extrapyramidal reactions
   d.   sedation

1.247   When highly emetogenic chemotherapy is to be administered, the patient generally receives a combination of antiemetics, rather than a single drug. The rationale for the use of multiple antiemetics is which of the following?
   a.   A combination of different antiemetic agents permits the use of lower doses of each agent and is therefore more economical.
   b.   Drugs such as prochlorperizine and granisetron are synergistic in their action.
   c.   The vomiting center is directly activated by multiple pathways.
   d.   all the above

1.248   The discovery of serotonin has greatly increased the efficacy of antiemetic protocols. Which of the following best describes the role of serotonin in nausea and vomiting?
   a.   Serotonin activates 5-HT3 receptors on visceral and vagal afferent pathways.
   b.   Serotonin acts on dopamine receptors in the brain.
   c.   When serotonin levels are reduced by serotonin antagonists, the patient is more at risk for delayed nausea and vomiting.
   d.   Serotonin levels are increased when toxic substances such as chemotherapy drugs stimulate the parafollicular cells of the gastrointestinal tract.

1.249   Mrs. Levy is noticeably anxious as she waits for her chemotherapy to be administered. This is her fourth cycle of CMF, cyclophosphamide orally (days 1–14), and methotrexate and 5-fluorouracil IV on days 1 and 8. She states that she felt nauseated yesterday and still feels sick today. Which of the following best describes the etiology of her nausea and the appropriate nursing action?
   a.   Her symptoms are likely due to something she ate. She will benefit from prochlorperzine.
   b.   The cyclophosphamide is probably causing her nausea. Prochlorperzine each day and IV granisetron and dexamethasone with her chemotherapy injection are appropriate.
   c.   Anticipatory nausea and vomiting occur in roughly 60% of patients on CMF, and she will benefit from behavorial modification and lorazepam.
   d.   She should be referred to the psycho-oncologist for desensitization because her symptoms are psychological in origin.

Analgesic Regimens

1.250   The drug used to treat respiratory depression related to opioid analgesics is:
   a.   naproxen
   b.   methadone
   c.   meperidine
   d.   naloxone

1.251   Which of the following is *not* a common side effect of opioids?
   a.   sedation
   b.   respiratory depression
   c.   increased motility
   d.   constipation

1.252   Antidepressants such as amitriptyline may be used to treat pain that is caused by:
   a.   tumor infiltration of nerves
   b.   narcotic withdrawal
   c.   brain metastases
   d.   surgery

1.253   Mrs. Villegas experiences extreme sedation as a result of her course of opioid analgesics. There are no other CNS problems, and she is in severe pain when the opioid dose is lowered. _____ may be indicated.
   a.   antihistamines
   b.   steroids
   c.   biphosphonates
   d.   psychostimulants

1.254   Steroids are sometimes used in the management of pain related to:
   a.   bowel obstruction
   b.   spinal cord compression
   c.   trigeminal neuralgia
   d.   tumor pressing on a vital organ

1.255   Scheduling of oral analgesics generally should be:
   a.   at fixed intervals
   b.   every 2 hours
   c.   as needed (prn)
   d.   related to a patient's activity level

1.256   The nursing diagnoses for patients receiving intraspinal opioids would include *all but* which of the following?
   a.   potential alteration in respiratory function
   b.   potential alteration in comfort related to pruritus, nausea, and vomiting
   c.   potential alteration in cardiac function
   d.   potential infection at the catheter site

Psychotropic Drugs

1.257   Cannabinoids such as Marinol are generally used as second-line antiemetics. Which of the following is a side effect of cannabinoids?
   a.   dysphoria
   b.   disorientation
   c.   impaired concentration
   d.   all of the above

1.258 Lorazepam is a benzodiazepine and is used in combination antiemetic therapy. The mechanism of action of lorazepam includes *all but* which of the following?
a. sedation
b. dopamine antagonism
c. CNS depressant
d. interference with afferent nerves from the cerebral cortex

1.259 Allison has shingles that was successfully treated, but she was instructed to take an antidepressant for approximately 2 weeks. The purpose of the antidepressant is which of the following?
a. treatment for postherpetic neuralgia
b. treatment for her depression
c. to inhibit uptake of the neurotransmitters into nerve terminals
d. a and c

1.260 Which of the following agents effectively counteracts opioid-induced drowsiness?
a. clonazepam
b. amitriptyline
c. methylphenidate
d. imipramine

1.261 Lorazepam is commonly used in combination antiemetic therapy. Side effects of this drug include *all but* which of the following?
a. addiction
b. drowsiness
c. amnesia
d. diarrhea

1.262 Mr. Goodie has complained of feeling more depressed over the last 2 weeks. He had been taking his Prozac faithfully, but stopped taking it a week ago when he was started on a new antidepressant, Parnate, a monoamine oxidase inhibitor, which he started 3 days ago. He now presents with mental status changes, including severe agitation and insomnia. The best explanation for his current symptoms includes which of the following?
a. He is experiencing normal reactions to the new antidepressant. These symptoms will subside over 3–4 days.
b. The Prozac is still in his system and is causing a drug interaction.
c. Once a patient is on a serotonin uptake inhibitor, a monoamine oxidase inhibitor is generally not sufficient to treat the depression.
d. Most antidepressants must be taken for 2 weeks to reach therapeutic levels.

1.263 Methylpenidate (Ritalin) is commonly added to opioid analgesics when used to treat chronic pain. What is the purpose of the methylpenidate in this instance?
a. to act as an antidepressant
b. to counteract the respiratory depression of the opioid analgesics
c. to counteract the sedation of the opioid analgesics
d. to act on the cortex and reticular activating system to decrease awareness of pain

1.264 In the weeks before death, many patients on opioid therapy experience agitation, confusion, and difficulty sleeping, especially at night. Which of the following medications is most therapeutic for patients experiencing these symptoms?
   a. amitriptyline for its anticholinergic effect
   b. lorazepam for its sedating effect
   c. promethazine because it potentiates the analgesic effect of opioids
   d. haloperidol, to combat confusion and agitation

Growth Factors

1.265 Colony-stimulating factors (CSFs) act on the stem cells to specifically mediate which of the following steps in hematopoiesis?
   a. cellular proliferation
   b. cellular differentiation
   c. stem cell maturation
   d. all of the above

1.266 Granulocyte (G) and granulocyte-macrophage (GM) colony-stimulating factors (CSFs):
   a. increase febrile episodes
   b. decrease myelosuppression
   c. increase mucositis
   d. decrease anorexia

1.267 Epidermal growth factor receptor has been found to correlate with a poor prognosis in which of the following?
   a. breast cancer
   b. bladder cancer
   c. glioblastoma
   d. all of the above

1.268 Which of the following is *not* considered a primary reason to administer CSFs to patients receiving chemotherapy?
   a. to permit administration of full doses of the chemotherapy agents
   b. to decrease infectious complications
   c. to shorten the period of febrile neutropenia
   d. to prevent neutropenia in all patients receiving chemotherapy

1.269 Which of the following is used primarily to boost production of red blood cells in response to hypoxia?
   a. erythropoietin
   b. thrombopoietin
   c. macrophage-CSF
   d. somatotropin

1.270 Mr. Prang, who is to receive a blood cell transplant, asks you to explain the function of HGFs in his treatment. Which of the following could be part of your response?
   a. HGFs cannot act alone to stimulate enhanced proliferation and maturation of neutrophils.
   b. HGFs provide a much more controlled response for mobilization.
   c. Although HGFs can enhance chemotherapy, chemotherapy alone yields more predictable results.
   d. all of the above

1.271   Epidermal growth factor receptors have recently been found to be an important prognostic indicator in breast cancer. Which of the following statements regarding the relationship between epidermal growth factor receptors and breast cancer is *false*?
  a.   The presence of the epidermal growth factor receptor means that a woman is most likely to be ER and PR positive.
  b.   The presence of the epidermal growth factor receptor means the patient has a poor prognosis.
  c.   Inhibiting growth factor receptors is therapeutic in women with breast cancer.
  d.   The presence of the epidermal growth factor has implications for selection of chemotherapy protocols.

1.272   Overexpression of the epidermal growth factor receptor (EGFR) is associated with a poor prognosis in which of the following cancer types?
  a.   breast cancer
  b.   bladder cancer
  c.   lung cancer
  d.   all of the above

1.273   The lesions associated with Kaposi's sarcoma (KS) tend to remain localized because the tumor is not capable of synthesizing its own angiogenic and vascular endothelial growth factors to support surrounding vessels.
  a.   true
  b.   false

ANSWER EXPLANATIONS

1.1   **The answer is d.** The neural activities that occur in transmission and modulation culminate in the mechanism of pain known as perception. Because perception varies considerably from one individual to the next, it is the mechanism that contributes to the great diversity in response to noxious stimuli/events. This process is the least understood of all those related to pain.

1.2   **The answer is b.** Fentanyl, 75 times more potent than morphine, is currently being administered via transdermal patches that are changed at prescribed intervals. This delivery system is an exciting new option for cancer patients who are experiencing pain, but it is not without its side effects, among them a prolonged effect after patch removal secondary to the long half-life of fentanyl.

1.3   **The answer is c.** Counterirritant cutaneous stimulation (e.g., massage, heat or cold therapy, transcutaneous electrical nerve stimulation) is thought to help relieve pain by somehow physiologically altering the transmission of nociceptive stimuli referred to in Melzack and Wall's gate control theory of pain. It is also thought that the relief achieved may outlast the actual application of the counterirritant.

1.4   **The answer is a.** Distraction (e.g., conversation, imagery, breathing exercises, watching television) directs attention away from the sensations and emotional reactions produced by pain and blocks awareness of the pain stimulus and its effects. It can be very helpful in reducing pain, but caregivers must remember that simply because a patient is effectively distracted from the pain does not mean that he or she is pain-free.

1.5   **The answer is d.** Of the five dimensions of the cancer pain experience described by Ahles et al., the cognitive dimension relates to the manner in which pain influences a person's thought processes, view of self, and the meaning of the pain.

1.6   **The answer is a.** Evidence suggests that children experience no more or less pain than adults, and patients in the general ward or in the early stages of their disease have less prevalence of pain than do those in a hospice or terminal care setting.

1.7   **The answer is c.** A great deal of valuable information is available in the field of pain management, but the lack of basic assessment skills, a lack of coordinated and detailed records, and inaccurate knowledge concerning pharmacological principles all create problems for successfully managing patients' pain. Existing legal statutes and government agencies have contributed to inadequate prescribing by physicians because of fear of regulatory scrutiny.

1.8   **The answer is c.** An assessment of behavioral parameters of pain should include the effect of the pain on activities of daily living (ADLs), such as eating, mobility, and social interactions, as well as activities/behaviors that increase or decrease the intensity of pain. A behavioral assessment also considers pain behaviors used, including grimacing or other nonverbal communication and the use of medications or other pain control interventions.

1.9   **The answer is a.** The husband is not becoming addicted but might be experiencing some degree of drug tolerance. This is normal, and it is not uncommon for drug doses to increase over time. He also might be having increased bone metastasis or other sites of pain; further assessment is required. Sleep is often the first sign of pain relief because patients may have been unable to rest comfortably with pain. Patients and caregivers often negatively influence the treatment of pain because of their fears about potent narcotics. They may increase the dose interval, withhold doses, or refuse certain medications or certain routes as they attempt to prevent dependence, addiction, somnolence, or sedation. The wife needs education regarding cancer pain and relief methods, as well as a great deal of support.

1.10   **The answer is c.** Fatigue is the most common side effect of cancer treatment. People with cancer may also experience fatigue as a symptom of the disease or as a result of physical deconditioning.

1.11   **The answer is b.** In contrast to weakness, fatigue has a voluntary component. Individuals with fatigue may push themselves to engage in highly valued activities despite their fatigue. Individuals suffering from weakness are unable to initiate or maintain specific muscular activities.

1.12   **The answer is c.** Because cancer patients often undergo multiple surgical procedures and because fatigue is a consistent side effect found in patients recovering from surgery, the cumulative effects of these procedures on patients suffering from cancer-related fatigue are very important.

1.13   **The answer is a.** Biologic response modifiers tend to produce fatigue that is more severe than that associated with surgery, radiation therapy, and the most commonly used chemotherapy regimens.

1.14   **The answer is b.** Fatigue may persist for months after the conclusion of treatment and may in fact worsen for those patients with advanced cancer. Assistive devices may still be necessary and appropriate.

1.15   **The answer is b.** Chronic fatigue, as opposed to acute fatigue, persists over time and is not readily relieved by rest. Weakness would have left Mary unable to walk her dog and swim, and depression would have been indicated if Mary had expressed a general sadness that resulted in her low levels of activity.

1.16   **The answer is c.** Choosing an objective indicator, giving Mark an endurance test, and asking Mark's family for information are all choices for gathering objective information—which your colleague says he wants. However, these things should be regarded as responses to fatigue rather than fatigue itself, and fatigue should be measured subjectively, according to the patient's perception of the problem.

1.17   **The answer is d.** Studies focused on reversing severe anemia caused by bone marrow suppression may not generalize to most patients receiving cancer treatments. Karen's much less severe anemia could be caused by many different factors and may be treated in a number of different ways, all of which may or may not improve the condition and her fatigue.

1.18   **The answer is d.** Pruritus, or itching, may be localized or generalized and may occur as a consequence of obstructive biliary disease or a treatment side effect such as dry desquamation following radiation therapy or as a reaction to opiate analgesics.

1.19   **The answer is b.** Pruritus, which frequently accompanies jaundice, is precipitated by irritation of the cutaneous sensory nerve fibers by accumulated bile salts. The use of deodorant soaps should be avoided because they tend to dry skin and intensify pruritus.

1.20   **The answer is d.** Vitamins A, C, D, and B complex can be given to reduce the effect of jaundice, but it is not a treatment for pruritus. Meticulous skin hygiene is needed to cleanse away the accumulated bile salts. Relief is sometimes obtained with oil-based lotions, antihistamines, and cholestyramine.

1.21   **The answer is a.** Pruritus, which frequently accompanies jaundice, is precipitated by irritation of the cutaneous sensory nerve fibers by accumulated bile salts. Therefore, an individual with liver cancer must have meticulous skin hygiene, and efforts to reduce itching should be implemented. Depending on the extent of liver dysfunction, deficits in clotting mechanisms may exist, occasionally necessitating the use of vitamin K to prevent bleeding. Most individuals with liver cancer are in a poor nutritional state and benefit greatly from a diet high in proteins and carbohydrates and low in fats.

1.22   **The answer is d.** Pruritus, or itching, may be localized or generalized and is associated with many medical conditions. Pruritus may occur in conjunction with thyroid disease, diabetes, anemia, polycythemia, leukemia, multiple myeloma, adenocarcinoma, Hodgkin's disease, non-Hodgkin's lymphoma, acquired immunodeficiency syndrome (AIDS), and Kaposi's sarcoma. It may also occur as a consequence of obstructive biliary disease or treatment side effects such as dry desquamation following radiation therapy, as a reaction to opiate analgesics, or an allergic dermatitis following chemotherapy.

1.23   **The answer is d.** Generalized pruritus may be an early sign of systemic disease as with Hodgkin's disease and T-cell lymphomas. In CNS malignancy, pruritus can present as a paraneoplastic syndrome.

1.24   **The answer is a.** Constitutional symptoms of fever, malaise, night sweats, weight loss and pruritus appear in about 40% of affected patients, and these manifestations, called B symptoms, are more common in patients with advanced disease.

1.25   **The answer is a.** Although some thinning can occur, true alopecia is rare. Severe itching and pruritus can be intense because of severe skin dryness. Rapid weight gain occurs as a result of capillary leak syndrome. The most severe nausea, vomiting, and diarrhea occur with IL-2 therapy, particularly high-dose regimens.

1.26   **The answer is a.** Environmental factors include keeping the room humidity at 30–40% and the room temperature cool.

1.27   **The answer is a.** Nail et al. studied the incidence of side effects from chemotherapy and the use of self-care activities. Sleeping difficulty as well as nausea and decreased appetite were reported by approximately 50% of the subjects.

1.28   **The answer is b.** The psychobiological-entropy hypothesis includes propositions that address the importance of achieving a balance between activity and rest.

1.29   **The answer is b.** Rest and napping are among the most frequently cited self-care strategies for relieving fatigue, but they are less effective in relieving fatigue than going to bed early.

1.30   **The answer is a.** Corticosteroids are frequently used in antineoplastic drug regimens and in antiemetic drug protocols and commonly cause sleep disruption, insomnia, restlessness, and increased motor activity.

1.31   **The answer is d.** Anticipatory nausea and vomiting are often brought about by the patient's previous experience with uncontrolled nausea and vomiting. Lorazepam acts as an antianxiety agent but also has some antinausea effects because it works well with other antiemetics. Sleep is an important adjunct to controlling nausea and vomiting with chemotherapy, and lorazepam is sedating.

1.32   **The answer is d.** Growth hormone and prolactin are elevated during sleep and enhance immune function, whereas corticosteroids and catecholamines are immunosuppressive and depressed during sleep.

1.33   **The answer is a.** It is often difficult to distinguish whether sleep disturbances are a function of the treatment and disease factors or are instead secondary to emotional factors. Affective factors unrelated to the cancer cannot be ignored as etiologic factors in sleep disturbance.

1.34   **The answer is a.** The newer hypnotics are not benzodiazepine derivatives, but act similarly without suppressing delta sleep, the stage during which physiologic restoration is thought to be the greatest.

1.35   **The answer is d.** Although it may be appropriate to suppress a dry, persistent, and debilitating cough, this should not be attempted at the expense of removal of secretions. The other strategies suggested promote comfort.

1.36   **The answer is d.** Dyspnea, although a subjective observation, is a general indication of inadequate respiration. Pleuritic chest pain may manifest as rapid, shallow breathing. Intercostal retractions on inspiration indicate obstruction of air inflow, and bulging interspaces on expiration are associated with outflow obstruction; either may be an indication of tumor. Stridor is a manifestation of extrathoracic airway obstruction. The use of accessory muscles for breathing; labored, prolonged expiration; and wheezing may indicate obstruction of intrathoracic airways.

1.37   **The answer is d.** Not all pleural effusions are malignant and etiology should be established before palliative treatment is initiated. When pleural effusions reaccumulate, as is often the case, pleurodesis is the recommended therapy.

1.38   **The answer is a.** Agents used for pleurodesis include bleomycin, talc, doxycycline, and minocycline. Tetracycline, formerly the most frequently used sclerosing agent, is no longer available in the injectable form.

1.39   **The answer is d.** Pleural fluid removal through an implanted port and interpleural catheter can be performed by the nurse on an outpatient basis. New technology using small-bore needles may permit management of malignant pleural effusions on an outpatient basis. These radiologically placed small-bore catheters are connected to a plastic bag with a one-way valve system for gravity drainage. In cases of recurrent effusion, a pleuroperitoneal shunt can be inserted to divert fluid from the chest cavity to the abdomen.

1.40   **The answer is a.** Dyspnea may be associated with destruction of lung tissue by tumor, pleural effusions, airway obstruction by endobronchial lesions, and increased mucus production. Radiation effects are not commonly part of the acute problem of dyspnea related to advanced lung cancer.

1.41   **The answer is a.** The purpose of the bleomycin is to obliterate the pleural space and prevent reaccumulation of fluid.

1.42   **The answer is b.** The cause of dyspnea is thought to be the decrease in cardiac output or the decrease in lung expansion by the pericardium. No adventitious sounds are heard with the disorder because pulmonary congestion is absent.

1.43   **The answer is a.** Side effects of BCG include cough that develops following treatment, which could possibly indicate a BCG infection. Fever is common, and fever over 101°F should be treated with acetaminophen. Most patients develop varying degrees of nausea and vomiting after BCG instillation and occasionally systemic hypersensitivity reactions, which can be treated with diphenhydramine.

1.44   **The answer is b.** Patients are monitored for prolonged flu-like symptoms and organ dysfunction (liver, kidney, and pulmonary abnormalities) that suggest potential BCG infection.

1.45   **The answer is c.** Fever is the cardinal symptom of infection. The neutropenic condition of marrow recipients masks the classic infection-related symptoms of inflammation, pus formation, and elevated white blood cell counts.

1.46   **The answer is c.** When the neutrophil count is less than 500, approximately 20% or more of febrile episodes have an associated bacteremia caused principally by aerobic gram-negative bacilli and gram-positive cocci.

1.47   **The answer is c.** The actions of endotoxins include release of endogenous pyrogens, resulting in a febrile response, alteration of the vascular endothelium, causing formation of microthrombi; activation of the complement, coagulation, and fibrinolytic systems; and release of bradykinin, histamine, and serotonin, producing vasodilation and increased capillary permeability.

1.48   **The answer is b.** In a study of 1130 patients with severe sepsis, only 55% had fevers greater than 38°C, 15% were hypothermic, and 30% were normothermic.

1.49   **The answer is c.** The hypersensitivity reactions with bleomycin include hypotension, rash, facial flushing, and bronchospasm, but in general most patients experience only a relatively high fever, chills, and a flu-like syndrome.

1.50 **The answer is c.** It has been demonstrated that unfiltered platelet concentrates accumulate high levels of cytokines, which can produce the signs and symptoms of a febrile transfusion reaction.

1.51 **The answer is c.** Nonhemolytic transfusion reactions are usually reversible with conservative therapy, and the transfusion may be resumed once the symptoms have subsided. Placing the patient in the Trendelenburg position and administering a fluid bolus are not ideal because of the dyspnea.

1.52 **The answer is c.** Treatment for tumor fever involves treating the underlying malignancy. Chemotherapy often leads to defervescence of the fever as the tumor burden is reduced. NSAIDs are very effective in controlling tumor fever and have been used as a diagnostic tool in patients with cancer who have fever of unknown origin.

1.53 **The answer is c.** Patients who are going to react to the Herceptin will usually react the first time with the loading dose, but then not again during subsequent dosing. The patients will generally do very well once they have the diphenhydramine and can continue their treatment.

1.54 **The answer is b.** Spirituality refers to that dimension of being human that motivates meaning-making and self-transcendence—or intra-, inter-, and transpersonal connectedness. Spirituality prompts individuals to make sense of their universe and to relate harmoniously with self, nature, and others—including any god(s) (as conceptualized by each person). Religion is the representation and expression of spirituality. Ethics involves reflecting systematically about right conduct and how to live as a good person.

1.55 **The answer is c.** Regardless of one's beliefs about religion, prayer (liberally defined) can be a resource to all; conversational and meditative types are usually more directly correlated with spiritual well-being than petitionary and ritualistic approaches to prayer.

1.56 **The answer is b.** The work of reconstructing a worldview to include new, wiser assumptions in response to trauma involves a process of balancing thinking about the painful subject with avoiding painful thoughts (approach versus avoidance). Using therapeutic techniques such as clarification and summarization, the nurse can assist a person in identifying and appreciating cognitive strategies that provide comfort and meaning.

1.57 **The answer is b.** In nursing literature that defines related terms such as spiritual distress, need, or well-being, spirituality is described as an integrating energy, a life principle, an innate human quality. In contrast to spirituality, religiosity often is viewed as a narrower concept.

1.58 **The answer is c.** Gotay found that praying, having faith, and hoping were used more often as coping strategies by women with advanced cancer than by their counterparts with early-stage cancer.

1.59 **The answer is c.** The rationale for nurses who opposed active euthanasia included personal and professional integrity, sanctity of life, and religious beliefs, and the nurses who supported active euthanasia typically cited patient autonomy, families' wishes, severe suffering, and terminal illness as reasons for supporting active euthanasia. It is important to note that private religiosity significantly influences oncology nurses' attitudes about end-of-life options.

1.60   **The answer is c.** Individuals assume that the world is meaningful and that they have worth. Traumatic events such as a cancer diagnosis can shatter these assumptions. When this happens, people work to reconstruct their worldview so that it includes assumptions about the event that are wiser and more mature. Cognitive strategies that individuals use for reconstructing the assumptions include making comparisons—for example "it could be worse." The individuals must construe their own meanings for life's traumas—the nurse cannot do this cognitive work for them.

1.61   **The answer is a.** Spirituality refers to that dimension of being human that motivates meaning-making and self-transcendence- or intra-, inter-, and transpersonal connectedness.

1.62   **The answer is a.** Individuals with low annual incomes are three to seven times more likely to die of cancer than those with high annual incomes.

1.63   **The answer is b.** In the late 1970s the question of the role of poverty in the differences in incidence, mortality, and survival of different ethnic groups was first raised. The disproportionate number of African Americans in the lower socioeconomic strata accounted for the increased incidence. One study that included only caucasians, who received the same level of care, found that indigent patients had poorer survival rates for each cancer type. Among male Veterans Administration patients with cancer, similar survival rates between black and caucasian Americans were found. All patients received the same treatment standard without regard to ability to pay for services.

1.64   **The answer is d.** A primary barrier to cancer care for many ethnic minority populations is access to health care, especially among the socioeconomically disadvantaged. Many programs focus on providing effective cancer screening for ethnic minority populations using culturally sensitive strategies.

1.65   **The answer is b.** Historically in the United States, cancer prevention services have not been reimbursed by payers at all levels. The growth of managed care and capitation and the increasing use of primary health care providers as gatekeepers are driving the coverage of preventive services. Quality-control efforts by health plans carefully monitor whether patients receive necessary preventive services. However, funding for preventive services remains inadequate, even in prepaid health systems.

1.66   **The answer is a.** A POS (point of service) plan allows members to access out-of-plan providers but imposes strict utilization strategies.

1.67   **The answer is d.** For middle- and upper-class families with adequate health insurance and relatively secure jobs, out-of-pocket expenditures for deductibles and copayments are not a concern, and with adequate insurance there are no gaps in coverage.

1.68   **The answer is c.** Increasingly, nurses are being called on to justify the resources that are needed to improve patient care. Feasibility studies and cost analysis studies, including cost-benefit analysis and cost-effectiveness analysis, are some techniques at the nurse's disposal. Feasibility studies determine whether a new program should be developed and implemented in a health care agency. Cost-benefit analysis assigns monetary value to all costs and benefits of a potential program or practice, resulting in a cost-benefit ratio. Cost-effectiveness analysis is all the costs, measured in dollars, necessary to achieve a certain benefit, calculated and expressed as cost per unit of effectiveness. This technique is used to compare relative costs of several alternatives.

1.69 **The answer is b.** Approximately 60% of uninsured Americans are in the active workforce but are employed by small companies that do not offer health coverage benefits. This category of worker will continue to increase as the number of small service-oriented companies increases and that of large manufacturing companies declines. The other factors are real, but less important.

1.70 **The answer is b.** The evaluation and selection of alternative care arrangements requires individual attention to the needs and goals of the patient. Two important considerations in this selection process are cost and the patient's financial resources, including insurance coverage and benefits, and the quantity and quality of care provided by alternative care settings or agencies.

1.71 **The answer is c.** The success of a coping strategy is determined by its outcome or intended outcome. The behavior of denial is "value neutral," meaning that it is not inherently adaptive or maladaptive. Its adaptiveness is determined by what it can or does achieve. Also, because this patient has "just been diagnosed," we may assume that not enough time has passed for us to determine whether the denial is adaptive or maladaptive.

1.72 **The answer is c.** Age is a sociodemographic factor that is predictive of psychological adjustment to cancer. Younger people report greater adjustment difficulties in comparison to older people.

1.73 **The answer is b.** When psychological boundaries are clear, they touch another boundary but do not get mixed up with the other person's priorities or goals. This is when caring is therapeutic.

1.74 **The answer is d.** A history of comorbidity (whether psychiatric or medical) and the presence of more advanced disease increases the individual's risk for poor psychosocial outcomes after a cancer diagnosis. Social networks have been found to have a protective effect with regard to psychosocial outcomes.

1.75 **The answer is b.** Three different role preferences have been identified among individuals with cancer. Between 12% and 20% of cancer patients expressed a desire to take an active role in making the final selection of treatment. A second group of 32–59% preferred passivity, allowing the physician to make the final decision about treatment. A third group of 28%–40% preferred to collaborate with the physician in making decisions.

1.76 **The answer is c.** Although it is possible to achieve complete remission in 93% of children with ALL, the same drug treatment—even with the addition of an anthracycline—produces remission rates of only 70–75% in adults with ALL.

1.77 **The answer is d.** According to stress theory, individuals come to the cancer experience with a history of stress responses. Those who have been unsuccessful in resolving past stress situations, who are dealing with several stressors simultaneously, and who perceive minimal social support in the situations are at higher risk for psychosocial distress.

1.78 **The answer is c.** The primary objective of psychosocial nursing intervention usually is to encourage coping responses by patients. These interventions may be focused on problem-solving choices (**a**, **b**, and **d**) or on emotional expression. Examples of emotion-focused interventions include fostering emotional expression through active listening; creating constructive release of affective responses through play therapy, music, or humor; and providing individual or group testing and counseling to facilitate insight into emotional needs and response patterns.

1.79   **The answer is a.** Denial or minimization may be an effective coping strategy, particularly in the early stages of the disease and at stressful points in the illness trajectory (such as during recurrence). Psychosocial responses cannot be clearly identified as either adaptive or maladaptive; this depends largely on the situation and on the adaptive potential of the particular response in that situation. A perception of uncertainty can result in an appraisal of danger or opportunity, depending on the individual's definition of the situation. Distancing behaviors by health professionals enhance patients' sense of loneliness and fear. Overinvolvement with patients can be countered through supportive collegial relationships.

1.80   **The answer is c.** Four dimensions that are typically represented in QOL include physical, functional, psychological, and social well-being.

1.81   **The answer is a.** The QOL dimension of social well-being includes social support, family functioning, and intimacy. Psychological well-being refers to emotional state, including both positive and negative moods.

1.82   **The answer is d.** When patients with low and high levels of information about their disease were compared, there was a significant correspondence between patient and spouse perceptions for patient with high information. When the individual with cancer knows little about his or her disease, the couple functions under highly restrictive conditions of denial, fear, isolation, and conjecture.

1.83   **The answer is b.** Social psychologists theorize that significant losses and changes cause individuals to search for meaning as a way of trying to make sense of such a negative experience.

1.84   **The answer is d.** The overwhelming demands and complexity of care for the individual with cancer can result in caregiver burden. When the individual with cancer knows little about his or her disease, the couple functions under highly restrictive conditions of denial, fear, isolation, and conjecture.

1.85   **The answer is c.** A detailed family assessment is important, particularly with regard to the status of the caregiver. Families are categorized as supportive, ambivalent, or hostile, and they generally continue to act as they did in previous crises.

1.86   **The answer is d**. Family units can be identified as supportive, hostile, or ambivalent, with their behavior described in terms of cohesion, adaptability, and communication. When crisis occurs or families are faced with the serious and difficult implications of cancer and its treatment, their behavior usually does not change and in some cases can intensify. Therefore, if a family was dysfunctional, hostile, or in conflict, it is very likely that their behavior will continue. The home health care nurse's primary concern is to support and care for the patient. The chances are high that the home health care nurse will be unable to change the behavior of the family members in conflict.

1.87   **The answer is c.** Each individual brings to the cancer experience unique personality traits and a personal socialization pattern different from all others. Understanding the uniqueness of the individual is achieved only through study of the commonalities of the personality and social psychological (psychosocial) aspects of illness.

1.88   **The answer is d.** Intensive family therapy may be helpful in selected situations. However, research indicates that the majority of cancer patients and significant others facing care are well adjusted without the need for intensive intervention.

1.89   **The answer is b.** Abnormal grief may manifest itself in exaggerated or excessive expressions of normal grief reactions, such as excessive anger, sadness, or depression. For most hospice programs, therapy for abnormal grief extends beyond the scope of the bereavement care services provided. The hospice program staff should be able to identify and recommend competent referrals for abnormal grief syndromes. It is therapeutic to review a person's life with a loved one. Listening to a family member share stories of their life with the loved one honors the meaning of their relationship and their life together. Funeral planning can be therapeutic and facilitate someone's loss as they do one last thing in a special way for their loved one. Delegating responsibilities that can be overwhelming or too painful might actually be an indicator of the grieving party being aware of their limitations and calling on their resources and support systems.

1.90   **The answer is b.** It is helpful to explore previous losses and coping mechanisms used.

1.91   **The answer is b.** Unresolved grief has been associated with multiple physical and emotional illnesses, including increased risk of suicide.

1.92   **The answer is c.** Adjusting to the environment in which the deceased is absent is crucial to the normal grief process.

1.93   **The answer is b.** The patient must desire palliative, not curative, treatment. Patients can receive treatments that are aimed at palliation, not cure. Blood is generally not given but can be, for palliative reasons, as can pamidronate.

1.94   **The answer is b.** Loss of a parent during adolescence has been documented as a critical event in the life of a child. Research has shown that during the illness, adolescents describe open information sharing among the family. After the death of the parent, however, adolescents assume the protector role in shielding the remaining parent from discussing distressful feelings. These adolescents frequently found the protector role extremely stressful.

1.95   **The answer is d.** A study of communication patterns between breast cancer patients and children within the family revealed that deteriorated relationships were correlated with a poor prognosis for the patient and with poor adjustment scores on the measurement instruments used. The frequency and magnitude of problems with fears related to prognosis, rejection, and refusal to discuss cancer were greatest in mother-daughter relationships.

1.96   **The answer is d.** Anticipatory mourning is considered to be a normal process associated with a chronic disease, whereby a grieving person begins to work through part of his or her grief before the patient dies.

1.97   **The answer is a.** There is a gradual decrease in the former smoker's risk of dying from lung cancer; eventually the risk is almost equivalent to that of a nonsmoker. The rate of decline of risk after cessation of smoking is determined by the cumulative smoking exposure prior to cessation, the age when smoking began, and the degree of inhalation.

1.98   **The answer is c.** Age has an influence on health behaviors.

1.99   **The answer is d.** All women starting at age 20 should perform BSE monthly. Women in Alexis's age category (20–40 years of age) should have a breast physical exam every 3 years, and women older than 40 years should have a breast physical examination every year.

1.100   **The answer is c.** Anxiety is most likely to occur when an individual experiences a nonspecific internal or external stimulus that is perceived as a threat to certain beliefs, values, and conditions essential to a secure existence.

1.101　**The answer is d.** In one study, anxiety levels (STAI scores) among the 85 patients studied were above the norms for acutely ill psychiatric patients. In addition to this finding, critical thinking was substantially reduced during hospitalization when compared with 6–8 weeks after discharge.

1.102　**The answer is c.** Loss of self-esteem is more commonly a symptom of depression. In general, nursing interventions that focus on anxiety are based on helping the patient to recognize various manifestations of anxiety, determining whether the patient desires to do anything about the response, and activating coping strategies to control anxiety levels.

1.103　**The answer is d.** In Hays's study of 100 patients during the last 10 days of their lives, patients who experienced more physical symptoms and more uncontrolled symptoms were more likely to require inpatient hospice services. In addition, patients whose families experienced increased anxiety and fatigue in response to the patient's uncontrolled symptoms also showed an increased use of inpatient hospice services.

1.104　**The answer is d.** Although it has been previously reported that the use of breast-preserving surgery (lumpectomy) has been shown to cause significantly less alteration in body image, sexual desire, and frequency of intercourse, recent studies showed no difference between women receiving lumpectomy and radiotherapy, and women undergoing mastectomy. What appears to be of significance is the opportunity or perceived opportunity to select the surgical technique employed. Thus, choices should be offered whenever possible.

1.105　**The answer is b.** Beau's lines indicate a reduction in or cessation of nail growth in response to cytotoxic therapy.

1.106　**The answer is a.** The TRAM flap procedure is sometimes known as the "tummy tuck" because the muscle and fat are tunneled from the abdominal muscle to the mastectomy site.

1.107　**The answer is a.** Recent studies have indicated the effectiveness of education and counseling as approaches to treatment of changes in sexual health. One problem with respect to such interventions is that effectiveness is often measured in terms of resumption of sexual intercourse rather than as the effect of the intervention on self-concept or on relationships with others. Another problem is that patients are generally not screened for participation. Screening increases the probability of identifying patients and partners with preexisting problems that may require more intensive therapy.

1.108　**The answer is a.** Among the factors that affect a cancer patient's sexuality are those related to the biologic/physiologic process of cancer, the effects of treatment, the alterations caused by cancer and treatment, and the psychologic issues surrounding the patient and family. Physiologic problems of infertility and sterility, changes in body appearance, and the inability to have intercourse are enhanced by psychologic and psychosexual issues of alteration in body image, fears of abandonment, loss of self-esteem, alterations in sexual identity, and concerns about self. Mutagenicity and psychosexual changes are not closely related.

1.109　**The answer is d.** If more than the anterior third of the vaginal wall is removed, the diameter of the introitus and the vaginal barrel can be severely compromised and intercourse may be restricted. In addition, because of its close proximity to the urethral meatus, the clitoris may be injured or have compromised function because of scarring and fibrosis after surgery.

1.110   **The answer is b.** For women receiving radiation therapy to the vagina, vaginal fibrosis and scarring with a loss of blood supply and elasticity is a major adverse effect. Frequent intercourse can minimize these effects. For patients who are not sexually active, the use of a vaginal dilator with water-soluble lubricants or prescribed estrogen cream starting 2 weeks after treatment are effective prophylactic measures to minimize functional loss.

1.111   **The answer is d.** Researchers found that 50% of patients experience lack of energy and fatigue severe enough to impede normal activities. The majority of women experience vaginal dryness and dyspareunia following BMT and TBI.

1.112   **The answer is d**. Body image includes those elements that refer to the physical self, including how we perceive our bodies, how our bodies actually look and how they function, the impact of sensory inputs (e.g., pain), and what we perceive as an "ideal" body or image.

1.113   **The answer is a.** In order of decreasing radiosensitivity are scalp, beard, eyebrows, eyelashes, axillary, pubic, and fine hair of the body.

1.114   **The answer is a.** Chemotherapy-induced alopecia occurs rapidly and usually starts 2–3 weeks following a dose of chemotherapy. After discontinuation of the epilating drugs, regrowth is visible in 4–6 weeks, but complete regrowth may take 1–2 years. In situations involving very high doses of alkylating agents, hair may not regrow.

1.115   **The answer is b.** Cyclophosphamide and methotrexate, the drugs that are commonly used in curable breast cancer, generally cause gradual thinning of hair.

1.116   **The answer is d.** Recommendations to minimize hair loss include using mild protein-based shampoos with conditioners, avoiding daily shampooing, allowing hair to dry naturally, and grooming hair with a wide-toothed comb. Minoxidil has not been shown to be effective in the prevention of hair loss.

1.117   **The answer is b.**

1.118   **The answer is b.** Radiation response is seen mostly in tissues and organs that are within or adjacent to the treatment field (i.e., they are site specific). Thus, an individual being treated in the abdominal field does not lose scalp hair from radiation.

1.119   **The answer is a.** Chemotherapy agents affect actively growing (anagen) hairs. Because anagen hair is the most rapidly proliferating cell population in the human body, alopecia is a common toxicity.

1.120   **The answer is c.** Chemotherapy agents associated with only mild hair loss include bleomycin, carmustine, epirubicin, 5-FU, methotrexate, mitoxantrone, and vinorelbine.

1.121   **The answer is b.** Cultural sensitivity is having respect for cultures—and the beliefs connected with those cultures—other than your own.

1.122   **The answer is a.** Make linkages with key members of the target community, involving members of the community in the development of educational materials, programs, and community outreach strategies.

1.123   **The answer is a.** Home remedies are first-line treatment in Hispanic cultures. To cure a hot or cold imbalance, the opposite quality of the causative agent is applied.

1.124   **The answer is a.** Among the high-risk behaviors in the Hispanic population are obesity, alcohol consumption, and sexual practices.

1.125   **The answer is c.** In Native American cultures, the singers are healers who treat illnesses and disharmony by laying on of hands, massage, sweatbaths, use of herbs and roots, and chanting.

1.126   **The answer is b.** In a culture of poverty, secondary prevention may be absent because of an orientation in which survival needs take precedence over screening and early detection. Delayed tertiary prevention is due to a lack of insurance, inability to pay for service, or limited care access.

1.127   **The answer is a.** The use of professional interpreters, if available, is the optimal choice. Family and/or friends may be used but the correct or complete message may not be relayed.

1.128   **The answer is a.** The basic unit of society is the family. Cultural values can determine communication with the family, the norm for the family size, and the roles of specific family members.

1.129   **The answer is a.** Education assists the patient in reducing his or her sense of helplessness and inadequacy. The most common means of reducing uncertainty is to provide preparatory information about the specific aspects of the cancer experience faced by the individual. Preparatory information also prevents or alleviates treatment-related symptoms.

1.130   **The answer is a.** Individuals use alternative methods for a variety of stated reasons, such as "I have nothing to lose" or "If it won't hurt me, why not try it?" Often they are confused by conflicting reports of cure rates of standard treatments and frightened by treatment risks and possibly side effects. Many unproven methods promise no side effects and draw on the patient's fantasy of cure involving "the body's natural defenses." By using an unconventional therapy, the patient hopes for an unconventional cure.

1.131   **The answer is c.** In theory, valid data on the efficacy of an alternative method is the best reason for a patient to choose that method, but then the method would no longer be "alternative." The fact remains that none of the various alternative methods discussed in this chapter has stood up to scientific scrutiny, especially the requirement of proven efficacy in human subjects. The reasons stated in the other choices are among the most likely to motivate the cancer patient to seek an alternative therapy.

1.132   **The answer is c.** Loss of control may be the most overwhelming and distressing feeling. Death at home can afford the patient and family control over their environment, as well as the comfort of being in the midst of familiar surroundings. Children can benefit from being involved in very concrete ways to better understand the dying process and facilitate their own grief.

1.133   **The answer is d.** The purpose of this legislation is to ensure that patients' wishes are carried out in the event they become mentally incapacitated or are incapable of making or communicating their decisions.

1.134   **The answer is d.** In studies of breast self-examination behavior, women who practiced breast self-examination more frequently were those who perceived an internal locus of control. This locus of control is often seen in combination with beliefs in high susceptibility and benefits.

1.135   **The answer is c.** Blunters are individuals who avoid threatening health information.

1.136   **The answer is a.** Disruption of family relationships is a key issue for adult children of cancer patients. Behavior problems may become a key issue in the younger child, and assuming the protector role is a documented response of many adolescents to the death of a parent. Other major issues for adult children include involvement in the parent's illness, unresolved relationship problems, and coping with illness demands.

1.137   **The answer is a.** In addition, the coexistence of signs and symptoms of disease and treatment that are similar to those of depression make the diagnosis of depression difficult.

1.138   **The answer is a.** Choice **b** is an affective response; other affective responses include worthlessness, hopelessness, and sadness. Choices **c** and **d** are cognitive responses; another cognitive response is a decreased ability to concentrate. Other behavioral responses include change in appetite, sleep disturbances, withdrawal, and dependency.

1.139   **The answer is c.** Critical to establishing a diagnosis of reactive (situational) depression in cancer patients is the evaluation of selected defining characteristics commonly attributed to depression among the psychiatrically ill. Some common characteristics of depression, however, may also occur in the cancer patient as a result of the disease, its treatment, or its side effects, or they may have existed in the patient before diagnosis. Therefore, the primary criteria for assessment of depression are that the characteristics are a change from previous functioning, are persistent, occur for most of the day and on more days than not, and are present for at least 2 weeks.

1.140   **The answer is b.** The other interventions listed are cognitive or behavioral in approach. Before these interventions are attempted, it is important for the nurse to acknowledge the patient's feelings associated with depression, including hopelessness, despair, anger, and guilt. The nurse can do this in many ways, starting with giving the patient permission to discuss those feelings, then demonstrating acceptance of them by attentive listening and by exploring methods for the patient to deal positively with them.

1.141   **The answer is d.** Hopelessness appears not to pervade the experience of the cancer patient, unlike anxiety and depression. Rather, it waxes and wanes with changes in perceived health, relationships, and spirituality.

1.142   **The answer is a.** Family responses of anxiety, depression, hopelessness, and altered sexual health in response to a diagnosis of cancer have been shown to be similar to those of the patients themselves.

1.143   **The answer is c.** Anxiety and depression can result from the disruption in lifestyle produced by fatigue. This may occur when fatigue experienced as a side effect of cancer treatment forces the individual to give up usual social roles or makes it impossible to reach desired goals.

1.144   **The answer is c.** *Self-concept* is defined as the total self-appraisal of appearance, background and origins, abilities, resources, atitudes, and feelings. The majority of empirical studies dealing with the relationship of cancer to self-concept have focused on women with gynecologic or breast cancer or on males with testicular or prostate cancer. Additional empirical data are needed on the issues of perception of significant others' responses to the physical and psychological sequelae of cancer and on the interaction of other variables, such as age, depression, and activity status, on the physical as well as psychosocial aspects of sexual health.

1.145   **The answer is b.** Up to 80% of cancer patients return to work after being diagnosed, and their performance differs little, if any, from others hired for similar assignments. "Job-lock" refers to survivors' fear of losing medical coverage were they to change jobs. Only a few states explicitly protect those with a history of cancer.

1.146   **The answer is d.** Four main considerations affect the adult cancer survivor's ability to achieve optimal physical, social, and psychological function: developmental considerations, disease trajectory considerations, physical function and cosmesis, and socioeconomic considerations.

1.147   **The answer is a.** Advanced disease at diagnosis is the most powerful predictor of cancer survival.

1.148   **The answer is a.** A living will may be applicable only when it pertains to a terminal illness but not for a patient whose health is declining for medical reasons other than those that can be classified as terminal or if the patient is in a vegetative state. In general, the power of attorney for health care is more useful than the living will. The living will does not identify another person who can act as the agent for a disabled patient. Verbal instructions are of little value if a family member or anyone else chooses to argue against what has been reportedly communicated verbally. Written instructions are necessary. An order that instructs not to intubate does not address any other interventions that might be suggested.

1.149   **The answer is c.** The observation over time of individuals with cancer and the calculation of their probability of dying over several time periods is called survival analysis.

1.150   **The answer is d.** The ability to conceive or father a child after BMT is related to age and treatment with TBI.

1.151   **The answer is b.** A review of the findings from 18 studies that included almost 1600 children born to 1078 mothers or fathers who had previously been treated for cancer indicated that there was no increase in fetal wastage or in congenital defects noted in the offspring when compared to the general population.

1.152   **The answer is a.** The target organs most commonly affected are the thyroid, ovaries, and testes. Late effects can include alterations in metabolism, growth, secondary sexual characteristics, and reproduction.

1.153   **The answer is b.** High doses of radiation to the hypothalamic pituitary axis can damage the hypothalamus and disrupt the production of growth hormone. Growth hormone deficiency with short stature is one of the most common long-term endocrine consequences of radiation to the CNS in children.

1.154   **The answer is a.** Radiation exposure during the first trimester represents the greatest risk to the fetus. In the second or third trimester, fetal death is unlikely, but growth retardation, sterility, and cataracts are common. Chemotherapy, particularly when received during the first trimester, has been related to congenital abnormalities, with approximately 10% of fetuses experiencing some type of anomaly.

1.155   **The answer is d.** Chemotherapy in the second and third trimester may cause premature birth or low birth weight, but congenital abnormalities are not increased over the normal pregnancy incidence.

1.156   **The answer is c.** Women over the age of 30 are less likely to regain ovarian function because they have fewer oocytes.

1.157   **The answer is d.** Those who do not believe that another pregnancy is contraindicated suggest a waiting period of 2–5 years after completion of all therapy inasmuch as recurrence is most likely during this time period. Further pregnancies after a diagnosis of breast cancer are considered controversial. Some authors suggest that all women refrain from any pregnancies, whereas others suggest that a pregnancy may actually protect against recurrence. Choice **b** is true but should not seriously affect an attempt at conception; choice **c** duplicates the initial reason.

1.158   **The answer is c.** Therapeutic abortion has not been shown to be beneficial in altering disease progression and should not be considered unless pregnancy will compromise treatment and thus prognosis. Therapeutic abortion is most likely to be recommended when the cancer is diagnosed at an advanced stage during the first trimester of pregnancy and the effects of combination chemotherapy are likely to damage the fetus.

1.159   **The answer is a.** During the first two trimesters, surgery or radiation therapy, without therapeutic abortion, is usually undertaken. Early-stage disease may be treated with radical hysterectomy and pelvic node dissection, whereas radiation therapy is the most common treatment in advanced disease. During the third trimester, fetal viability usually can be awaited and the baby delivered by cesarean section, after which appropriate cancer therapy can be given.

1.160   **The answer is d.** Certain malignancies, notably melanoma, non-Hodgkin's lymphoma (NHL), and leukemia, are known to spread from the mother to the fetus. If the mother has any of these cancers, the placenta should be carefully evaluated at delivery and the baby monitored for development of the disease.

1.161   **The answer is c.** Chemotherapy during the first trimester has been associated with fetal wastage, malformations, and low birth weight, although the incidence of fetal malformations is low and may be minimized or avoided with careful selection of agents. Maternal surgery can be safely accomplished with minimal risk to the fetus. Pelvic surgery is more easily accomplished during the second trimester. There is little risk to the fetus from short exposure to anesthetic agents after the first trimester, provided ventilation is adequate and hypotension is prevented. Low doses of radiation associated with diagnostic x-ray studies are not harmful if adequate fetal shielding is provided.

1.162   **The answer is d.** Only a few cancers spread from the mother to the fetus; melanoma, NHL, and leukemia are the most common.

1.163   **The answer is d.** The nerve-sparing procedure is recommended for patients with stage A or B disease who are eligible to undergo radical prostatectomy. Factors identified that promote sexual function after surgery are age less than 50, stage of disease, and the preservation of neurovascular bundles. In patients over 70, only 22% will regain potency postoperatively, even if both neurovascular bundles are spared.

1.164   **The answer is b.** Choices **a**, **c**, and **d**, while all associated with sexual dysfunction resulting from gastrointestinal surgery, primarily are psychosexual and not organic issues. For all patients the removal of rectal tissue appears to be the most common denominator to organic sexual dysfunction. If the rectum remains intact, there rarely is an associated sexual dysfunction without direct tumor invasion.

1.165   **The answer is a.** Permanent damage to erectile function with loss of emission and ejaculation may occur with perineal resection or radical prostatectomy. Retrograde ejaculation is common with transurethral and transabdominal resection and erectile dysfunction with transabdominal resection. Bilateral orchiectomy causes sexual dysfunction through gradual diminution of libido, impotence, gynecomastia, and penile atrophy.

1.166   **The answer is d.** Sexual identity, as well as sexual functioning, is often affected permanently by surgery of the vulva, vagina, uterus and uterine cervix, ovary and fallopian tube, or pelvic exenteration. Although vaginal cancer is less common than most other gynecologic malignancies, surgery for the majority of gynecologic cancers (except for carcinoma in situ) results in some abnormality and/or reconstruction of the vagina. In women, dysfunction related to pelvic exenteration (removal of all pelvic organs) with resulting ostomies is profound and is associated with changes in body image, sexual identity, and self-esteem. Simple hysterectomy, used to treat noninvasive cervical cancer, affects fertility and childbearing. Menopausal symptoms are most closely related to removal of the ovaries and fallopian tubes, which is not part of a radical hysterectomy.

1.167   **The answer is b.** Radiation therapy can cause sexual and reproductive dysfunction through primary organ failure (e.g., ovarian failure and testicular aplasia), through alterations in organ function (e.g., decreased lubrication and impotence), and through the temporary and permanent effects of therapy associated with reproduction (e.g., diarrhea and fatigue). In addition, radiation therapy can cause decreases in sexual enjoyment, ability to reach orgasm, libido, and frequency of intercourse and sexual dreams, as well as vaginal stenosis in women.

1.168   **The answer is d.** Radiation therapy can cause sexual and reproductive dysfunction through primary organ failure, through alterations in organ function, and through the temporary or permanent effects of therapy related to total dose, location, length of treatment, age, and prior fertility status.

1.169   **The answer is c.** Chemotherapy-induced reproductive and sexual dysfunction is related to the type of drug, dose, length of treatment, age, and sex of the individual receiving treatment and to the length of time after treatment, as well as to the use of single rather than multiple agents and drugs to combat side effects of chemotherapy. Combination chemotherapy with MOPP (mechlorethamine, Oncovin, procarbazine, and prednisone) has been shown to produce sexual dysfunction and to decrease fertility in both men and women. Androgen therapy affects sexual function in women; estrogen therapy affects sexual function in men. Chemotherapy may deplete the germinal epithelium that lines the seminiferous tubules in men.

1.170   **The answer is c.** Sexual dysfunction is not a normal side effect of chemotherapy. Although it is not uncommon in conjunction with breast cancer and surgery and it is more prevalent among younger women, sexual dysfunction can be treated, usually through therapy or a support group. The rest of these—ovarian failure, hot flashes, night sweats, and irregular menses—are common side effects of chemotherapy.

1.171   **The answer is d.** The traditional bilateral RPLND results in the loss of antegrade ejaculation with resultant infertility from retrograde ejaculation. The ability to experience a normal orgasm is not impaired.

1.172   **The answer is d.** The patient should be allowed to express his fears, concerns, and wishes regarding death; this can provide comfort and emotional healing. When coping with a difficult disease like lung cancer, it is the discovery of meaning in the disease that gives one a sense of mastery. The recurrence of lung cancer can be a greater crisis than the initial diagnosis. Often the fear of dying is not as profound as the fear of suffering in the process.

1.173   **The answer is b.** Suicide is the intentional taking of one's own life. Euthanasia refers to the act of assisting or enabling a sufferer's death, preferably without pain. Active euthanasia refers to direct intervention causing death, whereas passive euthanasia refers to letting a sufferer die by withholding or withdrawing life-sustaining care.

1.174   **The answer is a.** The most frequently addressed factors contributing to cancer-related suicide or euthanasia are pain and other symptom distress.

1.175   **The answer is c.** Hospice care pivots around the idea of palliative medical management. Palliative management involves a shift in treatment goals from curative toward providing relief from suffering. Euthanasia means active interventions to hasten a person's death and this is *not* the philosophy of hospice care.

1.176   **The answer is c.** The durable power of attorney is preferable. A living will gives advance directives for the final period of terminal illness, and the durable power of attorney covers any treatment situations at any stage in life. This document names an individual who will speak for the patient if the patient becomes incompetent to make decisions about health care.

1.177   **The answer is c.** This legislation required that all health care institutions receiving Medicare or Medicaid reimbursement ask patients they admit to the hospital whether they have an advance directive. If patients do not, the institution is obligated to provide written information about such directives.

1.178   **The answer is a.** The hospice team's goal is to help the family prepare for their loved one's death. Families need to be prepared for the actual time of the patient's death and what universal signs they can anticipate. Increasing sleep, a gradual decrease in need for food and drink, increased confusion or restlessness, decreasing temperature of extremities, and irregular breathing patterns may occur. Calling the oncologist would be indicating the need for intervention, when in fact the goal of care is purely palliative. The pain relief regimen should not be altered if the patient is comfortable, even if the patient is sleeping more and death is approaching.

1.179   **The answer is a.** In today's cost-driven health care climate, the biggest danger of euthanasia is that it will be used as a simple method of dispatching persons whose care costs too much or who are now considered to be a burden on society. For many theorists, the principle of nonmaleficence is not consistent with euthanasia. However, others argue that euthanasia is an appropriate and important form of caring for persons whose lives, by their own assessment, have become too burdensome to continue. It is possible, though less likely, that if euthanasia were permitted, over time caregivers would be encouraged to regard certain individuals' lives as not worthwhile or to refrain from proposing certain treatments for certain groups of individuals, such as the elderly.

1.180   **The answer is a.** National, state, and local governments have an impact on cancer control through legislation. Cancer control efforts are affected by the monies specifically appropriated to cancer control in the National Institutes of Health budget. The government can influence advancement in this area by setting national goals for cancer control, such as those in the Healthy People 2000 document.

1.181   **The answer is b.** Clinical trials are experimental medical trials that are implemented to determine whether there is any disease response to a new antineoplastic regimen. Patients and their families often turn to an experimental procedure when there are limited, if any, options remaining that might halt their disease progress. This choice suggests that the patient has not agreed to palliative care and is still pursuing curative treatment. Further assessment is indicated to make sure this is not the case, because a patient criterion for hospice care is that the patient is agreeable to palliative and not curative care. The remaining three options are actually patient criteria for hospice care: the patient has a primary caregiver; the patient resides in the hospice program's geographic area; and some programs require that the patient have a DNR status before admission to the hospice program.

1.182   **The answer is d.** The CPEN has developed several resources such as the Resource Guide to Cancer Patient Education Programs, a complete listing of planned educational programs of the NCI-designated centers. An annual conference offers members the opportunity to share information and to explore new developments in patient education.

1.183   **The answer is c.** Hospice care is a medically directed, interdisciplinary team–managed program of services that focuses on the patient/family as the unit of service. It has been the general experience of those who provide optimal palliative care that their patients do not need or desire euthanasia. Hospice in the United States began as an antimedical establishment and antiphysician movement. This antagonistic bias has unfortunately been a major factor in preventing hospice and palliative care principles from being applied to dying patients on a broader scale.

1.184   **The answer is a.** The ACS and the NCI are separate organizations. The ACS is a nationwide voluntary health agency dedicated to eliminating cancer as a health problem by preventing cancer, saving lives, and decreasing suffering through research, education, and service. Among its activities are publications, continuing education programs, conferences, scholarships, professorships, and programs for students.

1.185   **The answer is c.** The Food and Drug Act of 1906 called for the truthful labeling of ingredients used in drugs but did not ban false therapeutic claims on drug labels. The Sherley Amendment in 1912 made it a crime to make false or fraudulent claims regarding the therapeutic efficacy of a drug, but proof of intent to defraud the customer was needed. Finally, in 1962, Congress added that drugs must demonstrate efficacy in addition to safety before they can be marketed, and a process was created by which a substance can become approved for prescription use.

1.186   **The answer is b.** Potential hazards associated with the administration of antineoplastic agents have prompted the Occupational Safety and Health Administration (OSHA) to set guidelines for compounding, transporting, administering, and disposing of toxic chemotherapy agents.

1.187 **The answer is a.** Under COBRA, group medical coverage is ensured to those whose circumstances warrant reducing or changing work hours or leaving the job. The employee is eligible for extended benefits for up to 18 months, and spouse and dependents receive these benefits for 36 months.

1.188 **The answer is d.** The CIS is a toll-free telephone service sponsored by the NCI that answers questions about cancer prevention, control, diagnosis, treatment, and rehabilitation. CIS counselors use the NCI's computerized database, PDG (Physician's Data Query), to provide state-of-the-art information to callers. The CIS also functions as a change agent in providing varied techniques to quit smoking, including basic strategies for behavior change.

1.189 **The answer is a.** A random donor platelet concentrate may expose the recipient to multiple tissue antigens, leading to platelet refractoriness. A single donor platelet concentrate is taken from one donor or one HLA-matched donor; patients are therefore not exposed to multiple antigens. This may be important with patients who are severely immunosuppressed, such as those who have undergone bone marrow transplantation.

1.190 **The answer is a.** These are signs of ABO incompatibility, which is an acute hemolytic transfusion reaction. Choice **b** is a mild allergic reaction; choice **c** is a febrile, nonhemolytic reaction. Choice **d** characterizes a delayed hemolytic reaction.

1.191 **The answer is c.** Vitamin K might be administered to a patient experiencing hypocoagulability, but not the hypercoagulability caused by DIC. All of the other therapies may provide short-term relief of DIC symptoms. Treatment of the underlying malignancy is vital in treating the patient with DIC, inasmuch as the tumor is the ultimate stimulus.

1.192 **The answer is c.** A serious transfusion complication in patients who are significantly immunosuppressed is the risk of developing graft versus host disease. It is generally recommended that all blood products given to the severely immunocompromised host be exposed to pretransfusion irradiation. Blood is irradiated to inhibit proliferation of lymphocytes without impairment of platelets, red cells, or granulocytes.

1.193 **The answer is d.** Leukocytes remaining in donor blood collected for transfusion are responsible for many of the complications related to transfusion therapy including immunologic effects, nonhemolytic febrile reactions, and transmission of viral infections.

1.194 **The answer is d.** Nonanemic patients can donate up to 6 units of blood prior to surgery. Blood usually can be donated from 42 days to 72 hours prior to surgery.

1.195 **The answer is d.** Blood products must be irradiated to destroy T lymphocytes, which can cause GVHD in the marrow recipient. Patients whose platelets become refractory to random platelet transfusions can receive HLA-matched platelets from family or community donors, and platelets that have undergone plasmapheresis from marrow donors yield optimal increments. Alloimmunization and platelet refractoriness contribute to a 1% case fatality rate from hemorrhage complications.

1.196 **The answer is b.** The causes of anemia frequently seen in patients with cancer include decreased red cell production secondary to myelosuppressive therapy (e.g., chemotherapy and radiation therapy) and the primary disease process.

1.197 **The answer is d.** The most common side effect from erythropoietin is hypertension; therefore, the patient's blood pressure should be monitored frequently. Lung cancer commonly metastasizes to the brain and presents as headache. Severe anemia is why Stanley is getting the erythropoietin, which can stop working after a while.

1.198   **The answer is d.** Tumor invasion into the bone marrow can occur by metastatic invasion or the presence of the primary tumor that is intrinsic to the bone marrow. The decrease in production of normal marrow elements is due to crowding and the metabolic end products that are toxic to normal cells. Myelophthisis refers to tumor invasion of the bone marrow, not the effects of radiation.

1.199   **The answer is c.** Home care assessment for HPN begins with a visit coincidental with the arrival of equipment. The nurse should review orders for HPN with the supplying agency. The assessment should include the type and status of the venous access device, the patient's and family's knowledge of the management of HPN, and an evaluation of the home for safety factors. Adequate refrigeration should be available in the home for a 2- to 3-week supply of solutions. An electric infusion pump with a battery backup is normally part of the equipment. Choices **a** and eventually **d** are handled by the family; **b** is done by the home infusion therapy company personnel.

1.200   **The answer is a.** Total parenteral nutrition for prolonged periods or home TPN is indicated only in situations in which enteral feeding is not feasible because of advanced disease or severe toxicities of cancer therapies. Patients with enterocutaneous fistulas are not able to use the enteral route for nutrition because oral intake stimulates fistula output and can lead to metabolic and electrolyte disturbances.

1.201   **The answer is c.** Enteral feeding, especially in the upper gastrointestinal tract, maintains the normal stimulation of enzymatic and mucosal activity in the gut, which is not accomplished with parenteral nutrition. The other statements may be true, but they are not the best answer.

1.202   **The answer is d.** Nutritional approaches are the most commonly used questionable treatments and include macrobiotic, metabolic, and megavitamin therapy.

1.203   **The answer is a.** Because Mr. Smith seems to be very healthy otherwise, enteral nutrition is the preferred route, assuming that his GI tract is functioning. Total parenteral nutrition (TPN) for brief periods (7–10 days) may be indicated in a severely malnourished patient who cannot be fed via the enteral route. Home TPN or prolonged TPN is indicated only in situations in which enteral feeding is not feasible because of advanced disease or severe toxicities.

1.204   **The answer is a.** Terminally ill patients are not candidates for parenteral nutrition. The largest group of cancer patients receiving home parenteral nutrition are those with severe enteritis following curative radiation treatment. Patients with head and neck cancer generally have enteral nutrition but may also benefit from total parenteral nutrition (TPN).

1.205   **The answer is d.** Adding fiber to the formula helps to prevent diarrhea, as will giving the formula at room temperature, diluting it more, and giving it as a continuous infusion.

1.206   **The answer is c.** Enteral feedings, especially in the upper gastrointestinal tract, maintain the normal stimulation of enzymatic and mucosal activity in the gut, an important attribute when oral feeding is resumed.

1.207   **The answer is c.** Research involving women receiving adjuvant chemotherapy for breast cancer indicates that exercise may relieve fatigue. Patients who participated in a supervised aerobic, interval training exercise program showed an improvement in fatigue measured as a component of mood, nausea, and functional capacity.

1.208   **The answer is d.** Three scenarios in which limb salvage is not a treatment option are (1) when the surgeon is unable to attain adequate surgical margin, (2) when the neurovascular bundle is involved, and (3) when the patient is younger than 10 years. In the latter case, limb salvage is contraindicated because of the resultant limb length discrepancy, although recent advances in expandable prostheses enable more children afflicted with bone cancer to retain their limbs during surgery.

1.209   **The answer is d.** Many patients may ultimately use all three speech methods at different times in the rehabilitation period: artificial larynx immediately after surgery; esophageal voice therapy a month or so after surgery; and, after a few months, surgical voice restoration or TE puncture.

1.210   **The answer is c.** TE puncture enables the patient to divert exhaled pulmonary air through a surgically constructed fistula tract directly into the esophagus.

1.211   **The answer is c.** Liquids are the most difficult thing for the patient to swallow without aspirating.

1.212   **The answer is a.** Due to the absence of thoracic fixation after laryngectomy, the patient's ability to lift heavy objects is compromised.

1.213   **The answer is d.** Although care does consist of holistic and direct physical care, the ultimate goal is to enable the family and/or patient to provide the care. Choices **b** and **c** apply more to hospice care and not necessarily to home care. The patient and family are encouraged to assume responsibility for the care of the patient.

1.214   **The answer is c.** The success of any cancer survival program depends on the commitment of the health care team to provide ongoing evaluation and planning for change in the lives of survivors. Under such a dynamic program, preventive and restorative goal-setting become critical to a long-term survivorship trajectory that is characterized by minimal debilitation and a wellness orientation. Particular attention is also paid to the ongoing and long-range implications of financial burden imposed by cancer.

1.215   **The answer is c.** Rehabilitation refers to the process by which individuals, within their environments, are assisted to achieve optimal functioning within the limits imposed by cancer. The goals are to improve the quality of life for those experiencing cancer and to help the individual regain wholeness.

1.216   **The answer is d.** Severity or duration of disease is the factor most closely related to the cancer patient's rehabilitation needs. The physical needs frequently occurring with a variety of cancers includes general weakness, limited activities of daily living, and issues related to limited mobility.

1.217   **The answer is c.** The PICC catheter requires daily flushing and central line dressing changes as frequently as every 3–7 days. Although some PICC catheters have more than one lumen, any lumen can be used for blood withdrawal. The major advantage is that the catheter can be placed by specially trained nurses in the home so the patient can avoid going to the hospital or doctor's office.

1.218   **The answer is d.** In the case of implanted ports, the cause of drug extravasation is usually a misplaced or displaced needle. Another mechanism for drug extravasation from ports involves retrograde subcutaneous leakage from percutaneously inserted catheters obstructed by a fibrin sheath.

1.219   **The answer is d.** It is not uncommon for a catheter to be properly placed, without evidence of catheter damage, and still have an absent or intermittent blood return. The catheter or port is still safe to use, provided it flushes easily without subjective complaints. Fibrin sheaths can form at the catheter insertion site and float, like a sleeve, around the outside of the catheter. If the sheath extends beyond the lumen, it can cause withdrawal occlusions. Lysis of the sheath may be achieved by instilling urokinase 5000–10,000 units into the catheter with an extended dwell time of 1–24 hours.

1.220   **The answer is d.** The Ommaya reservoir is surgically implanted through the cranium. It is placed underneath the skin with the catheter extending from the reservoir to the ventricle. It provides permanent intraventicular access for patients in whom repeated translumbar puncture is impractical. Cerebrospinal fluid is gently aspirated and sent for cytology or laboratory studies. The chemotherapy drug is administered slowly.

1.221   **The answer is a.** PICCs are ideal for short-term access (1 week to several months).

1.222   **The answer is c.** Epidural ports are flushed with 1–2 ml of sterile, preservative-free saline after use. Never flush epidural lines with heparin.

1.223   **The answer is c.** Signs and symptoms of a venous thrombosis are related to impaired blood flow and include: edema of the neck, face, shoulder, or arm; prominent superficial veins; neck pain; tingling of the neck, shoulder, or arm; and skin color or temperature changes. A venogram with contrast media is used to assess for a venous thrombosis.

1.224   **The answer is d.** When giving a vesicant, it is always better to have a blood return throughout the injection, so a smaller-gauge needle is not preferable in that situation. For patients with small veins, choose an Angiocath that is thin-walled with an over-the-needle cannula.

1.225   **The answer is d.** A patient undergoing BCT requires a catheter that is stiffer than the traditional CVC used for ABMT because of the need for high volume and pressure during pheresis.

1.226   **The answer is c.** Aggressive antiviral therapy with intravenous acyclovir is the standard therapy.

1.227   **The answer is a.** The early proliferation of MALT lymphoma is reversible by eradication of the bacteria with antibiotics, whereas the later tumor is not and requires conventional anticancer therapy.

1.228   **The answer is d.** It is important for the patient and/or family to know at what temperature to store the medication because consideration needs to be given to the stability of the drug. A knowledge of signs and symptoms is important because the nurse will not be present at most infusions. Withdrawal of heparin and heparin administration are required following drug administration to keep the VAD patent. Infusion therapy agencies with pharmacies will prepare and deliver the antibiotics and the supplies on schedule.

1.229   **The answer is d.** Anecdotal reports and clinical observations suggest that use of masks and garment covers is declining. Cost-benefit analysis does not convince that such methods eliminate or reduce infection. Hand washing, scrupulous hygiene, and protective isolation may be the most cost-effective and meaningful conventions for infection control.

1.230   **The answer is b.** Immunosuppressive medications are aimed at removing or inactivating T lymphocytes that attack target organs. Cyclosporine and methotrexate inhibit T lymphocytes that are believed to be responsible for acute GVHD and are the first-line therapy.

1.231   **The answer is c.** Veno-occlusive disease is almost exclusive to BMT and is the most common nonrelapse life-threatening complication of preparative-regimen–related toxicity for bone marrow transplantation. Patients at risk for developing VOD include those with hepatitis and infections before BMT and those who receive repeated doses of chemotherapy prior to transplant in addition to high-dose irradiation in pretransplant conditioning regimens. An additional risk factor is the use of antimicrobial therapy with acyclovir, amphotericin, or vancomycin and mismatched or unrelated allogeneic marrow grafts.

1.232   **The answer is b.** Side effects of trimethoprim include rash, nausea, vomiting, hepatotoxicity, and myelosuppression. Side effects of dapsone include hemolytic anemia, hypersensitivity reactions, blood dyscrasias, hepatic toxicity, and peripheral neuropathy.

1.233   **The answer is c.** Amphotericin B is the drug of choice for treatment of systemic fungal infections. However, it is associated with significant side effects and toxicity, including fever, chills, rigors, nausea, vomiting, hypotension, bronchospasms, and occasionally seizures.

1.234   **The answer is a.** Premedication with acetaminophen and the addition of hydrocortisone sodium succinate to the IV solution generally reduces the reactions associated with the amphotericin. IV meperidine can be used to ameliorate fever and chills that frequently accompany the initial administration of amphotericin.

1.235   **The answer is c.** Treatment strategies for GVHD include systemic immunosuppressive therapy; topical steroids, which may or may not be beneficial; and fluoride therapy for patients at risk for caries secondary to xerostomia.

1.236   **The answer is d.** Aspirin has been demonstrated to increase the risk of bleeding. The clinical risk for bleeding associated with nonsteroidal anti-inflammatory drugs is much less than that for aspirin; however, they should be used cautiously in patients with already-low platelet counts.

1.237   **The answer is b.** Nonsteroidal anti-inflammatory drugs (NSAIDs) act on the peripheral nervous system by preventing the conversion of arachidonic acid to prostaglandin. These medications have a maximum ceiling effect for analgesic potential, and their indication for use in cancer patients should be pain that is mild to moderate in intensity.

1.238   **The answer is c.** Medications such as phenothiazines, tricyclic antidepressants, heparin, cimetidine, thiazide diuretics, and estrogen may suppress platelet activity, but aspirin is the medication most commonly associated with platelet dysfunction.

1.239   **The answer is c.** Aspirin and other nonsteroidal anti-inflammatory drugs inhibit the platelet secretory process, diminish collagen-induced aggregation and epinephrine-induced aggregation, and inhibit platelet function.

1.240   **The answer is c.** An example of how chemoprevention may potentially be applied to high-risk populations is the use of nonsteroidal anti-inflammatory drugs for the prevention of colorectal cancer.

1.241   **The answer is d.** The NSAIDs inhibit cyclo-oxygenase in peripheral tissues, which prevents arachidonic acid from converting to prostaglandin. The loss of the cytoprotective effect of prostaglandin on the GI epithelium causes the occurrence of the GI side effects.

1.242   **The answer is b.**

1.243   **The answer is b.**

1.244   **The answer is c.** Despite effective antiemetic regimens, 93% of patients receiving a high dose of cisplatin experience delayed nausea and vomiting up to 6–7 days.

1.245   **The answer is c.** The combinations of dopamine antagonists with steroids have been found to provide complete control of nausea and vomiting in up to 100% of patients undergoing high-dose cisplatin-base regimens. The combination of ondansetron and dexamethasone has been found to be more efficacious than ondansetron alone in controlling emesis.

1.246   **The answer is c.**

1.247   **The answer is c.** The vomiting center lies close to the respiratory center on the floor of the fourth ventricle and is directly activated by the visceral and vagal afferent pathways from the gastrointestinal tract, chemoreceptor trigger zone (CTZ), vestibular apparatus, and the cerebral cortex.

1.248   **The answer is a.** Serotonin is released from the enterochromaffin cells in the small intestine. Serotonin activates 5-HT3 receptors on visceral and vagal afferents, sending a message to the chemotherapy trigger zone (CTZ) and the vomiting center.

1.249   **The answer is b.** Anticipatory nausea and vomiting occur in 25% of patients as a result of classic operant conditioning from stimuli associated with chemotherapy, usually 12 hours before administration. Nausea commonly occurs in patients receiving oral cyclophosphamide.

1.250   **The answer is d.** Naloxone is the drug of choice in the treatment of respiratory depression related to opioid overdosing. The amount of naloxone a patient receives should be titrated to changes in respiratory rate. Rapid injections of naloxone should be avoided in opioid-tolerant patients, so as not to precipitate an abstinence syndrome that may include intense pain.

1.251   **The answer is c.** All of these are common side effects, except increased motility; opioids commonly decrease motility.

1.252   **The answer is a.** Antidepressants (e.g., amitriptyline, desipramine, imipramine) control pain by inhibiting the uptake of neurotransmitters into nerve terminals. They are used in the treatment of many types of nonmalignant pain, such as migraine headaches, but are also believed to be useful in neuropathic pain that is due to tumor infiltration of nerves, often described as having a continuous, burning quality.

1.253   **The answer is d.** Psychostimulants may be indicated when the dose of the opioid causes extreme sedation, produces no other side effects, and the dose cannot be lowered.

1.254   **The answer is b.** Steroids are extremely efficacious for managing the pain caused by epidural cord compression. Some side effects of steroid use, such as mood elevation and increased appetite, may also be desirable in some patients. However, the use of these drugs as adjuvant analgesics early in the course of a patient's pain problem is not recommended.

1.255   **The answer is a.** Except in a few circumstances, oral pain medication should be on a fixed-interval basis. Although the evidence is not conclusive, most caregivers agree that round-the-clock scheduling is most effective in treating pain.

1.256   **The answer is c.**

1.257   **The answer is d.**

1.258   **The answer is b.**

1.259   **The answer is d.** Antidepressants are useful for patients with a neuropathic component to their pain. These drugs act by inhibiting the uptake of neurotransmitters into nerve terminals.

1.260   **The answer is c.** Two psychostimulants used most often for opioid-induced sedation are amphetamines and methylphenidate. Amphetamines are a more powerful CNS stimulant than is methylphenidate. They both decrease the central depression caused by other drugs.

1.261   **The answer is d.**

1.262   **The answer is b.** There have been reports of serious, sometimes fatal, reactions in patients receiving Prozac in combination with a monoamine oxidase inhibitor (MAOI) and in patients who have recently discontinued Prozac and then started on an MAOI. Some patients present with extreme agitation and progress to delirium and coma. Since Prozac and its major metabolite have a very long half-life, at least 5 weeks should be allowed before starting a MAOI.

1.263   **The answer is c.** Methylphenidate counteracts the sedation that accompanies opioid analgesics.

1.264   **The answer is d.** Haloperidol can be used to treat opioid-induced acute confusional states (e.g., hallucinations, agitation from delirium).

1.265   **The answer is d.** CSFs mediate all these steps.

1.266   **The answer is b.** Granulocyte (G) and granulocyte-macrophage (GM) colony-stimulating factors (CSFs) decrease myelosuppression, febrile episodes, and number of hospital days when given in conjunction with chemotherapy. Both mucositis and anorexia are complications of chemotherapy and have no relationship to biotherapy.

1.267   **The answer is d.** High levels of epidermal growth factor receptors (EGF) on cells from cancers of the breast and bladder indicate a worse prognosis. High levels of EGF are noted on many epithelial carcinomas, and mutant EGF receptors have been found on high-grade glioblastomas.

1.268   **The answer is d.** CSFs are appropriate when febrile neutropenia is expected in more than 40% of patients, such as results from high-dose chemotherapy. It is not appropriate as routine prevention of neutropenia.

1.269   **The answer is b.** HGFs provide a much more controlled response for mobilization. HGFs stimulate enhanced proliferation and maturation of neutrophils.

1.270   **The answer is a.** The reticulocyte count is a useful indicator of bone marrow function with regard to RBC production. Once the cell becomes committed to the erythroid line, its development is induced by erythropoietin (EPO).

1.271   **The answer is a.** There is an inverse correlation between epidermal growth factor receptors and ER status, with ER-negative tumors tending to have a higher level of epidermal growth factor receptor than ER-positive tumors.

1.272   **The answer is d.** EGFR is associated with poor prognosis for breast, bladder, colon, lung, and esophageal cancers.

1.273   **The answer is false.** The KS cell is capable of synthesizing its own angiogenic and growth factors, including vascular endothelial factor which ensures the continued growth of surrounding vessels and KS cells.

STUDY NOTES

STUDY NOTES

CHAPTER **2**

PROTECTIVE MECHANISMS

ALTERATIONS IN MOBILITY

2.1   Assessment of cerebellar function focuses on the ability to:
    a. coordinate movement
    b. maintain normal muscle tone
    c. maintain equilibrium
    d. all of the above

2.2   After surgery for resection of prostate cancer, Jeffrey develops several complications. The most significant complication to treat is:
    a. wound infection
    b. wound dehiscence
    c. a new neurological deficit
    d. none of the above

2.3   Which of the following is *not* a typical complication of allograft bone reconstruction?
    a. rejection
    b. infection
    c. fracture
    d. nonunion

2.4   Mr. Pen has metastatic prostate cancer to bone and is receiving Lupron, an LHRH agonist, as his primary therapy. One and one-half weeks into his treatment, he calls complaining of worsening bone pain and difficulty in walking. He is concerned that the Lupron is not working. Your most appropriate response would be which of the following?
    a. He is probably correct. The increase in pain may be because the Lupron is not working and he may need to talk to his doctor about switching therapy.
    b. The pain is probably caused by release of calcium from lytic lesions in the bone.
    c. The Lupron causes an initial increase in testosterone levels and a "flare" in symptoms.
    d. There is a rapid decrease in testosterone levels that causes intense pains in the area of the tumor.

2.5   Mrs. James has metastatic breast cancer that has spread to her bones and has recently begun pamidronate (Aredia) in conjunction with paclitaxel therapy. She does not fully understand why she is being offered Aredia therapy. Your teaching would involve *all but* which of the following?
   a. Aredia should help to make the paclitaxel work better because they are synergistic.
   b. Aredia will help to manage her bone pain.
   c. Aredia will reduce her hypercalcemia and risk for fractures.
   d. Aredia may help to prevent the development of osteolytic metastases.

2.6   A patient's physical performance classification is established before treatment and is intended to accomplish *all but* which of the following?
   a. determine whether or not the individual is a candidate for a research study
   b. influence the type of treatment planned
   c. establish the individual's quality of life using numerical values
   d. provide prognostic information

2.7   Mrs. Geoffry has lung cancer metastatic to her bones. She has recently completed 3 weeks of radiation to her thoracic spine. She phones you with complaints of recent onset of repeatedly dropping things and radicular pain. Which of the following best describes the etiology of her symptoms and appropriate nursing action?
   a. Her symptoms are most likely due to delayed effects of radiation and she should be cautioned against dropping items and instructed to take an analgesic for pain.
   b. Her symptoms are related to her cancer in her bones and will get better in a few weeks because that is when the radiation will have its peak effect.
   c. Her symptoms are new and are most likely indicative of spinal cord compression at the level of her thoracic spine. She should see her physician immediately for evaluation.
   d. Her symptoms are probably related to metastatic disease in her brain and she should be evaluated immediately.

2.8   The mechanism by which tumor spreads from the primary site to bone is which of the following?
   a. direct extension to adjacent bones
   b. arterial embolization
   c. direct venous spread
   d. all of the above

2.9   Mrs. Ellis has breast cancer with metastatic disease in her bones, including her right hip. Which of the following is considered an indication for surgical stabilization of the hip?
   a. lesions greater than 2.5 cm involving 50% or greater of the cortex
   b. pain in the hip, despite lack of weight bearing
   c. radiologic evidence of bony deterioration following radiation therapy
   d. all of the above

2.10   Mrs. George has multiple myeloma and has been confined to bed because of a pathological fracture. Her daughter calls the nurse because her mother is sleeping more and is more difficult to arouse. The patient's symptoms are most likely due to which of the following?
   a. hyperviscosity syndrome due to multiple myeloma
   b. hypocalcemia due to multiple myeloma
   c. steroid psychosis
   d. all of the above

2.11   Alfred is a 14-year-old who is undergoing an above-the-knee amputation for sarcoma. The advantages of an immediate prosthetic fitting include *all but* which of the following?
   a.   better emotional adjustment
   b.   increased motivation to ambulate
   c.   less incidence of contracture and phantom limb pain
   d.   a prosthesis helps to shape the stump

2.12   As part of your preoperative teaching for a patient who is having an allograft implant following resection of a malignant tumor, you would include *all but* which of the following?
   a.   The patient will need to take immunosuppressive drugs for up to 6 months following transplant.
   b.   Joint stability and function are improved by suturing allograft soft tissue attachments to host tissue.
   c.   Allograft tissue can be custom sized in the operating room.
   d.   The patient will need to limit weight bearing and may need to wear a brace for up to 12 months.

2.13   Which of the following chemotherapy agents is *not* commonly associated with palmar-plantar erythrodysesthesia syndrome?
   a.   topotecan
   b.   doxorubicin hydrochloride liposomal
   c.   capecitabine
   d.   cytarabine

2.14   Incidence of bone cancer is most common in people with:
   a.   a family tendency in bone cancer
   b.   prior high-dose radiation cancer therapy
   c.   preexisting bone conditions
   d.   all of the above

2.15   Bone tumors originate in the blood vessels of the bone, in the bone marrow, or in collagen-producing cells. An example of a bone tumor that originates in the bone marrow is:
   a.   Ewing's sarcoma
   b.   osteogenic sarcoma
   c.   chondrosarcoma
   d.   angiosarcoma

2.16   Mr. Riley is being assessed after presenting with bone pain in his leg. One characteristic of the pain associated with the presence of a bone tumor is that it:
   a.   has a sudden, unexplainable onset
   b.   is exacerbated with activity
   c.   is worse on awakening
   d.   has a gradual onset

2.17   All of the following are goals in the treatment of primary malignant bone cancer *except*:
   a.   preservation of maximum function
   b.   early detection and intervention in children felt to be at high risk
   c.   eradication of tumor
   d.   avoidance of amputation

2.18   All of the following are considered to be indications for limb-salvage surgery *except*:
    a. a locally aggressive chondrosarcoma
    b. the absence of soft-tissue invasion
    c. a tumor that typically metastasizes late
    d. a child younger than 10 years

2.19   After amputation, Mr. Riley reports pain in the missing leg. The nurse should be aware that this phantom limb pain:
    a. generally resolves in several months
    b. is likely to worsen with aging
    c. indicates a patient's inability to cope with loss
    d. usually occurs immediately following surgery

2.20   The rationale for the use of preoperative chemotherapy in patients with osteogenic sarcoma includes *all but* which of the following aspects?
    a. It treats micrometastases.
    b. It decreases the size of the primary tumor, possibly facilitating limb-salvage surgery.
    c. It enhances the effect of postoperative radiation.
    d. It evaluates the effectiveness of the chemotherapy.

2.21   The most common sites of occurrence for chondrosarcoma are the:
    a. femur, tibia, patella, and metatarsal
    b. vertebrae and scapula
    c. ribs, scapula, long bones, and pelvic bones
    d. mandible and maxilla

2.22   Treatment of metastases to the bone may include surgery, chemotherapy, and/or radiotherapy. When radiation therapy is used, the primary goal often is to:
    a. eliminate the need for surgical intervention
    b. palliate pain
    c. decrease the likelihood of further metastases
    d. treat the primary cancer

NEUTROPENIA

2.23   Infection in the neutropenic patient is a serious complication of chemotherapy and can be fatal in what percentage of patients?
    a. 20%
    b. 30%
    c. 40%
    d. 50%

2.24   Kate is being treated with chemotherapy for Hodgkin's disease and is monitored weekly for myelosuppression. This is appropriate because neutropenia:
    a. is the most common dose-limiting side effect of chemotherapy
    b. is potentially the most lethal side effect of chemotherapy
    c. is most severe with antimetabolites and vinca alkaloids
    d. a and b

2.25   Mr. Howards, who is receiving high-dose chemotherapy, has developed neutropenia. The usual symptoms of infection will very likely be absent or muted in this patient because:
   a.   most infections are due to organisms that are part of the body's normal flora
   b.   the WBCs drop rapidly and recovery time is slow
   c.   neutrophils are necessary to produce an inflammatory response
   d.   the immunoglobulins are reduced

2.26   Patients who are neutropenic may or may not have a high fever despite the presence of overwhelming infection. The best explanation for this is which of the following?
   a.   Severe vasoconstriction causes hypothermia.
   b.   Neutropenia prevents the inflammatory response.
   c.   Infection causes a paradoxical lowering of the temperature.
   d.   There is decreased vascular resistance and heat dissipates.

2.27   The most common site of infection in the granulocytopenic patient is which of the following?
   a.   perineal region
   b.   respiratory tract
   c.   urinary tract
   d.   gastrointestinal tract

2.28   Which of the following are *not* considered to be early signs of septic shock in the neutropenic patient?
   a.   restlessness, anxiety, confusion
   b.   high temperature and shaking chills
   c.   tachycardia
   d.   nausea, vomiting, and diarrhea

2.29   Mr. Jackson's busulfan therapy for chronic myelogenous leukemia will be stopped if his white blood count is less than:
   a.   1000 WBC/mm^3
   b.   3000 WBC/mm^3
   c.   10,000 WBC/mm^3
   d.   20,000 WBC/mm^3

2.30   Mrs. Carsen develops a chemotherapy-induced infection and is started on an antibiotic because of fever. You explain that she will take the antibiotic:
   a.   until cultures indicate eradication of the causative organism
   b.   for a minimum of 7 days
   c.   until the neutrophil count is greater than 500/mm^3
   d.   any of the above

2.31   Cytokines are small protein hormones synthesized by a variety of leukocytes. The primary function of cytokines is to:
   a.   provide long-term protection against microorganisms
   b.   initiate and regulate inflammatory and immune responses
   c.   process and convert antigens to lymphocytes
   d.   stimulate the immune response

2.32   Which of the following are *not* considered to be cytokines?
a.   interferons
b.   interleukins
c.   growth factors
d.   natural killer cells

2.33   Your patient is scheduled for chemotherapy and has a WBC of 2100 cells/mm^3 with 28% polymorphonuclear neutrophils (PMNs), 18% bands, and 42% lymphocytes. He is informed that his treatment will be delayed. The reason for this is most likely which of the following?
a.   His white count is too low.
b.   His absolute neutrophil count (ANC) is less than 1000.
c.   His ANC is less than 500.
d.   None of the above; his ANC is adequate for treatment.

2.34   Alfred is a patient with colon cancer who is scheduled to have a vascular access port placed before beginning continuous infusion of 5-fluorouracil. He has recently experienced diarrhea and fever of unknown origin. His hemogram reveals a hemoglobin of 11.0 grams, a WBC of 2000/mm^3 with an ANC of 750, and platelets of 92,000/mm^3. His surgeon has delayed his port placement for another week. The likely cause of this delay is which of the following?
a.   Diarrhea is a common cause of fever of unknown origin.
b.   Platelets less than 100,000/mm^3 are associated with bleeding during surgery.
c.   Neutropenia is the primary risk factor for infection with vascular access catheters.
d.   Anemia is associated with postoperative complications.

2.35   The administration of colony-stimulating factors as prophylaxis following highly myelosuppressive chemotherapy is intended to accomplish primarily which of the following?
a.   maintain an elevated white count above 10,000 cells/mm^3
b.   prevent pancytopenia
c.   minimize infection and stomatitis
d.   decrease the number of days that the white count is at its nadir

2.36   What percentage of neutropenic patients develop an infection?
a.   15%
b.   30%
c.   45%
d.   60%

2.37   Of all the chemotherapy patients who are neutropenic and develop an infection as a result of their neutropenia, what percentage will have documented bacteremia?
a.   10%
b.   20%
c.   30%
d.   40%

2.38   The most common and lethal side effect of chemotherapy is:
a.   respiratory distress
b.   electrolye imbalance from nausea, vomiting, and diarrhea
c.   myelosuppression
d.   increased liver function tests

THROMBOCYTOPENIA

2.39 Thrombopoietin:
a. is the factor that stimulates the proliferation of CFU-MK cells
b. stimulates multipotential progenitor cells that later result in increased numbers of cells from multicell lineages including platelets
c. stimulates the differentiation of megakaryocytes into platelets
d. a and c

2.40 Thrombocytopenia in cancer patients can be caused by any of the following factors *except:*
a. an abnormal distribution of platelets that results in increased platelet sequestration
b. rapid platelet destruction characterized by a shortened platelet life span
c. overstimulation of normal coagulation causing rapid platelet thrombosis
d. decreased production of platelets in the bone marrow due to tumor involvement

2.41 The anemia associated with multiple myeloma is believed to be caused by:
a. the effects of radiation
b. a normochromic iron deficiency
c. the replacement of erythrocyte precursors with plasma cells
d. erythrocyte destruction by WBCs

2.42 The decrease in production of normal marrow elements due to the "crowding out" of normal cells by metastatic cancer cells in the marrow is referred to as:
a. myelodysplasia
b. macroglobulinemia
c. myelophthisis
d. microcellular anemia

2.43 Ms. Drake has myelodysplastic syndrome (MDS). She reports being asymptomatic "forever" and asks you why she still has to endure ongoing monitoring. The best explanation you can offer is that:
a. T cell abnormalities increase the risk of opportunistic infections.
b. Compliance with the prescribed treatment will delay or prevent the onset of symptoms.
c. All patients with MDS eventually develop anemia, thrombocytopenia, and/or neutropenia.
d. All patients with MDS eventually develop acute leukemia.

2.44 A cumulative and delayed thrombocytopenia has been associated with *all but* which of the following chemotherapeutic agents?
a. methotrexate
b. mitomycin
c. lomustine
d. streptozocin

2.45 Mr. Tom has a malignant brain tumor and has been receiving 5-fluorouracil and BCNU every 6 weeks. His blood counts today reveal a white count of 3,000 cells/mm3, hemoglobin of 10 g/100 ml, platelet count of 50,000 cells/mm^3. His treatment is delayed today. The best explanation for delaying his treatment is which of the following?
a. He is moderately to severely immunosuppressed.
b. He is moderately anemic.
c. He is moderately at risk for bleeding due to thrombocytopenia.
d. He is severely at risk for bleeding due to thrombocytopenia.

2.46   When platelets decrease to 10,000 cells/mm^3, the patient is most at risk for which of the following?
   a.   spontaneous central nervous system bleeding
   b.   gastrointestinal bleeding with black tarry stools
   c.   fatal respiratory tract hemorrhage
   d.   all of the above

2.47   During the physical exam of a new patient you notice that he has small red eruptions on his upper and lower extremities. He appears pale and states that he is exhausted most of the time. You are concerned and call the doctor. You know his physical exam is suspicious for which of the following?
   a.   severe anemia and bleeding
   b.   disseminated intravascular coagulopathy (DIC)
   c.   thrombocytopenia
   d.   leukemia

2.48   Allen has prostate cancer with metastasis to the bone. He has had chemotherapy and some radiation therapy to control his disease. He comes to the clinic for further chemotherapy. His blood counts are as follows: WBC 2700 cells/mm^3, hemoglobin 8.7 g/100 ml, and platelets 88,000 cells/mm^3. His thrombocytopenia is most likely due to which of the following?
   a.   tumor invasion of the bone marrow
   b.   acute or delayed effects of chemotherapy
   c.   delayed effects of radiation therapy
   d.   all of the above

2.49   The most common cause of thrombocytopenia in patients with cancer is:
   a.   chemotherapy
   b.   hypersplenism
   c.   decreased megakaryocytopoiesis
   d.   immune-mediated thrombocytopenia

2.50   Jenny has chronic lymphocytic leukemia. She has immature platelets in the bone marrow and a platelet count of 45,000 cells/mm^3. She has evidence of petechiae, purpura, and ecchymosis. Her condition is most likely associated with which of the following platelet disorders?
   a.   thromobocytopenia
   b.   idiopathic thrombocytopenia purpura (ITP)
   c.   thrombocytosis
   d.   hypocoagulopathy

2.51   Research involving the use of Interleukin-11 is specifically aimed at which of the following blood components?
   a.   granulocytes
   b.   erythrocytes
   c.   platelets
   d.   all of the above

2.52 Which of the following is not a side effect of interleukin-11?
  a. fatigue
  b. arthralgias
  c. myalgias
  d. hyperthermia

2.53 Your patient just started a new regimen of chemotherapy including vincristine and methotrexate 1 week ago. He is elderly and has had some problems with constipation. Other significant problems include a platelet count of 20,000 cells/mm^3 and stomatitis. Nursing action would include which of the following?
  a. stool softener and a laxative each day as needed
  b. rectal exam to rule out impaction
  c. rectal suppository followed by a tap water enema
  d. all of the above

2.54 Which of the following chemotherapeutic agents is *not* considered to be platelet sparing?
  a. ifosphamide
  b. mitoxantrone
  c. mitomycin
  d. vincristine

2.55 Mr. Czar has an enlarged spleen and has been started on corticosteroid therapy. The primary purpose of this therapy is which of the following?
  a. Steroids have a capillary-stabilizing effect.
  b. Steroids help to control platelet sequestration.
  c. Steroids help to minimize bleeding potential.
  d. all of the above

2.56 Your patient with leukemia is septic and is suffering from severe thrombocytopenia. Despite many platelet transfusions, his platelet count is only 30,000 cells/mm^3. Which of the following is the most logical explanation for why multiple platelet transfusions are less effective in some situations?
  a. The patient must be bleeding somewhere.
  b. The platelets must not have been stored properly.
  c. Fever and infection destroy platelets.
  d. The leukemia cells destroy platelets.

2.57 Your patient has received multiple transfusions of random-donor platelets and is experiencing no increment in his platelet count. What is this process called?
  a. HLA resistance
  b. alloimmunization
  c. hyperimmunization
  d. autoimmunization

ALTERATIONS IN SKIN INTEGRITY

2.58   After the administration of doxorubicin, you notice that swelling has occurred at the injection site. The patient complains of some burning. In addition, you determine that there is a lack of blood return. These clues alert you that the patient may be experiencing:
a. venous flare
b. erythema
c. extravasation
d. all of the above

2.59   Mrs. Kelly is about to receive radiation therapy for the first time. She says, "I have such sensitive skin. I'm worried about what effect radiation could have on my skin." You tell Mrs. Kelly that acute radiation effects:
a. result from the depletion of actively proliferating parenchymal or stromal cells
b. are characterized by dilation, local edema, and inflammation
c. are usually temporary
d. all of the above

2.60   Which of the following is *not* true regarding radiation-induced skin reactions?
a. Higher doses given over shorter periods of time to larger volumes will result in more severe acute skin reactions.
b. Electrons produce greater skin reactions than photons.
c. Placing tissue-equivalent material on the skin creates a skin-sparing effect during radiation therapy, minimizing dose at the level of the skin.
d. When treatment is targeted at areas of skin apposition, increased reaction secondary to warmth and moisture can be expected.

2.61   Following radiation therapy to the chest, your patient plans a trip to Bermuda. You instruct her to use a sunscreen with an SPF of 15 or more because radiation has undoubtedly affected her skin via:
a. skin-sparing effect during radiation therapy
b. slower rate of melanin production in new epidermal cells in the radiation field
c. faster rate of melanin production in new epidermal cells in the radiation field
d. destruction of lymphocytes in the irradiated epidermis

2.62   The signs and symptoms of an extravasation from chemotherapy can be subtle. Which of the following might be considered a definite sign of infiltration of a vesicant agent?
a. a bleb formation at the injection site
b. swelling that occurs in more deeply accessed veins
c. loss of a blood return
d. a and b

2.63   A 60-year-old female reports a flesh-colored, raised, firm papule on the top of her nose. It is examined and found to be a squamous cell carcinoma (SCC). How do SCCs differ from most BCCs?
a. They tend to be less aggressive than BCCs, even though they have faster growth rates.
b. Their margins are well demarcated, as compared to those of the BCCs.
c. They tend to have greater metastatic potential.
d. a and c

2.64   In the days *immediately* following abdominal surgery:
   a.   one should not be surprised to see a temporary suppression of wound healing; healing will become more proliferative after 21 days
   b.   chemotherapy agents can be used to best advantage
   c.   granulation tissue is usually formed in the first 3–25 days following surgery, providing the characteristic strength of the wound
   d.   b and c

2.65   A graft or flap is most often used in the surgical treatment of a nonmelanoma cancer when:
   a.   the lesion is large or located in an area with insufficient tissue for closure
   b.   risks of bleeding are high and vasculature must be maintained
   c.   the extent of the tumor must be accurately assessed and margins are relatively unclear
   d.   the lesion is small, superficial, or recurrent

2.66   Side effects of radiation to the skin are least likely to include:
   a.   mild erythema and moist desquamation
   b.   fibrosclerotic changes that make skin smooth, taut, and shiny
   c.   permanent tanning
   d.   complete or patchy alopecia

2.67   Rachel is a new surgical nurse assisting in a center that frequently performs oncologic surgeries. She has noticed that surgical wound closure seems to be much more unsuccessful in cancer surgeries. She points this out to you and asks, "Why do you think that happens?" You explain that:
   a.   irradiated tissue is fibrotic and prone to dehiscence
   b.   healthy tissue often cannot be reached surgically because the ulcers are so deep
   c.   radiation injury extends beyond the ulcer to surrounding tissues
   d.   all of the above

2.68   When your patient begins radiation treatments after her lumpectomy, she notices redness and tenderness over her breast. Her breast also itches, and the skin is scaly and dry. She comes to you when her breast has become very tender and expresses concern. You tell her that:
   a.   some patients have these reactions to the radiation treatments; if the symptoms persist, she will need to take a few days off from radiation
   b.   she should rub the skin with baby oil just prior to her radiation treatments
   c.   all patients have reactions to the radiation treatments and it's nothing to worry about
   d.   her radiation dosage is obviously too high and she needs to see the radiation oncologist

2.69   Mrs. Kelly is experiencing hyperpigmentation. You explain to her that this may be a reaction to:
   a.   L-asparaginase
   b.   bleomycin
   c.   paclitaxel
   d.   cisplatin

2.70   High-risk factors for cutaneous melanoma (CM) include all of the following *except:*
   a.   skin pigmentation
   b.   a persistently changed or changing mole
   c.   the presence of a precursor lesion such as dysplastic nevi
   d.   oral contraceptives

2.71   Mr. Finkle reports a "rash of some kind" in his mouth. He reports that he likes spicy foods but says that his wife predicts the rash has been caused by his habit of smoking a pipe. The type of irritation you might be most likely to discover on inspecting Mr. Finkle's mouth is:
   a.   snuff keratosis
   b.   nicotine stomatitis
   c.   leukoplakias
   d.   erythroplakia

2.72   Ms. Allison has a skin lesion that appears to be possibly cancerous. The action *least likely* to be part of your response is:
   a.   documenting the size, location, and description of the lesion
   b.   teaching Ms. Allison appropriate routine self-examination of the skin
   c.   referring Ms. Allison to a physician for diagnosis
   d.   following Ms. Allison up for recurrent disease

2.73   Which of the following statements about dysplastic nevi (DN) is *not* correct?
   a.   DN may be familial or nonfamilial.
   b.   Most persons affected by DN have about 25–75 abnormal nevi.
   c.   DN develop from precursor lesions of CM known as congenital nevi.
   d.   A distinctive feature of DN is a "fried egg" appearance with a deeply pigmented papular area surrounded by an area of lighter pigmentation.

2.74   The phase of CM tumor growth that is characterized by focal deep penetration of atypical melanocytes into the dermis and subcutaneous tissue is the:
   a.   radial phase
   b.   vertical growth phase
   c.   nodular phase
   d.   acral lentiginous phase

2.75   Which of the following statements about primary prevention of skin cancers is false?
   a.   UV radiation is strongest during the mid-part of the day.
   b.   For most people, sunscreen is not required on overcast days.
   c.   Certain medications (e.g., oral contraceptives) can make individuals photosensitive.
   d.   Surfaces such as sand and water can reflect more than one-half of the UV radiation onto the skin.

NEUROPATHIES

2.76   Davis is taking vincristine. You are able to discern from his conversation that although he is familiar with some of vincristine's adverse effects, he seems unfamiliar with its neurotoxic effects. Thus, you tell him that vincristine is well known for potential:
   a.   encephalopathy
   b.   peripheral neuropathy
   c.   acute cerebellar dysfunction
   d.   leukoencephalopathy

2.77   Which of the following chemotherapy agents is *not* associated with peripheral neuropathies?
    a. cytarabine
    b. cisplatin
    c. methotrexate
    d. carboplatin

2.78   A patient receiving docetaxel has recently complained that she has some trouble walking without stumbling. After examining the patient, the physician changes her chemotherapy. What is the most logical explanation for switching her chemotherapy?
    a. She probably has a brain tumor and the chemotherapy is not working.
    b. The docetaxel is causing a cerebellar dysfunction.
    c. The docetaxel could be causing the progressive peripheral neuropathy.
    d. The cancer could be impinging on the spinal nerves.

2.79   Which of the following chemotherapy drugs is *not* associated with arthralgias and myalgias?
    a. paclitaxel
    b. docetaxel
    c. ifosfamide
    d. vinorelbine

2.80   Which of the following is *not* considered a risk factor for ifosfamide-induced encephalopathy?
    a. hepatic insufficiency
    b. previous taxane therapy
    c. low serum albumin
    d. high serum creatinine

2.81   Mr. Rogers has a metastatic cancer of unknown origin. He originally went to his doctor because of ataxia and lower extremity weakness. His doctor described his symptoms as being related to a paraneoplastic syndrome. Which of the following statements best describes the cause of the patient's weakness?
    a. Cerebellar function is impaired because of the effect of the tumor.
    b. The cancer is in the brain and is pressing on the cerebellum.
    c. Chemotherapy is the most likely cause of the weakness.
    d. Muscle wasting is common in metastatic cancer.

2.82   Your patient has a possible brain tumor involving the frontal lobe. He is unable to coordinate skilled movements, but is not paralyzed. This process is called:
    a. dysphasia
    b. apraxia
    c. aphasia
    d. dysreflexia

2.83   Which of the following symptoms may accompany peripheral neuropathy associated with chemotherapy?
    a. ataxia
    b. diminished temperature sense
    c. diminished touch sense
    d. all of the above

2.84   Which of the following chemotherapeutic agents is *not* commonly associated with peripheral neuropathy?
   a.   cisplatin
   b.   doxorubicin hydrochloride liposomal
   c.   vincristine
   d.   paclitaxel

2.85   The cause of peripheral neuropathies caused by chemotherapy is best described by which of the following?
   a.   Sensory and motor axons are injured.
   b.   Demyelination reduces nerve conduction velocity.
   c.   Deep-tendon reflexes are lost.
   d.   Nerve cells are damaged by the cytotoxic effects of the drugs.

2.86   Which of the following is *most likely* to increase the risk of peripheral neuropathy from chemotherapy?
   a.   diabetes
   b.   alcoholism
   c.   severe malnutrition
   d.   all of the above

2.87   Jonas has finished his last course of chemotherapy including cisplatin, etoposide, and paclitaxel. He comes for an office visit complaining of colicky abdominal pain, constipation, urinary retention, and impotence. You are concerned because you know that his symptoms are most likely due to which of the following?
   a.   tumor recurrence
   b.   a paraneoplastic syndrome
   c.   the effect of chemotherapy on autonomic fibers
   d.   opstipation from chemotherapy

2.88   Which of the following is *not* considered to increase the risk of vincristine-induced peripheral neuropathy?
   a.   vincristine 2 mg intravenous twice a month
   b.   age greater than 60
   c.   hepatic dysfunction
   d.   concomitant etoposide therapy

2.89   Which of the following statements regarding the effect of cisplatin on hearing loss is *not* true?
   a.   The drug causes loss of the hairs in the inner ear.
   b.   Hearing loss begins with asymptomatic loss of high-frequency tones.
   c.   Tinitus is the first symptom to appear.
   d.   Loss of medium-frequency sounds is always permanent.

2.90   Annie has just completed her 10 treatments of weekly paclitaxel. Over the last few weeks, she has complained of difficulty buttoning her clothes and asks how soon it will get better. Your most appropriate response would be which of the following?
   a.   Her symptoms will probably get worse before they get better.
   b.   This means she cannot receive more paclitaxel.
   c.   Most symptoms will improve 2–3 weeks after treatment ends.
   d.   Her symptoms will improve but may never completely resolve.

2.91 The risk of ototoxicity from cisplatin therapy is increased by *all but* which of the following?
a. continuous infusion therapy
b. aminoglycoside therapy
c. dehydration
d. rapid drug delivery

2.92 Metabolic encephalopathy manifested as blurred vision, seizures, motor system dysfunction, and irreversible coma has been reported in up to 30% of patients receiving which drug?
a. high-dose cisplatin
b. etoposide continuous infusion
c. ifosfamide
d. cytarabine

2.93 Mr. Jones is an elderly gentleman who has been receiving 5-fluorouracil and leucovorin weekly as treatment for his colon cancer. His wife phones you to say that he is unsteady on his feet and complains of intermittent double vision. You encourage her to bring him in right away because you suspect which of the following?
a. acute cerebellar dysfunction due to the 5-fluorouracil
b. leukoencephalopathy from the cumulative effect of the drugs
c. dehydration due to severe diarrhea from the 5-fluorouracil
d. metastatic disease to the brain causing ataxia and diplopia

ALTERATIONS IN MENTAL STATUS

2.94 The single most important adjunctive treatment to combat the effects of vasogenic cerebral edema is the use of glucocorticoids. Which of the following is *not* a therapeutic mechanism of action of glucocorticoids?
a. inhibition of the capillary permeability factor produced by tumor cells
b. increase cerebral blood flow
c. suppress antidiuretic hormone
d. reduce the rate of cerebral fluid formation

2.95 After his emergency treatment for carotid hemorrhage, Mr. Jessup begins to experience tingling in his extremities on the ipsilateral side, as well as progressive motor loss and changes in the level of consciousness. You suspect, therefore, that he might have:
a. Cushing's syndrome, in response to progressive tumor
b. intermittent pulmonary failure with cardiac episodes, secondary to carotid artery ligation
c. cerebral ischemia secondary to carotid artery ligation
d. none of the above

2.96 A patient, who is receiving high-dose cytosine arabinoside (HDCA) for AML begins to experience slight difficulty with articulation of words. She smiles apologetically and says, "I guess I didn't get enough sleep. My mouth is pretty dry, too." Your response is to:
a. do an oral examination, offer mouth care, and continue HDCA therapy
b. withhold her HDCA dose and do a neurological evaluation
c. withhold her medication and check her renal function tests
d. interview the patient to identify factors contributing to sleeplessness, which is also contributing to dry mouth

2.97   Mrs. Ely has breast cancer and is receiving treatment for metastatic disease to bone, liver, and skin. She feels markedly fatigued, slightly constipated, and at times confused. Her symptoms are likely due to which of the following?
   a.   brain metastasis
   b.   liver failure
   c.   symptoms classic for chemotherapy
   d.   hypercalcemia

2.98   Which of the following signs and symptoms could be associated with hypercalcemia?
   a.   impaired concentration
   b.   extreme restlessness
   c.   irritability and confusion
   d.   all of the above

2.99   In severe hypercalcemia, a patient exhibits which of the following symptoms?
   a.   hypotension, dysrhythmias, severe diarrhea, stupor
   b.   atrioventricular block and asystole, hypertension, and coma
   c.   extreme agitation, hypertension, and constipation
   d.   diarrhea, hypotension, and coma

2.100 A patient with breast cancer has meningeal carcinomatosis that commonly manifests as:
   a.   headache
   b.   cranial nerve palsie
   c.   radiculopathies
   d.   all of the above

2.101 Which of the following is considered to be a classic sign of increased intracranial pressure (ICP)?
   a.   headache at the base of the brain
   b.   change in level of consciousness
   c.   agitation
   d.   forgetfulness

2.102 The most frequently observed symptoms of HIV-associated CNS lymphomas include:
   a.   nerve inflammation and fever resulting from cryptococcosis or toxoplasmosis
   b.   increased metabolism and pulse due to decreased serum protein/albumin levels
   c.   "B" symptoms, including fever, chills, weight loss, and diarrhea
   d.   confusion, lethargy, memory loss, and alterations in personality or behavior

2.103 Which of the following treatments is most closely associated with progressive demyelination, which may be important in the early stage of delayed injury to the brain?
   a.   methotrexate alone
   b.   radiation alone
   c.   methotrexate combined with radiation
   d.   methotrexate combined with both radiation and surgery

2.104 The most frequently described neuropsychologic late effects of CNS treatment for cancer include a deterioration in general intellectual performance. If we can assume that neuropsychologic changes in the brain are related to neuroanatomic abnormalities that result from cranial radiation, then one plausible explanation for the deterioration of intellectual performance is:
   a. injury to subcortical white matter
   b. destruction of the hypothalamus
   c. the formation of myelin membranes on nerve axons
   d. the overstimulation of thyroid tissue

2.105 Allison has been on tapering doses of steroids over the past week following the completion of her radiation therapy to her head for metastatic breast cancer. She has been doing fine, but currently has been sleeping more and seems confused about her surroundings. The cause of changes in her mental status is *most likely* due to:
   a. increasing intracranial pressure
   b. hypercalcemia due to metastatic breast cancer
   c. delayed side effects of radiation therapy
   d. steroid psychosis

2.106 Judith is an elderly woman with colon cancer metastatic to the liver. She has been responding well to leucovorin and 5-fluorouracil and radiation therapy. Her only problem has been nausea about 30 minutes after her radiation therapy. For this she takes prochlorperazine 10 mg po with lorazepam 1 mg every 6 hours. Her husband is calling because he is concerned that she is sleeping so much more than usual. He states that she sleeps all the time since she started the radiation. Your advice should be:
   a. Stop the prochlorperazine and the lorazepam because they are making her too sleepy.
   b. The radiation is associated with fatigue and she should sleep.
   c. Report her symptoms to the doctor because she probably is in the early stages of liver failure.
   d. Stop the lorazepam because it is broken down in the liver.

2.107 Which of the following is not considered to be a side effect of dronabinol?
   a. excessive salivation
   b. euphoria
   c. dysphoria
   d. orthostatic hypotension

2.108 A common manifestation of CNS lymphoma is:
   a. a change in personality
   b. syndrome of inappropriate antidiuretic hormone (SIADH)
   c. frontal headache
   d. spinal cord compression

2.109 The most common acute sign of malignant cerebral edema is:
   a. headache
   b. nausea/vomiting
   c. seizure
   d. disorientation

2.110   In most instances of CNS tumors, the first, earliest, and most sensitive indicator of dysfunction is a change in:
   a.   level of consciousness
   b.   cognitive ability
   c.   motor and sensory function
   d.   all of the above

INFECTION

2.111   Which of the following is considered to be the cardinal symptom of infection?
   a.   pus formation
   b.   inflammation
   c.   fever
   d.   elevated white blood cell count

2.112   What percentage of infections that occur in persons with cancer arise from endogenous microbial flora?
   a.   20%
   b.   40%
   c.   60%
   d.   80%

2.113   Mr. Smith has recently undergone a splenectomy for Hodgkin's disease. Part of your teaching involves informing him regarding the special precautions he needs to take as a result of being asplenic. These include which of the following?
   a.   Risk of infection is approximately 30% greater than normal.
   b.   Risk of overwhelming infection and death is 50 times greater than normal.
   c.   Risk of bleeding due to trauma is 10 times greater than normal.
   d.   He is no longer able to produce sufficient antibodies and should never be exposed to a live virus.

2.114   Despite current shifts in the patterns of infection, the primary cause of infection in granulocytopenic patients continues to be:
   a.   gram-positive organisms
   b.   gram-negative organisms
   c.   fungal infections
   d.   mycobacterial infections

2.115   Mrs. Carsen develops a chemotherapy-induced infection and is started on an antibiotic. You explain that she will take the antibiotic:
   a.   until cultures indicate eradication of the causative organism
   b.   for a minimum of 7 days
   c.   until the neutrophil count is greater than $500/mm^3$
   d.   any of the above

2.116 Melanie is about to undergo treatment with cyclophosphamide and doxorubicin. She is at risk for developing hemorrhagic cystitis. What preventive measures can be taken?
   a. Protection of the bladder focuses on controlled hydration.
   b. Intravenous acrolein may produce sulfhydryl complexes and subsequent detoxification.
   c. She is instructed to drink 8–10 glasses of fluid a day to prevent hemorrhagic cystitis.
   d. She should receive amifostine therapy daily.

2.117 The body's first line of defense against bacteria, which is commonly altered by cancer, is:
   a. granulocytes
   b. the skin
   c. macrophages
   d. the acid pH of fluid

2.118 The specific white blood cell that constitutes 55–70% of circulating white blood cells and responds quickly to bacterial invasion is the:
   a. polymorphonuclear neutrophil
   b. monocyte
   c. macrophage
   d. lymphocyte

2.119 What is the name given to the microbes that normally live in the body and lead to over 80% of infections in cancer patients?
   a. exogenous organisms
   b. intracellular organisms
   c. extracellular organisms
   d. endogenous organisms

2.120 Meticulous skin care is required when caring for the patient with reactivated varicella zoster virus to:
   a. minimize spread to other areas of the body
   b. prevent a secondary bacterial infection
   c. promote drainage of the vesicles
   d. provide the primary source of pain relief

2.121 The single most important measure to prevent infection when caring for the patient with granulocytopenia is:
   a. promptly instituting empiric antibiotics
   b. washing the hands meticulously
   c. providing optimal nutrition
   d. restricting the presence of live flowers and plants

2.122 Tricia develops a disseminated candidal infection that spreads from her mouth to part of her esophagus. Treatment would probably include:
   a. amphotericin B
   b. heparin
   c. ketoconazole
   d. fluconazole

2.123 Ms. Daniels has developed profound immunosuppression that has resulted in neutropenia, along with a denuding of the mucosa in the GI tract. This combination puts her at particular risk for:
a. *Candida* infection
b. *Aspergillus* infection
c. Epstein-Barr virus infection
d. *Pneumocystis carinii* pneumonia

2.124 Ms. Camara develops neutropenia. You are monitoring her regularly for signs of infection. Which of the following are you *most* concerned about?
a. viral infection
b. fungal infection
c. infection from gram-positive organisms
d. infection from gram-negative organisms

2.125 The leading cause of liver cancer throughout the world is:
a. chronic hepatitis B virus
b. chronic hepatitis C virus
c. chronic cirrhosis
d. chronic hepatitis A virus

2.126 A 52-year-old male presents with signs and symptoms of lymphoma. Subsequent assessment and diagnostic tests confirm stage IIB Hodgkin's disease. Mortality in this individual, if it occurs as a result of HD, is *most likely* to result from:
a. spinal cord compression
b. superior vena cava obstruction
c. failure of the liver or kidneys
d. infection or hemorrhage

2.127 Mr. Jackson's wife and children come with him for subsequent follow-up examinations after his allogeneic BMT. Although things are going very well, you instruct his family not to take what during the first year following Mr. Jackson's BMT because of possible shedding with subsequent infection in Mr. Jackson?
a. amoxicillin and ampicillin
b. Sabin oral polio vaccine
c. chemotherapeutic agents
d. the "flu shot"

2.128 You have been working with Mr. Prang, who received a blood cell transplant; Mrs. Adams, who has been treated with autologous BMT; and Ms. Creighton, who is receiving allogeneic BMT. Now, in post-transplant care, you are aware that, by decreasing the length of the nadir and with aggressive use of prophylaxis:
a. Ms. Creighton will be at less risk of infection than Mr. Prang
b. Mrs. Adams will be at less risk of infection than Ms. Creighton
c. Mr. Prang will still be at greatest risk for infection than the other two
d. a and c

2.129 Evidence that Kaposi's sarcoma (KS) may be linked to infection by cytomegalovirus (CMV), as well as by HIV, is that:
   a. CMV is found in a large percentage of homosexual men and AIDS patients.
   b. The genetic makeup of CMV is almost identical to that of HIV.
   c. CMV has been demonstrated to produce immunodeficiency in non-AIDS patients, including those receiving organ transpants.
   d. CMV has been found only in the fluids and organs of AIDS patients.

2.130 In caring for patients with AIDS-related Kaposi's sarcoma, nurses should be aware of both the special psychosocial (e.g., homosexuality, drug use) and physical aspects of the disease. For example, regarding physical aspects of the disease it is important to remember that:
   a. Tumor lysis syndrome is a common side effect that requires immediate attention.
   b. Confusion, lethargy, and memory loss occur frequently in KS patients.
   c. Side effects of chemotherapy tend to be more severe in the AIDS population.
   d. Risk must be established before effective care can begin.

2.131 The occurrence of non-Hodgkin's lymphoma (NHL) in AIDS patients appears to be related to:
   a. the destruction of helper T cells as a result of infection by cytomegalovirus (CMV)
   b. decreased levels of serum protein/albumin as a result of internal coalesced lesions
   c. opportunistic infections of the CNS related to toxoplasmosis
   d. the proliferation of B lymphocytes as a result of EBV and HIV infection

HEMORRHAGE

2.132 The most important measure in the early detection of bleeding is:
   a. accurate screening, beginning with a platelet count
   b. observation for subtle diagnostic signals, such as skin petechiae
   c. a family history, focusing on possible congenital bleeding disorders
   d. diagnostic testing of the complete cardiovascular system

2.133 Ms. Edwards, a cancer patient, is being assessed for abnormal bleeding. She is to receive a prothrombin time test. This test is a measure of:
   a. the ability of platelets to aggregate
   b. the concentration of functional factor in plasma
   c. platelet plug formation
   d. diminished or absent coagulation factors

2.134 The typical response of the body to a reduction in the platelet count, such as that caused by bleeding, is:
   a. an increase in the fibrinolytic activity of remaining platelets
   b. a release of ADP into the bloodstream, which increases the oxygen-carrying capacity of available platelets
   c. sequestering of red blood cells in the spleen
   d. increased production of megakaryocytes in the bone marrow

2.135 Circulating platelets perform several vital functions, including all of the following except:
   a. fibrinolysis, or the lysis of fibrin clots and vessel repair
   b. the release of plasminogen activators required for clot formation
   c. furnishing a phospholipid surface for the biochemical phase of hemostasis
   d. the formation of a mechanical hemostatic plug at the site of vessel injury

2.136 Bleeding with cancer is most often due either to the mechanical pressure of tumors on organs or to:
   a. interference with vasculature
   b. damage to the spleen
   c. hypocoagulability of the blood
   d. infection

2.137 Acute bleeding that occurs as a result of tumor-induced structural damage to vasculature is best managed by:
   a. radiotherapy combined with chemotherapy
   b. oral or parenteral iron supplements to reduce anemia
   c. mechanical pressure (e.g., nasal packing during epistaxis)
   d. direct and steady pressure at the site of bleeding

2.138 The single most significant measure for predicting bleeding in an individual with cancer is:
   a. tumor site
   b. platelet count
   c. abnormal platelet function
   d. an imbalance in coagulation factors

2.139 Mr. Jessup, who has a tracheostomy, is having a carotid hemorrhage. Besides controlling the bleeding, what should you do first to prevent aspiration of the blood?
   a. suction his throat and oral cavity
   b. deflate the cuff and remove the tracheostomy tube to clear the airway
   c. inflate the tracheostomy cuff
   d. transport him immediately to the operating room for ligation of the carotid artery

2.140 You are monitoring Liza to ensure that she does not develop complications associated with leukostasis. The most common and most lethal complication is:
   a. intracerebral hemorrhage
   b. cerebellar toxicity
   c. blast crisis
   d. disseminated intravascular coagulation

2.141 The individual who has recently had an ultrasound-guided percutaneous needle biopsy of the liver must be monitored closely for symptoms of:
   a. spinal cord compression
   b. hematemesis
   c. headache
   d. hemorrhage

2.142 Patients with liver cancer are more at risk for bleeding due to:
   a. a decrease in vitamin K absorption
   b. varices from portal hypertension
   c. increase in prothrombin time (PT) and partial thromboplastin time (PTT)
   d. all of the above

2.143 A patient with a brain tumor is suspected of having possible hemorrhage. The test most likely needed to determine this is:
   a. noncontrast CT
   b. CT with contrast
   c. MRI
   d. cerebral angiography

2.144 Postoperative care of an individual who has undergone palliative surgery for pancreatic cancer includes all of the following *except*:
   a. administration of pancreatic enzyme supplements
   b. providing a diet that is low in fat, is high in protein, and includes a glass of red wine with lunch and dinner
   c. observing for hemorrhage, hypovolemia, and hypotension
   d. examining stools for steatorrhea

2.145 One of the common sequelae of liver cancer is:
   a. esophageal varices
   b. visual disturbances
   c. fat intolerance
   d. urinary retention

2.146 The risk of carotid artery rupture after radical neck dissection is associated with all of the following *except*:
   a. coverage of the artery with a skin flap
   b. infection of the surrounding area
   c. a small trickle of blood from the area
   d. persistent tumor in the area

2.147 An example of a postoperative situation requiring immediate nursing intervention is:
   a. a smooth suture line with no sign of swelling
   b. hematoma formation beneath a skin flap
   c. evidence of cranial nerve damage
   d. clearing of airway secretions by coughing

2.148 Patients with cancers may at times have bleeding, despite normal platelet counts and coagulation factors. An example is bleeding caused by:
   a. platelet sequestration
   b. disseminated intravascular coagulation (DIC)
   c. decreased platelet adhesiveness
   d. hypocoagulability

2.149 There are numerous steps in the cascade of events leading to blood clot production. Which of the following substances results from both the intrinsic and the extrinsic pathway and is necessary for conversion of prothrombin to thrombin?
   a. factor XII
   b. factor VII
   c. thromboplastin
   d. fibrinogen

ANSWER EXPLANATIONS

2.1　**The answer is d.** Assessment of cerebellar function focuses on the ability to coordinate movement and to maintain normal muscle tone and equilibrium.

2.2　**The answer is c.** Complications related to surgical intervention, besides standard surgical risks, include neurological deficits, infection, and wound dehiscence. The most significant complication to treat is a new neurological deficit in which the neurological function often does not return.

2.3　**The answer is a.** The bone is frozen, which diminishes its immune response. Bone allograft recipients do not require immunosuppressive agents.

2.4　**The answer is c.** LHRH agonists initially increase testosterone levels, but after several days of therapy, testosterone levels fall to castration level. The surge of testosterone production after initiation of an LHRH agonist is called a "flare." During a flare, patients need to be aware that symptoms can worsen and require prompt medical intervention.

2.5　**The answer is a.** Pamidronate treatment in women with breast cancer and bone metastases led to reductions in the occurrence of hypercalcemia, severe bone pain, symptomatic impending fractures, and need for radiotherapy compared with untreated controls. Clinical trials are under way to evaluate the role of pamidronate in preventing the development of osteolytic metastases.

2.6　**The answer is c.** Performance scales that measure a person's functional status are used frequently in the eligibility criteria for cooperative group clinical trials and also periodically to evaluate the effects of treatment and disease. It may be helpful to interpret a person's quality of life, but it is not a primary objective of performance status.

2.7　**The answer is c.** Individuals with spinal metastasis may have radicular pain, paresthesias, heaviness of limbs, leg buckling, and episodes of dropping items. Compression of the spinal cord is likely and needs immediate treatment to prevent progressive neurological injury.

2.8　**The answer is d.** The three mechanisms by which a tumor spreads from the primary site to bones are (1) direct extension to adjacent bones, (2) arterial embolization, and (3) direct venous spread through the pelvic and vertebral veins.

2.9　**The answer is a.** Lesions greater than 2.5 cm in diameter that involve 50% of the cortex are at risk for fracture and need prophylactic stabilization.

2.10　**The answer is a.** Mental status changes can be an initial sign of hypercalcemia, hyperviscosity syndrome, or drug toxicity.

2.11　**The answer is d.** Advantages to immediate fitting include better emotional adjustment, increased motivation to ambulate early, and decreased stump edema, phantom limb pain, and contracture.

2.12　**The answer is a.** The bone is frozen, which diminishes its immune response. Bone allograft recipients do not require immunosuppressive agents, which are often given to organ recipients.

2.13　**The answer is a.** The hand-foot syndrome is characterized by an often painful rash and swelling of the palms of the hands and soles of the feet. Patients can have difficulty walking, especially if the cause is capecitabine. Topotecan has similar effects as capecitabine but less dermatologic toxicity.

2.14   **The answer is d.** All three factors play a role in the development of bone cancer: familial tendency, prior cancer therapy in the form of high-dose irradiation, and some preexisting bone conditions such as Paget's disease.

2.15   **The answer is a.** Ewing's sarcoma is an example of a bone tumor that originates in the bone marrow reticulum. Other examples in this category are reticulosarcoma and lymphosarcoma.

2.16   **The answer is d.** The most common presenting symptom in bone cancer is pain (sometimes described as "dull" or "aching") that has had a gradual onset and may have been present for several months before evaluation is sought. Abrupt onset of pain is possible, although not common, and most likely indicates a pathologic fracture.

2.17   **The answer is b.** Avoidance of amputation, preservation of maximum function, and eradication of tumor are all goals in the treatment of primary malignant bone cancer. Although there is evidence of a familial tendency for some of the bone cancers, early intervention in these cases is not common practice.

2.18   **The answer is d.** Three scenarios in which limb salvage is not a treatment option are (1) when the surgeon is unable to attain adequate surgical margin, (2) when the neurovascular bundle is involved, and (3) when the patient is younger than 10 years. In the latter case limb salvage is contraindicated because of the resultant limb length discrepancy, although recent advances in expandable prostheses make it possible for more children afflicted with bone cancer to retain their limbs during surgery.

2.19   **The answer is a.** Although phantom limb sensations (i.e., itching, pressure, tingling) are often experienced shortly after surgery, phantom limb pain (i.e., cramping, throbbing, burning) usually does not occur until 1–4 weeks after surgery. For most individuals, phantom limb pain resolves in a few months; pain for 5–10% of those who have limbs amputated worsens over the years. This worsening may be a sign of a neuroma or of locally recurrent cancer in the stump.

2.20   **The answer is c.** Currently chemotherapy is given preoperatively. The rationale for preoperative chemotherapy is to treat micrometastasis, decrease the size of the primary tumor (thereby increasing the likelihood of limb-salvage surgery) and assess the effectiveness of the chemotherapeutic agents for 2–3 months. The route of the chemotherapy is either intravenous or intra-arterial.

2.21   **The answer is c.** Chondrosarcoma is a tumor arising from either the interior medullary cavity of the cartilage (central chondrosarcoma) or from the bone through malignant changes in benign cartilage tumors (peripheral chondrosarcoma). The most frequent sites for this cancer are the pelvic bones, long bones, scapula, and ribs. Less common sites include the bones of the hands and feet.

2.22   **The answer is b.** Radiation to the involved sites is used primarily to relieve pain, improve bone strength, and improve neurological deficits.

2.23   **The answer is d.** Infection in the neutropenic patient is always considered a potentially life-threatening emergency. Fatality rates in untreated individuals during the first 48 hours of infection can exceed 50%.

2.24   **The answer is d.** Myelosuppression is not only the most common dose-limiting side effect of chemotherapy but also potentially the most lethal. Antimetabolites, vinca alkaloids, and antitumor antibiotics are most damaging to cells that are in a specific phase of the cell cycle; thus, myelosuppression is less severe with these agents.

2.25 **The answer is c.** The patient with neutropenia is unable to mount an inflammatory response. Fever is usually the first sign of infection. Choices **a**, **b**, and **d** are all true, but they explain why the neutropenic patient is at greater risk for infection rather than why the usual signs and symptoms of infection are often absent.

2.26 **The answer is b.** Granulocytopenic patients may not manifest clinical evidence of infection because granulocytopenia prevents the mounting of an inflammatory response. Progression to systemic infection and septic shock is usually rapid.

2.27 **The answer is b.** The respiratory tract is the most common site of infection in neutropenic patients. A high incidence of pneumonia in immunocompromised patients warrants thorough assessment of the respiratory tract. The mouth and orophayrnx are also high incidence sites for infection.

2.28 **The answer is a.** Any change in blood pressure, mental status, or urinary output in high-risk patients alerts the nurse to the probability of early shock. Restlessness, anxiety, and confusion are signs of late-phase shock.

2.29 **The answer is d.** Busulfan is taken daily in the chronic phase of CML. Blood counts begin to drop 10–14 days after therapy is begun. To prevent prolonged or severe myelosuppression, treatment is stopped if the WBC is less than 20,000/mm^3.

2.30 **The answer is d.** Antibiotics are used to treat chemotherapy-induced infections until (1) cultures indicate eradication of the causative organism, (2) for a minimum of 7 days, or (3) the neutrophil count is greater than 500/mm^3.

2.31 **The answer is b.** Cytokines initiate and regulate a number of inflammatory and immune responses.

2.32 **The answer is d.** Cytokines include interferons, interleukins, growth factors, and colony-stimulating factors.

2.33 **The answer is b.** The ANC is determined by multiplying the percentage of PMNs and bands by the total number of WBCs. The individual in this example is considered neutropenic because the ANC is less than 1000.

2.34 **The answer is c.** The incidence of catheter-related bacteremia is influenced by specific therapy, degree of catheter use, patient population, catheter insertion technique, and care and maintenance procedures. However, neutropenia remains the primary risk factor for patients with an infection who have a vascular access catheter.

2.35 **The answer is d.** Infections, due to invasion and overgrowth of pathogenic microbes, increase in frequency and severity as the ANC decreases. Risk for severe infections increases when the nadir persists for more than 7–10 days. The purpose of colony-stimulating factors is to reduce the number of days that the nadir is below 500 cells/mm^3.

2.36 **The answer is d.** Approximately 60% of neutropenic individuals develop an infection.

2.37 **The answer is c.** Almost 30% have documented bacteremia, another 30% have documented infection without bacteremia, and the rest have an apparent infection with no microbiologically documented pathogen.

2.38   **The answer is c.** Myelosuppression is the most common and lethal side effect of chemotherapy. Since hematopoietic cells divide rapidly, they are vulnerable to chemotherapy, potentially resulting in dangerously low levels of red blood cells, white blood cells, and platelets. When this occurs, patients are at risk for bleeding, infection, and circulatory compromise.

2.39   **The answer is d.** Thrombopoietin is the factor that stimulates the proliferation of CFU-MK cells and the differentiation of megakaryocytes into platelets.

2.40   **The answer is c.** The other choices all result in lowered platelet count. Choice **a** is often associated with splenomegaly, an enlarged spleen; **b** is frequently due to an autoimmune response in which antibodies are formed against the person's own platelets; **d** may also be the consequence of cancer therapy on bone marrow. A fourth cause of thrombocytopenia is platelet dilution, often caused by the use of stored platelet-poor blood.

2.41   **The answer is c.** A multifactorial model for multiple myeloma-associated anemia has been postulated, including the replacement of erythrocyte precursors with plasma cells.

2.42   **The answer is c.** Invasion and replacement of bone marrow by tumor may affect hematopoiesis. This process, called myelophthisis, can result in anemia, thrombocytopenia, granulocytopenia, and impaired natural killer cell activity.

2.43   **The answer is c.** All patients with MDS eventually develop life-threatening anemia, thrombocytopenia, and/or neutropenia. Regular evaluation of patients with MDS is important to monitor the need for supportive therapy with red blood cells, platelets, or antibiotics. MDS can transform to acute leukemia; however, this does not occur in all patients with MDS.

2.44   **The answer is a.** A cumulative and delayed onset of thrombocytopenia has been observed with carmustine, fludarabine, lomustine, mitomycin-c, streptozocin, and thiotepa.

2.45   **The answer is c.** When platelets are lower than 50,000 cells/mm^3, there is a moderate risk of bleeding. As the platelets continue to decrease below 10,000 cells/mm^3, a severe risk exists for fatal bleeding.

2.46   **The answer is d.** As the platelets continue to decrease below 10,000 cells/mm^3 a severe risk exists for fatal gastrointestinal, central nervous system, and respiratory tract hemorrhage.

2.47   **The answer is c.** Manifestations of thrombocytopenia are easy bruising; bleeding from gums, nose, or other orifices; and petechiae on the upper and lower extremities.

2.48   **The answer is d.** A decreased production of platelets may be due to tumor invasion of the bone marrow or to acute or delayed effects of chemotherapy or radiation. Pancytopenia is usually present.

2.49   **The answer is c.** The most common cause of thrombocytopenia in patients with cancer is a disorder involving decreased megakaryocytopoiesis.

2.50   **The answer is b.** ITP occurs most frequently in individuals with lymphoproliferative disorders such as chronic lymphocytic leukemia. It rarely is associated with solid tumors.

2.51   **The answer is c.** Interleukin-11 has shown a potent ability to elevate platelet counts after chemotherapy.

2.52   **The answer is d.** The clinical utility of interleukin-11 as treatment for thrombocytopenia may be limited by patient complaints of fatigue, arthralgias, and myalgias.

2.53   **The answer is a.** Rectal manipulation may place the thrombocytopenic patient at risk for bleeding. The use of suppositories or enemas is contraindicated. Stool softener and a laxative are important for preventing constipation in the patient who is receiving vincristine.

2.54   **The answer is c.** Mitomycin causes a cumulative and often delayed thrombocytopenia.

2.55   **The answer is d.** Transient control of platelet sequestration has been achieved with corticosteroid therapy. Steroids have a capillary-stabilizing effect that is important in minimizing the bleeding potential of thrombocytopenia.

2.56   **The answer is c.** Fever and infection enhance the consumption of platelets and can increase the occurrence of hemorrhage. Patients with fever or sepsis may require more frequent platelet transfusions to maintain adequate platelet counts.

2.57   **The answer is b.** Platelet survival is greatly decreased when alloimmunization to the platelet transfusion develops. Alloimmunization results when repeated transfusions of random-donor platelets fail to provide a therapeutic increment in the platelet count.

2.58   **The answer is c.** Symptoms that could indicate extravasation include swelling; stinging, burning, or pain at the injection site (not always present); redness (not often seen initially); and lack of blood return. Lack of a blood return alone is not always indicative of an extravasation. An extravasation can occur even if a blood return is present. This patient is presenting the classic signs of extravasation, and the possibility of a flare reaction is inappropriate.

2.59   **The answer is d.** Acute radiation effects result from the depletion of actively proliferating parenchymal or stromal cells and is characterized by vascular dilation, local edema, and inflammation. They are usually temporary and occur after higher doses are given over shorter periods of time to larger volumes of tissue.

2.60   **The answer is c.** Factors that determine the degree, onset, and duration of radiation-induced skin reactions include the following, among others: Higher doses given over shorter periods of time to larger volumes result in more severe acute skin reactions; electrons produce greater skin reactions than do photons; placing tissue-equivalent material on the skin reduces the skin-sparing effect of radiation therapy, allowing for maximum dose at the level of the skin. Finally, when treatment is targeted at areas of skin apposition, increased reaction secondary to warmth and moisture can be expected.

2.61   **The answer is b.** Following radiation therapy, the skin's ability to protect itself from UV rays is decreased as a result of destruction of melanocytes in the irradiated epidermis and the slower rate of melanin production in new epidermal cells in the radiation field.

2.62   **The answer is d.** The one obvious sign of drug infiltration is a bleb formation at the injection site or swelling that occurs in more deeply accessed veins. The absence of a blood return does not confirm an extravasation. The needle bevel or cannula tip may be positioned against the vein wall, preventing appropriate and obvious blood return.

2.63   **The answer is c.** SCC is more aggressive than BCC because it has a faster growth rate, less well-demarcated margins, and a greater metastatic potential. SCC appears as a flesh-colored or erythematous raised, firm papule. It is usually confined to areas exposed to UVR.

2.64   **The answer is c.** During the proliferative phase of wound healing, which lasts from 3 to 25 days following surgery, granulation tissue is formed and provides the characteristic strength of a wound. Most chemotherapy agents act by interfering with protein synthesis. Thus, wound healing could be disrupted by the administration of most chemotherapeutic agents in the early phases of wound healing.

2.65   **The answer is a.** A graft or flap is indicated when a lesion is large or located in an area in which insufficient tissue for primary closure would result in deformity, for example, after excision of large carcinomas of the eyelid and lip. Function is preserved in this manner. A skin flap consists of skin and subcutaneous tissue that are transferred from one area of the body to another. A flap contains its own blood supply, whereas a graft is avascular and depends on the blood supply of the recipient site for its survival.

2.66   **The answer is d.** Except in cases of whole-body irradiation or irradiation to the head, alopecia should not occur.

2.67   **The answer is d.** Surgical wound closure is often unsuccessful for the following reasons: irradiated tissue is fibrotic and unyielding, making it prone to dehiscence; healthy tissue often cannot be reached surgically because the ulcers are so deep; and radiation injury extends beyond the ulcer to surrounding tissues.

2.68   **The answer is a.** All patients have some skin reactions to radiation treatments. The fact that the skin is reddened is normal; however, the fact that it is painful means she needs a break.

2.69   **The answer is b.** Hyperpigmentation occurs with bleomycin. Other drugs inducing this reaction include cyclophosphamide, busulfan, carmustine, nitrogen mustard, 5-FU, and etoposide. The other drugs listed as choices in this question have in common the HSRs (type I reactions).

2.70   **The answer is d.** Multiple etiologic and risk factors are associated with skin cancers. High-risk factors for CM include a persistent changed or changing mole and the presence of irregular pigmented precursor lesions, including dysplastic nevi, congenital nevi, and lentigo maligna. Other possible risk factors for CM include UV radiation, age, hormonal factors, immunosuppression, and a previous history of melanoma. There is no conclusive evidence regarding the use of oral contraceptives and the increased risk of CM. High-risk factors for nonmelanoma cancers include ultraviolet (UV) radiation, especially UV-B and UV-A, and skin pigmentation.

2.71   **The answer is b.** Nicotine stomatitis is a diffuse white condition that contains numerous red dots. This lesion usually covers the entire hard palate and is almost always associated with pipe smoking. It has minimal or no malignant potential. Complete resolution should occur with cessation of smoking.

2.72   **The answer is b.** If a skin lesion is detected, the nurse has three responsibilities: accurate documentation of size, location, and description of the lesion; referral of the patient to a physician for diagnosis; and follow-up for recurrent disease.

2.73   **The answer is c.** DN are precursor lesions of cutaneous melanoma (CM) that develop from normal nevi, usually after puberty. It has been reported that 50% of CM evolve from some form of DN. They may be familial or nonfamilial, with the risk of CM in a family member with DN approaching 100% in melanoma-prone families. DN are often larger than 5 mm and can number from 1 to 100, with most affected persons having 25–75 abnormal nevi. They appear typically on sun-exposed areas, especially on the back, but also may be seen on the scalp, breasts, and buttocks. Pigmentation is irregular, with mixtures of tan, brown, and black or red and pink. A distinctive feature is a "fried egg" appearance.

2.74   **The answer is b.** Melanoma has been classified into several types, including lentigo maligna (LMM), superficial spreading (SSM), nodular, and acral lentiginous. Each type is characterized by a radial and/or vertical growth phase. In the radial phase, tumor growth is parallel to the skin surface, risk of metastasis is slight, and surgical excision is usually curative. The vertical growth phase is marked by focal deep penetration of atypical melanocytes into the dermis and subcutaneous tissue. Penetration occurs rapidly, increasing the risk of metastasis.

2.75   **The answer is b.** Sunscreen should always be applied on overcast days because 70–80% of UV radiation can penetrate cloud cover.

2.76   **The answer is b.** Vincristine is well known for potential peripheral neuropathy.

2.77   **The answer is c.** Methotrexate is associated with cerebellar dysfunction, such as unsteady gait and seizures, but not with peripheral neurophathies. Cytarabine, cisplatin, and carboplatin are all associated with peripheral neurophathies, particularly at higher doses.

2.78   **The answer is c.** Docetaxel can produce mild sensory neuropathy. At a cumulative dose of 600 mg/m^2 severe and disabling neuropathy can develop. Symptoms include paresthesia, numbness, loss of sensory qualities, and decrease in deep-tendon reflexes.

2.79   **The answer is c.** Ifosfamide can cause cerebellar and cranial dysfunction, but not myalgia or arthralgia.

2.80   **The answer is b.** Risk factors associated with ifosfamide encephalopathy include duration of administration, hepatic insufficiency, previous cisplatin use, presence of bulky disease, low serum albumin, and high serum creatinine.

2.81   **The answer is a.** Subacute cerebellar degeneration is a group of paraneoplastic neurologic disorders caused by antibodies that attack nerve cells, such as Purkinje cells, resulting in this neurologic syndrome.

2.82   **The answer is b.** Apraxia is the condition in which an individual cannot coordinate skilled movements, but is not paralyzed.

2.83   **The answer is d.** Patients who develop peripheral neuropathy as a side effect of chemotherapy may develop sensory abnormalities such as diminished temperature and touch sense in addition to the numbness and tingling commonly experienced. Proprioceptive losses in the lower extremities can lead to ataxia.

2.84   **The answer is b.** Doxorubicin hydrochloride liposomal is not commonly associated with peripheral neuropathies.

2.85   **The answer is d.** The sensory and motor axons are injured. Demyelination reduces nerve conduction velocity, leading to loss of deep-tendon reflexes, but the cause is the effect of the drug on the microtubules in the axon transport system, which results in axonal degeneration.

2.86   **The answer is d.** Individuals at greatest risk for peripheral neuropathies from chemotherapy are those with preexisting peripheral neuropathy, such as diabetes, alcoholism, or severe malnutrition.

2.87   **The answer is c.** Damage to the autonomic fibers can occur from chemotherapy and cause dizziness, constipation, abdominal colicky pain, ileus, impotence, urinary retention, and SIADH.

2.88   **The answer is a.** Factors that increase the risk of neurotoxicity with vincristine are frequent drug administration (such as weekly); dose greater that 2 mg; age greater than 60 years; concomitant isoniazid, teniposide, or etoposide therapy; and severe liver dysfunction as the drug undergoes hepatic metabolism and clearance.

2.89   **The answer is d.** With continued drug use, symptomatic loss of medium-frequency sound occurs and may be permanent.

2.90   **The answer is d.** Although mild symptoms may appear 1–3 days after high-dose paclitaxel, resolving 3–6 months after drug discontinuance, more severe symptoms, such as loss of fine motor movements, may resolve only partially.

2.91   **The answer is a.** Rapid drug delivery, simultaneous administration of aminoglycosides, and dehydration seem to increase the potential for ototoxicity.

2.92   **The answer is c.** Neurotoxicity characterized by metabolic encephalopathy manifested as blurred vision, seizures, motor system dysfunction, urinary incontinence, cranial nerve dysfunction, or irreversible coma has been reported in 5–30% of patients treated with ifosfamide.

2.93   **The answer is a.** 5-Fluorouracil may cause an acute cerebellar dysfunction, which is usually more common in the elderly. It is characterized by rapid onset of gait ataxia, limb incoordination, dysarthria, nystagmus, and diplopia.

2.94   **The answer is c.** Glucocorticoids rapidly reduce the rate of edema fluid formation by the tumor by inhibiting the capillary permeability factor produced by tumor cells. The aim of steroid therapy is to reduce intracranial pressure and increase cerebral blood flow.

2.95   **The answer is c.** Numbness or tingling of the extremities on the ipsilateral side, diplopia, blindness, progressive motor loss, and changes in the level of consciousness alert the nurse to possible cerebral ischemia secondary to carotid artery ligation.

2.96   **The answer is b.** The cytosine arabinoside (HDCA) should be withheld because dysarthria is a symptom of cerebellar toxicity from the drug. HDCA can cause cerebellar toxicities that may be irreversible. A full neurological examination should be done before each dose, even in the absence of symptoms.

2.97   **The answer is d.** Symptoms of hypercalcemia in order of reported frequency are fatigue, anorexia, weight loss, bone pain, constipation, polydipsia, muscle weakness, nausea and vomiting, mental changes, and polyuria.

2.98   **The answer is d.** Initial CNS dysfunction can present as personality changes, impaired concentration, mild confusion, drowsiness, and lethargy. Personality changes occur subtly and often are unnoticed by the family or individual. Extreme restlessness, irritability, overt confusion, and progressive deterioration in congitive function may develop.

2.199 **The answer is b.** Atrioventricular block and asystole may occur when the serum calcium level reaches 18 mg/dl or more. Hypertension may occur due to the direct effect of hypercalcemia on arterial smooth muscle.

2.100 **The answer is d.** Clinical manifestations of meningeal carcinomatosis are headache, mental status changes, gait disturbances, hydrocephalus, cranial nerve palsies, back pain, radiculopathies, weakness, and paresthesias.

2.101   **The answer is b.** Change in the level of consciousness is a classic sign of elevated ICP.

2.102   **The answer is d.** The cell of origin for primary CNS lymphoma is the same as that causing NHL elsewhere in the body. The transformed cell, which multiplies in an area that does not allow expansion (i.e., the brain), is the cause of most presenting symptoms, including confusion, lethargy, memory loss, and alterations in personality or behavior. Seizures may also develop. Symptoms are very similar to those caused by other mass lesions in the CNS, for which toxoplasmosis is the usual explanation.

2.103   **The answer is c.** Progressive demyelination (disruption of the myelin membrane that insulates nerve axons) may be due to a synergistic relationship between radiation and methotrexate. The myelin-producing glial cells in the CNS are proliferative during early childhood and therefore are radiosensitive. Damage to or a reproductive loss of glial cells from radiation can disrupt the myelin membrane. Methotrexate appears to contribute to this effect.

2.104   **The answer is a.** Brain atrophy and decreased subcortical white matter are the most frequent abnormalities that have been observed in long-term survivors who received whole-brain radiation. Because both abnormalities affect brain function, it is reasonable to see a connection between these neuroanatomic late effects and a deterioration in general intellectual performance. Other treatment-related changes in the brain, including demyelination of nerves, calcifications, and thickening of capillary walls, no doubt also are associated with intellectual deterioration.

2.105   **The answer is a.** The purpose of the steroids is to minimize swelling of the brain tissue caused initially by the tumor and the radiation. When it is stopped, the swelling may resume and the patient becomes more somnolent.

2.106   **The answer is d.** Prochlorperazine and lorazepam can both make a person sleepy, but the prochlorperazine is low dose and she needs it for her nausea. The lorazepam is broken down in the liver and is generally not a good choice in elderly patients as an antianxiety or antinausea drug.

2.107   **The answer is a.** Side effects from dronabinol (THC) that are particularly bothersome in middle-aged and older adults include dry mouth, sedation, orthostatic hypotension, ataxia, dizziness, and euphoria or dysphoria.

2.108   **The answer is a.** CNS lymphoma commonly causes neurologic dysfunction, apathy, confusion, and/or personality changes. It does not typically cause the headaches that are common to brain tumors, spinal cord compression, or SIADH.

2.109   **The answer is c.** Malignant cerebral edema produces diffuse signs and symptoms reflecting its more global effects on brain functioning, as opposed to the focal signs and symptoms caused by direct destruction of tissue by tumor. Subtle early changes in the patient's status are vague and usually are observed only by someone who knows the patient well. Seizure is the most common acute-onset sign. Headache, another common early symptom, is due to distortion and traction of pain-sensitive structures by the edema.

2.110   **The answer is a.** In most instances the first, earliest, and most sensitive indicator of dysfunction is a change in the level of consciousness. Mental status and cognitive ability, as well as motor and sensory function and cranial nerve function, are also assessed.

2.111 **The answer is c.** Fever is the cardinal symptom of infection. The neutropenic condition of marrow recipients masks the classic infection-related symptoms of inflammation, pus formation, and elevated white blood cell counts.

2.112 **The answer is d.** It is estimated that 80% of the infections that occur arise from endogenous microbial flora (GI or respiratory tract).

2.113 **The answer is b.** The spleen has two major roles in infection management. The spleen serves as a mechanical filter, removing bacteria from the bloodstream, and it also participates in antibody production. The risk of overwhelming sepsis and death in persons with asplenia, especially those with Hodgkin's disease, is at least 50 times greater than that in the normal population.

2.114 **The answer is b.** The most significant consequence of gram-negative infection is the potential for endotoxic or systemic shock.

2.115 **The answer is d.** Antibiotics are used to treat chemotherapy-induced infections until (1) cultures indicate eradication of the causative organism, (2) for a minimum of 7 days, or (3) the neutrophil count is greater than 500/mm^3.

2.116 **The answer is c.** To help prevent hemorrhagic cystitis during therapy with cyclophosphamide, patients are encouraged to drink 8–10 glasses of fluid a day and to void frequently.

2.117 **The answer is b.** The skin is the first line of defense against invading bacteria and subsequent infection. When a break in the skin occurs, environmental microbes and those that normally inhabit hair follicles and sebaceous glands can enter the body and cause infection.

2.118 **The answer is a.** Polymorphonuclear neutrophils comprise 55–70% of white blood cells and are the first to respond to invading bacteria. The primary function of PMNs is the destruction and elimination of microorganisms through phagocytosis, the process of engulfing and ingesting foreign matter.

2.119 **The answer is d.** Undisturbed, endogenous microbial flora exist as a carefully balanced synergistic microenvironment within the host. Alterations in normal flora predispose persons with cancer to serious opportunistic or nosocomial infection. More than 80% of infections developing in cancer patients arise from endogenous organisms, nearly half of which are acquired during hospitalization.

2.120 **The answer is b.** Diagnosis of VZV infection is based on a history of chickenpox, characteristic dermatomal distribution of vesicular lesions, and positive culture results. Because skin lesions (vesicles) can become confluent, meticulous skin care is required to prevent secondary bacterial infection.

2.121 **The answer is b.** Meticulous hand washing, by every person who enters the room or comes in contact with the individual at risk, is the single most important preventive measure against infection in the patient with granulocytopenia. Neutropenic individuals are advised of their risk and are encouraged to remind family, visitors, and staff about hand washing precautions.

2.122 **The answer is a.** A course of low-dose IV amphotericin B is indicated for nonresponsive infection and in severe esophageal and disseminated candidal infection.

2.123 **The answer is a.** Profound immunosuppression with resulting neutropenia concomitant with denuding of the mucosa in the GI tract places marrow recipients at risk for *Candida* infection.

2.124   **The answer is b.** Fungal infections are difficult to treat in the neutropenic and immuno-compromised patient, and recovery of the marrow is the best hope for survival.

2.125   **The answer is a.** Chronic hepatitis B virus infection is the leading cause of hepatocellular carcinoma throughout the world.

2.126   **The answer is d.** In this early stage, only infection or hemorrhage could be the cause of death. All the others would not occur at this stage.

2.127   **The answer is b.** Family members of BMT recipients should not be given the Sabin oral polio vaccine during the first year because of possible virus shedding and subsequent infection in the recipient. If the vaccine is given, the patient needs to be isolated from that family member for 8–12 weeks.

2.128   **The answer is b.** By decreasing the length of the nadir and with aggressive use of prophylaxis, the risk of infection with autologous BMT and BCT is lower than with allogeneic BMT. Recipients of allogeneic BMT remain immunosuppressed for 6 months to 2 years, depending on the presence and degree of GVHD.

2.129   **The answer is a.** One study found the DNA of cytomegalovirus in the nucleus of cells of KS lesions, which suggests a viral cause of KS. Serologic testing demonstrates that as many as 94% of all homosexual men have been infected by CMV, as evidenced by antibodies to CMV. CMV has also been isolated from the body fluids and organs of patients with AIDS, which suggests the possible role of latent CMV infection in AIDS-related KS. CMV indeed may produce a similar effect in patients receiving immunosuppressing drugs, but it has not been demonstrated. CMV may be found in the fluids and organs of individuals who do not have AIDS.

2.130   **The answer is c.** Because side effects of chemotherapy tend to be more severe in the AIDS population, the nurse should be aggressive in the assessment of potential complications, alert the physician promptly when complications occur, implement appropriate nursing interventions, and remember that these patients have an underlying illness that predisposes them to other opportunistic infections and malignancies.

2.131   **The answer is d.** AIDS-associated NHLs are typically intermediate- to high-grade B-cell malignancies. They appear to be associated with a rise in polygonal B-cell lymphoproliferation that results from EBV and HIV infection. AIDS-NHL has been associated with persistent generalized lymphadenopathy, suggesting polyclonal B-cell activation. One possibility is that once HIV infection occurs, EBV may trigger lymphocyte proliferation that remains unchecked as a result of HIV-induced immune dysfunction. This proliferation, in turn, may allow the expression of two oncogenes, resulting in a polygonal or monoclonal NHL.

2.132   **The answer is b.** Because diagnostic signals may be subtle (e.g., skin petechiae that may be noticed while bathing the person, traces of blood during brushing of teeth), it is important for the nurse to be keenly observant. A family history and various screening tests may be valuable in assessment, but they do not substitute for observation.

2.133   **The answer is d.** This screening test is called prothrombin time (PT). Choice **a** is the platelet aggregation test; **b** is the specific factor assays test; and **c** is the bleeding time test.

2.134   **The answer is d.** Megakaryocytes mature in the bone marrow and fragment to form platelets, which are then released into the bloodstream. Under normal circumstances any reduction in platelet count—from bleeding, malignancy, chemotherapy or radiotherapy, or other causes—causes an increase in the production of megakaryocytes and platelets in the bone marrow. This activity is controlled by a regulatory hormone called thrombopoietin.

2.135 **The answer is b.** Plasminogen activators are enzymes that are present in most body fluids and tissues. They are responsible for the conversion of plasminogen to plasmin in the presence of thrombin. It is plasmin that is responsible for the lysis (and not the formation) of fibrin clots.

2.136 **The answer is a.** All the other choices can be factors in bleeding, but erosion and rupture of vessels precipitated by tumor invasion or pressure is the other major cause of bleeding in persons with cancer. Any tumor involvement of vasculature tissue or any tumor lying in close proximity to major vessels is seen as a threat of bleeding. Bleeding may also be the result of radiotherapy or radical cancer surgery and various platelet and coagulation abnormalities.

2.137 **The answer is c.** If acute bleeding does occur, direct methods to halt the hemorrhage should be instituted immediately. Choices **a** and **b** are preventive methods; choice **d**, although immediate and direct, applies to an exposed bleeding site. Another example of the use of mechanical pressure to stop acute bleeding is the insertion of an occlusion balloon catheter into the bronchus.

2.138 **The answer is b.** Although all the other choices are factors in bleeding as well, platelet count is the single most important factor in predicting bleeding in the individual with cancer. Patients with platelet counts below 20,000 cells/mm³ have a greater than 50% chance of bleeding. Low platelet count (thrombocytopenia) is also the most frequent platelet abnormality associated with cancer.

2.139 **The answer is c.** The nursing actions during a carotid hemorrhage focus on maintenance of the airway and control of bleeding. If the patient has a tracheostomy, the cuff should be inflated to prevent aspiration. Firm pressure should be applied to the neck using a towel or dressing material. If an internal carotid bleed is suspected, a vaginal pack or fluff dressing should be used to tightly pack the oral cavity and oropharynx. The patient is then transported to the operating room for ligation of the carotid artery.

2.140 **The answer is a.** Leukostasis occurs as the leukemic blast cells accumulate and invade vessel walls, causing rupture and bleeding. Patients with extremely high numbers of circulating blasts (WBC >50,000/mm³) are at increased risk for leukostasis. Intracerebral hemorrhage is the most common and most lethal manifestation of this complication.

2.141 **The answer is d.** Because most liver tumors are highly vascular, the person having an ultrasound-guided percutaneous needle biopsy of the liver must be monitored closely for intra-abdominal hemorrhage. In general, this procedure is rapid, safe, and commonly used; however, some clinicians strongly believe that needle biopsies should be avoided at all costs if there is any potential for curative resection, because of the potential for seeding and spreading the cancer during the procedure.

2.142 **The answer is d.** Patients with liver cancer are more at risk for bleeding because of a decrease in vitamin K absorption, an increase in PT and PTT times, and varices from portal hypertension.

2.143 **The answer is a.** Noncontrast CT is necessary to determine the presence of calcium or hemorrhage. Contrast is then administered to delineate the margins and extent of blood-brain barrier disruption. MRI is the more definitive and preferred imaging study for the individual with a CNS tumor. Cerebral angiography may be used to confirm that the lesion in question is a vascular malformation or an aneurysm, rather than a neoplasm.

2.144   **The answer is b.** Hemorrhage, hypovolemia, and hypotension pose the greatest threats to an individual who has just undergone surgery for cancer of the pancreas. As soon as possible after pancreatectomy, small feedings are started with a diet that is usually bland, low in fat, and high in carbohydrates and protein. Restrictions include caffeine, alcohol, and overindulgence. The stool should be examined daily for the characteristic signs of steatorrhea: frothy, foul-smelling stool with fat particles floating in the water.

2.145   **The answer is a.** As liver cancer advances, serious complications arise, usually involving many body systems. Portal vein obstruction may lead to necrosis, rupture, and hemorrhage. Esophageal varices and unrelenting ascites are also common sequelae of either primary or secondary liver cancer.

2.146   **The answer is a.** Skin flaps are usually made to cover and protect the carotid artery. However, skin flap necrosis leaves the artery unprotected, and infection and persistent tumor raise the risk of rupture. Carotid artery blowout usually is preceded by a small trickle of blood from the area.

2.147   **The answer is b.** Hematoma formation can affect the adherence of skin flaps, resulting in flap necrosis. Excessive bleeding may require a return to the operating room for ligation of the bleeding vessel. Choices **a** and **d** are desirable; as for choice **c**, cranial nerve damage may have occurred during surgery and cannot be affected by nursing action.

2.148   **The answer is c.** Choices **b** and **d** are coagulation abnormalities; choice **a** is a quantitative abnormality. Qualitative abnormalites such as choice **c** refer principally to alterations in platelet function, which may include a decreased procoagulant activity of platelets, decreased platelet adhesiveness and decreased aggregation in response to ADP, thrombocytosis associated with myeloproliferative disorders, and the coating of platelets by fibrin degradation products as a result of the increased activation of coagulation factors.

2.149   **The answer is c.** Thromboplastin is needed for conversion of prothrombin to thrombin, and its formation results from both pathways of the clotting cascade—the intrinsic and the extrinsic pathways.

STUDY NOTES

STUDY NOTES

GASTROINTESTINAL AND URINARY FUNCTION

ALTERATIONS IN NUTRITION

Dysphagia

3.1   What is the best treatment approach for radiation esophagitis?
     a. symptom relief and supportive care
     b. dietary manipulation
     c. topical anesthesia and systemic analgesia when needed
     d. all of the above

3.2   Mr. Bill has completed 2 weeks of radiation therapy and concomitant chemotherapy for carcinoma of the trachea. He complains of dysphagia, odynophagia, and intermittent epigastric pain. He is *most likely* suffering from which of the following?
     a. tracheitis
     b. bronchitis
     c. esophagitis
     d. cholangitis

3.3   Mr. Bill complains of intense pain in his throat and difficulty swallowing. The nurse practitioner suggests using sucralfate suspension. The sucralfate is intended to accomplish which of the following?
     a. promote comfort and possibly healing by binding to exposed mucosa
     b. promote comfort by numbing exposed nerve endings
     c. promote healing by reducing infection
     d. pain control only

3.4   Which of the following chemotherapy agents is likely to potentiate the problem of esophagitis in patients also receiving radiation therapy to the esophagus?
     a. cyclophosphamide
     b. 5-fluorouracil
     c. paclitaxel
     d. procarbazine

3.5   Complications and side effects of radiotherapy for esophageal cancer include all of the following *except:*
a. esophageal stricture
b. radiation pneumonitis
c. skin reaction
d. diarrhea

3.6   An elderly woman presents with a thyroid mass and symptoms of dyspnea and dysphagia. Assessment indicates carcinoma of the thyroid with metastases to the lung. Her symptoms of dyspnea and dysphagia are *most likely* to be the result of:
a. involvement of the parathyroid gland and associate hypercalcemia
b. compressive effects of the tumor on the larynx and esophagus
c. infection caused by irritation of the oral mucosa
d. a high concentration of iodine in the follicular cells of the thyroid

3.7   Dysphagia is the most common presenting complaint of persons with which of the following?
a. tracheal cancer
b. esophageal cancer
c. epiglottal cancer
d. laryngeal cancer

3.8   Your patient has aspiration pneumonia from a tracheoesophageal fistula. He is terminal and in hospice care. The physician has ordered scopolamine (0.6 mg IM) three to four times a day as needed. You explain to the patient and family that the purpose of the scopolamine is which of the following?
a. to decrease the amount of secretions
b. to manage his nausea
c. to decrease anxiety
d. to help manage dyspnea

3.9   Your patient has difficulty swallowing without aspirating following a hemilaryngectomy for a supraglottic carcinoma. You consult a swallowing specialist, who recommends which of the following to help the patient relearn swallowing without aspiration?
a. try liquids first, then semisolids
b. try crackers or toast followed by a sip of liquid
c. try semisolids first, then solids followed by liquids
d. none of the above until he can manage his own secretions

Anorexia

3.10 Loss of appetite is a common problem in individuals with cancer. Which of the following is *most likely* to contribute to anorexia?
a. cytokines
b. circulating lipids and lactic acid
c. serotonin and bombesin
d. all of the above

3.11   Angela has metastatic cancer. Among her many complaints is that she is having trouble eating and is steadily losing weight. Her doctor prescribes megestrol acetate 400 mg per day. Your teaching includes which of the following?
   a.   The purpose of the megestrol acetate is to increase her appetite.
   b.   The purpose of the megestrol acetate is to treat her cancer.
   c.   The side effects of megestrol acetate are edema and hyperglycemia.
   d.   If she has congestive heart failure, she should not take megestrol acetate.

3.12   Vinny has started radiation therapy to his left leg for a sarcoma. He complains of anorexia and slight nausea following his radiation treatment. Your explanation would include which of the following?
   a.   Because the radiation port does not include his stomach, it is not likely that his symptoms are related to the radiation.
   b.   The likelihood is that the tumor is secreting substances that cause him to feel ill. He should feel better as the tumor shrinks.
   c.   The waste products of tissue destruction are likely the cause of his symptoms.
   d.   The Cori cycle is producing excess urea.

3.13   Anorexia is characterized by which of the following?
   a.   abnormalities of carbohydrate, protein, and fat metabolism
   b.   visceral and lean body mass depletion
   c.   muscle atrophy
   d.   all of the above

3.14   Which of the following is *not* considered to be a reflection of immune status in an individual suffering from anorexia?
   a.   hypoalbuminemia
   b.   decreased macrophage mobilization
   c.   depressed lymphocyte function
   d.   impaired phagocytosis

3.15   Which of the following places an individual at significant high risk for protein-calorie malnutrition?
   a.   loss of 10% body weight within the previous 6 months
   b.   an unintentional weight loss of more than 1 kilogram a week
   c.   a macrobiotic diet
   d.   all of the above

3.16   A newly diagnosed, unresectable lung cancer patient complains that he has not had an appetite for many weeks and is concerned because he is losing weight. What is the *most likely* cause of his weight loss?
   a.   Anorexia and cachexia are common manifestations of lung cancer.
   b.   He is probably depressed over his situation and should improve with treatment.
   c.   The chemotherapy and radiation cause weight loss.
   d.   Liver disease is most likely causing his loss of appetite.

3.17   Mr. Dillon is dying from lung cancer and has had no appetite for some time. His family states they are uncomfortable with their loved one starving to death and want him to be force-fed. Which of the following is *not* an appropriate rationale for intervention?
    a.   If the family wants the patient to have enteral or parenteral nutrition, this is a therapeutic option.
    b.   Artificial nutrition can lead to congestive heart failure, nausea, vomiting, and diarrhea.
    c.   Anorexia is an adaptive, protective mechanism that leads to a gentler death.
    d.   Dehydration and starvation are not uncomfortable ways to die.

3.18   Your patient is suffering from anorexia and says nothing tastes good. Which of the following medications has been found to be most helpful in combating anorexia?
    a.   steroids
    b.   hydrazine sulfate
    c.   dronabinol
    d.   megestrol acetate

3.19   The etiology of anorexia-cachexia syndrome is best explained by which of the following?
    a.   the nutritional demands of the tumor
    b.   reduced food intake due to tumor by-products
    c.   multiple metabolic and physiologic abnormalities
    d.   loss of appetite due to food intolerances

Mucositis

3.20   Mucositis is observed more often when:
    a.   5-FU is combined with other mucositis-producing drugs, such as methotrexate and doxorubicin
    b.   5-FU is given alone
    c.   bleomycin is used to abruptly replace 5-FU
    d.   none of the above

3.21   Which of the following is considered an effective measure to minimize oral stomatitis?
    a.   oral cryotherapy during chemotherapy treatment
    b.   sucralfate oral suspension
    c.   frequent oral hygiene
    d.   all of the above

3.22   Which of the following factors is considered a risk factor for stomatitis with cancer treatment?
    a.   dehydration
    b.   preexisting dental problems
    c.   diagnosis of leukemia
    d.   all of the above

3.23   A patient who has been treated with radiation to the mouth and oropharynx has developed mucositis. Effective management of this side effect incorporates all of the following *except:*
    a.   encouraging the patient to avoid alcohol and cigarettes
    b.   administering a Benadryl solution as a mouthwash or spray
    c.   removing the plaque-like tissue that forms with mucositis
    d.   administering Maalox to coat and soothe the mucosa

3.24   Which of the following will increase the risk of mucositis to a patient receiving radiation to the base of the tongue?
    a.   metal tooth fillings
    b.   tobacco usage
    c.   alcohol consumption
    d.   all the above

3.25   The dose-limiting toxicity of 5-fluorouracil (5-FU) when given as a continuous infusion is:
    a.   myelosuppression
    b.   mucositis
    c.   nausea and vomiting
    d.   cerebellar ataxia

3.26   Your bone marrow transplant patient has an oral herpetic lesion and asks you how she could have gotten it. Which of the following statements would *not* be accurate concerning oral herpes simplex virus (HSV) infections?
    a.   Most oral infections are due to reactivation of latent infections.
    b.   HSV infections in this population present as soft-tissue ulcerations rather than vesicles.
    c.   The incidence in this population is about 50%.
    d.   This population is more at risk for dissemination of HSV infection than other immunocompromised patients.

3.27   Hydrogen peroxide is an effective oral agent for the care of the patient with mucositis, but is *not* recommended for long-term oral care for which of the following reasons?
    a.   its destructive effects on new granulation tissue
    b.   the risk of tooth decalcification
    c.   the overgrowth of the white papillae of the tongue and increased risk of fungal infections
    d.   all of the above

3.28   An important nursing intervention during the postoperative period following surgery for pituitary adenoma pertains to the operative site and involves:
    a.   stimulation of salivary flow with hard candy to avert sialadenitis
    b.   the administration of antiemetics to counteract the effects of radioisotopes
    c.   oral inspection and meticulous mouth care to maintain integrity of the mucous membranes
    d.   monitoring for signs of shock related to the profound derease in available catecholamines

3.29   Patients with acute myelocytic leukemia frequently have gingival hypertrophy with swelling, necrosis, and infection of the gums. All of the following treatments are appropriate. Which one will be *most* effective in relieving the problem?
    a.   oral care with a solution of one quart water with one teaspoon each of salt and sodium bicarbonate
    b.   antifungal mouth rinses
    c.   local or systemic analgesics as needed
    d.   initiating chemotherapy

Xerostomia

3.30   Your patient is receiving chemotherapy and begins to complain of a dry mouth and thick, ropy saliva. The condition is beginning to interfere with his appetite and speech. Which of the following will *not* be part of your patient education plan regarding this reaction?
   a.   This reaction is permanent, and although not life-threatening, it can eventually lead to oral caries and candidal infections.
   b.   Xerostomia is a dysfunction of the salivary gland that occurs following chemotherapy.
   c.   Xerostomia is a decrease in the quality and quantity of saliva.
   d.   Saliva substitutes, frequent rinses with ice water, and sugarless gum may provide relief.

3.31   Which is *not* part of your treatment plan for the patient experiencing xerostomia?
   a.   Oral care before meals helps to freshen the mouth and stimulate appetite.
   b.   Increasing fluid intake during meals and snacks helps to lubricate food and ease swallowing.
   c.   Lemon glycerin is an excellent substitute for the more irritating commercial mouthwashes.
   d.   Vegetable or corn oil swished in the mouth may be a cost-effective alternative for artificial lubrication.

3.32   What can be used to dissolve and break up thick saliva?
   a.   sugar-free lemon candy and sugar-free gum
   b.   papain (found in papaya) and amylase (found in pineapple)
   c.   sialagogues
   d.   pilocarpine

3.33   After treatment, Michelle complains of a dry mouth and within 3 weeks develops a thick, ropy saliva. The side effect Michelle is experiencing is:
   a.   xerostomia
   b.   mucositis
   c.   trismus
   d.   desquamation

3.34   Mr. Allen is having radiation therapy as primary treatment for a pyriform sinus lesion. In your teaching regarding xerostomia, you are likely to discuss which of the following?
   a.   Xerostomia is likely to be permanent.
   b.   He can expect excessive saliva formation for at least 3 months following radiation.
   c.   He will receive medication to minimize the severity of the xerostomia.
   d.   Receiving chemotherapy will worsen the severity of the xerostomia.

3.35   Four weeks after radiation therapy ends, Mr. Allen complains that the xerostomia is not improving. The physician prescribes oral pilocarpine. Your teaching includes which of the following points?
   a.   The pilocarpine is used to suppress the exocrine gland production.
   b.   Side effects include diaphoresis, lacrimation, and increased gastric secretion.
   c.   Photosensitivity worsens over time.
   d.   all of the above

3.36 Xerostomia, a decrease in saliva secretion, is a side effect of:
   a. oral surgery
   b. bone marrow transplantation
   c. cisplatin administration
   d. head and neck irradiation

3.37 Which of the following statements about xerostomia is *not* correct?
   a. It is characterized by dry mouth due to destruction of the saliva glands.
   b. Xerostomia is due to radiation therapy.
   c. Oral pilocarpine is used to increase saliva production.
   d. Xerostomia is rarely permanent.

3.38 Besides a dry mouth, the primary problem with xerostomia is:
   a. lack of pH balance in the mouth
   b. enamel decalcification
   c. diminished protection from fungal infections
   d. increased tracheal and esophageal irritation

Nausea and Vomiting

3.39 Mr. Jones is receiving cisplatin therapy for testicular cancer and requires a serotonin antagonist and a steroid daily during his treatment. The rationale for this combination is based on which of the following?
   a. Cisplatin is often associated with cumulative and delayed nausea.
   b. The steroid is used to boost the immune system.
   c. The steroid enhances the antiemetic effect of the serotonin antagonist.
   d. a and c

3.40 Eric is treated with ^{131}I for his tumor. The side effect he is *least likely* to experience is probably:
   a. radiation-induced pulmonary fibrosis
   b. nausea and vomiting
   c. bone marrow suppression
   d. salivary gland inflammation

3.41 Nausea and vomiting have been effectively treated with:
   a. meditation
   b. exercise
   c. oral ginger
   d. all of the above

3.42 Which of the following antineoplastic agents is commonly associated with delayed nausea?
   a. doxorubicin
   b. cisplatin
   c. cyclophosphamide
   d. all of the above

3.43 Anticipatory nausea and vomiting during the 12-hour period prior to chemotherapy occurs in approximately what percentage of patients?
   a. 15%
   b. 20%
   c. 25%
   d. 30%

3.44 Degree and severity of nausea and vomiting from chemotherapy vary. Which of the following is *not* considered to be a factor in predicting the degree and severity of chemotherapy-induced nausea and vomiting?
   a. rate of chemotherapy infusion
   b. previous emetic control
   c. drug sequencing
   d. age

3.45 Which of the following chemotherapy agents is *not* associated with a moderate to high incidence of emesis?
   a. vincristine
   b. methotrexate
   c. doxorubicin
   d. topotecan

3.46 Serotonin antagonists represent a new class of drugs used to prevent and manage chemotherapy-induced nausea and vomiting. Which of the following best describes the characteristics of these agents compared to the dopamine antagonists?
   a. Unlike the phenothiazines, serotonin antagonists are not associated with extrapyramidal reactions.
   b. Serotonin antagonists work both centrally and peripherally, whereas the dopamine antagonists work only centrally.
   c. Dexamethasone potentiates the effects of dopamine antagonists.
   d. a and b

3.47 Protracted nausea and vomiting following chemotherapy and total body irradiation is a consistent problem for the bone marrow transplant patient. Which of the following is *most responsible* for the protracted nature of these symptoms?
   a. GVHD
   b. CMV esophagitis
   c. GI infections
   d. all of the above

3.48 Your patient is to have total body irradiation (TBI) as part of a bone marrow transplant. In teaching the patient about the possible side effects, you would emphasize *all but* which of the following?
   a. TBI penetrates the sanctuary sites where cells may be hidden.
   b. TBI is delivered in a single dose.
   c. Nausea and vomiting is common.
   d. Xerostomia and loss of taste are temporary.

3.49 Dimethyl sulfoxide (DMSO) is the preservative used during blood cell transplantation. Aside from its objectionable odor, there are other side effects. Which of the following is *not* an anticipated side effect of DMSO either during or immediately after infusion?
   a. hyperpyrexia
   b. nausea and vomiting
   c. chilling and cramping
   d. cough, dyspnea, and chest tightness

3.50   John has a lung tumor with a single brain lesion for which he has received a full course of radiation therapy. He has been doing well on paclitaxel and carboplatin, until he experiences vomiting that seemed to come on without warning. Select the *most appropriate* advice to give this patient.
    a. His vomiting is most likely due to the chemotherapy, and he should take an antiemetic and call back if he does not feel better.
    b. He is probably experiencing delayed nausea and vomiting from the combination of the radiation and the chemotherapy. An antiemetic is appropriate.
    c. His symptoms could be related to increased intracranial pressure, and he should come to the emergency room as soon as possible.
    d. His symptoms could be due to chemotherapy or to increased intracranial pressure, and he should be advised to take dexamethasone, which is appropriate in either case.

3.51   Your 28-year-old patient is receiving doxorubicin and cyclophosphamide for her breast cancer. She complains of feeling jittery and nervous following her chemotherapy. She is taking ondansetron 24 mg plus dexamethasone 10 mg and prochlorperazine 15 mg according to her schedule. Which of the following interventions is *most appropriate* and why?
    a. Eliminate the dexamethasone from her protocol because it is making her jittery.
    b. Discontinue the prochlorperazine because she is allergic to it.
    c. Administer diphenhydramine 25 mg with the prochlorperazine because she is young and likely to be sensitive to it.
    d. Discontinue both the dexamethasone and the prochlorperazine because either one can cause jitteriness and a hypersensitivity reaction.

Taste Alterations

3.52   You decide to do some research to find out how and why chemotherapy causes an effect on nutrition. In your reading, you learn *all but* which of the following?
    a. Chemotherapy can indirectly cause food aversions.
    b. Chemotherapy can alter the intestinal absorptive surface.
    c. Chemotherapy does not interfere with specific metabolic reactions.
    d. Chemotherapy may cause excitation of the true vomiting center.

3.53   Which of the following medical terms is used to describe taste abnormalities in cancer?
    a. hypogeusia
    b. dysgeusia
    c. hyposmia
    d. all of the above

3.54   Which of the following is *not* considered to be a cause of altered taste and smell in individuals with cancer?
    a. deficiencies in zinc, copper, nickel, and niacin
    b. direct tumor invasion
    c. hypercalcemia
    d. cancer-associated circulating factors

3.55   Jim complains that food does not taste the same and that everything tastes like cardboard. He especially dislikes the taste of red meat. This is best explained by the fact that persons with cancer commonly experience:
    a. an increased threshold for sweet, sour, and salt and a decreased threshold for bitter foods
    b. a decreased threshold for sweet, sour, and salt and an increased threshold for bitter foods
    c. difficulty digesting their food
    d. intolerance to bland foods

3.56 Lou is a 67-year-old plumber who is receiving radiation to his posterior hypopharynx. Your teaching would include which of the following points regarding the effects of radiation on taste?
a. He can expect to experience alterations of taste about 2–3 weeks into treatment.
b. The most severely affected taste qualities are salt and bitter.
c. Sweet taste is generally least affected.
d. all of the above

3.57 Common symptoms of carcinoma of the nasal cavity and paranasal sinuses include all of the following *except*:
a. diplopia
b. hyperesthesia of the cheek
c. taste changes
d. headache pain

3.58 Because of the changed configuration of the aerodigestive tract, the person who has undergone a laryngectomy can expect change in all of the following functions *except*:
a. speaking
b. eating
c. taste
d. smell

3.59 An example of a chemotherapeutic agent that may cause a metallic taste during administration, leading to taste changes, is:
a. etoposide
b. cyclophosphamide
c. doxorubicin
d. dacarbazine

3.60 Cancer patients often experience a general reduction in taste perception (hypogeusesthesia) and/or a perverted sense of taste (dysgeusia). One of the conditions implicated in this is:
a. sustained hyperglycemia
b. permanent damage to the chemoreceptor trigger zone
c. an increase in circulating lipids and peptides
d. vitamin and mineral deficiencies

Electrolyte Imbalances

3.61 Janie has ovarian cancer and is beginning her cancer treatment with enthusiasm. In addition to chemotherapy, she wants to begin a macrobiotic diet and take dietary supplements. You want to encourage her and guide her in the right direction. Which of the following would *not* be appropriate advice to give this patient?
a. Alternative therapies have not been proved to be effective and she should not take any vitamins or dietary supplements.
b. Macrobiotic diets tend to be deficient in protein, calories, iron, and vitamin B_{12}.
c. Megadose vitamin supplements tend to be excessively high in the B complex, C, A, D, and E vitamins.
d. Megadose vitamins can cause liver damage, kidney stones, and coagulation abnormalities.

3.62 Mr. Johns is undergoing chemotherapy for high-grade testicular cancer. He complains of being jittery, and his lab tests reveal low magnesium, albumin, and calcium. He is *most likely* experiencing which of the following complication of chemotherapy?
a. anorexia and weakness due to chemotherapy
b. low magnesium due to cisplatin therapy
c. low calcium due to uremia syndrome
d. a paraneoplastic syndrome

3.63 Mary has lung cancer and wants to try alternative approaches to nutrition to help to improve her immune system. She is leaning toward a macrobiotic diet and asks if there are any adverse effects associated with this type of diet. The major problem with a macrobiotic diet is which of the following?
a. colitis and electrolyte imbalance
b. deficiencies in vitamin B_{12}
c. protein deficiencies
d. b and c

3.64 Health food stores are replete with vitamin supplements to treat everything from fatigue to terminal cancer. Your patient wants to be as healthy as she can be and wants you to teach her about megavitamin supplementation as an adjunct to her cancer treatment. Trying to give accurate, objective, and scientific information, which of the following would you include as potential hazards of vitamin therapies?
a. vitamin therapy usually includes high doses of B complex, C, A, D, and E vitamins
b. cardiac abnormalities and liver damage
c. kidney stones and coagulation abnormalities
d. all of the above

3.65 Paracentesis is a procedure commonly used to manage peritoneal ascites. While caring for patients and teaching them about the procedure, it is important to remember that:
a. the procedure is therapeutic
b. the procedure can lead to severe protein depletion and electrolyte imbalance
c. patients can experience postural hypotension
d. b and c

3.66 Which of the following metabolic disorders is common in patients who receive cisplatin therapy?
a. hypokalemia
b. hypomagnesemia
c. hypophosphatemia
d. hypocalcemia

3.67 Individuals with cancer may experience fluid and electrolyte imbalances related to hyper-uricemia. In this conditlon:
a. a sudden decrease in levels of serum uric acid causes renal failure
b. tumor lysis releases calcium deposits in the renal tubules, which leads to renal failure
c. tumor lysis causes the syndrome of inappropriate antidiuretic hormone secretion (SIADH)
d. urate crystals may be deposited in the kidneys, causing renal failure

3.68   Which of the following tests is used to determine protein status?
a. midarm muscle circumference
b. skinfold thickness measurement
c. daily weight
d. orthostatic vital signs

3.69   An analysis of biochemical data often yields information regarding nutritional status. Decreased levels of urinary creatinine may be an indicator of:
a. decreased mortality
b. fat depletion
c. increased gastrointestinal absorption
d. decreased lean body mass

Weight Changes

3.70   Betty will be having a mastectomy. In planning ahead and helping her to get ready for the surgery, you tell her that:
a. because of the bed rest required in recovery, surgery will decrease her energy requirements
b. nutritional problems resulting from her surgery will probably extend well past the immediate perioperative period
c. surgery on her breast cancer should not have any direct implication for her nutritional needs
d. surgery can increase her energy requirements to 1.5 times what she normally needs

3.71   The three classic signs of a pancreatic tumor located in the head of the pancreas are progressive jaundice, pain, and:
a. profound weight loss
b. projectile vomiting
c. confusion
d. hyperkalemia

3.72   Betty is one of your patients who is receiving adjuvant chemotherapy for breast cancer. She is near her ideal weight when she begins treatment. Which of the following is something you might explain to her during her nutritional assessment?
a. The majority of women with breast cancer who do not receive chemotherapy lose weight.
b. The majority of women with breast cancer who receive chemotherapy gain weight.
c. Gaining weight, or overnutrition, is not known to be harmful for women undergoing treatment.
d. none of the above

3.73   Your patient Sean has been participating in professional athletics for several years. At 170 pounds, he weighs far more than he should for his height of 5 feet 6 inches, but he does not appear to be overweight. In trying to determine whether you should counsel Sean to reduce his caloric and fat intake, you decide to use _____ to determine his percentage of body fat.
a. a body mass index
b. a resting metabolic nomogram
c. a skinfold measure
d. REE

3.74   In trying to determine how much weight Charles has lost over what span of time, you learn that he is 5 feet 10 inches tall and weighed 170 pounds 1 year ago. Three months ago, he weighed 160 pounds, and now he weighs 132 pounds. What is the percentage of Charles's weight change in the past 3 months?
   a.   17%
   b.   20%
   c.   22%
   d.   7%

3.75   You are attempting to choose an instrument to gain a more complete diet history from Charles. He has already told you that he doesn't pay much attention to what he eats, and he has a hard time remembering what he had for lunch (or if he had lunch) yesterday. Charles is very upset about his recent diagnosis, and this has changed his eating habits considerably. However, he is willing to cooperate with you, and he understands the importance of being honest in the things he tells you. Keeping in mind that Charles is in the hospital now, but he will not be for most of his treatment, you choose:
   a.   a calorie count
   b.   24-hour dietary recall
   c.   a food frequency record
   d.   a diet diary

3.76   Postoperative care of an individual who has undergone palliative surgery for pancreatic cancer includes all of the following *except*:
   a.   administration of pancreatic enzyme supplements
   b.   providing a diet that is low in fat, is high in protein, and includes a glass of red wine with lunch and dinner
   c.   observing for hemorrhage, hypovolemia, and hypotension
   d.   examining stool for steatorrhea

3.77   Of women who receive adjuvant chemotherapy for breast cancer, many will gain weight and even become obese. What percentage of women on adjuvant chemotherapy for breast cancer gain weight?
   a.   30–40%
   b.   40–70%
   c.   40–50%
   d.   60–90%

Cachexia

3.78   William asks you for an appetite stimulant. Keeping in mind that he is on an extensive chemotherapy regimen, is diabetic, and has not had problems with nausea or vomiting, which of the following drugs is the *best possible* intervention for him?
   a.   corticosteroids
   b.   megestrol acetate
   c.   metoclopramide
   d.   THC

3.79 Cancer-associated nutritional problems, rather than treatment-related nutritional problems, are best reversed by:
a. extensive verbal counseling
b. self-care actions
c. medications
d. successful treatment of the tumor

3.80 At what stage does nutritional intervention have the best chance to alter patient outcome?
a. early, when the tumor burden is small
b. later, when the malignancy is aggressive
c. during treatment
d. after treatment has ended

3.81 Charles is one of your patients with lung cancer. Because he is diabetic and already well under his ideal weight, one of your major concerns is to provide Charles with adequate nutrition and prevent cachexia. You are dismayed to learn that he "lost his appetite" when he recently received his diagnosis and almost entirely stopped eating. Which of the following is probably *not* a factor that would have contributed to the loss of appetite?
a. circulating cytokines
b. cancer-induced sepsis
c. psychological distress
d. bombesin

3.82 When you give David a complete assessment, you find that he is suffering from anorexia, skeletal muscle atrophy, and asthenia. His hepatic glucose production is at normal levels, perhaps even a bit higher. What is your diagnosis?
a. primary cachexia
b. secondary cachexia
c. starvation
d. marasmus

3.83 With cachexia, the total body fat and skeletal muscle components can drop as much as _____ and _____, respectively.
a. 20%; 30%
b. 50%; 40%
c. 85%; 75%
d. 60%; 80%

3.84 The most frequently occurring and well-defined paraneoplastic syndromes (PNSs) are:
a. renal PNSs
b. neurological PNSs
c. endocrine PNSs
d. hematologic PNSs

3.85 Mr. Thomas has been steadily losing weight and progressively deteriorating from his pancreatic cancer. He is experiencing severe muscle wasting and energy loss. The appropriate term for this condition is:
a. cancer cachexia
b. malnutrition
c. inanition
d. undernutrition

3.86   Mr. Thomas has pancreatic cancer and feels as if he cannot get out of bed at times and that if he tried he would probably be up for only a few minutes due to an overwhelming loss of strength. This loss of strength is referred to as which of the following?
  a.   asthenia
  b.   marasmus
  c.   protein-calorie malnutrition
  d.   anorexia-cachexia syndrome

Ascites

3.87   The cancer *most often* associated with malignant ascites is:
  a.   ovarian cancer
  b.   pancreatic cancer
  c.   breast cancer
  d.   esophageal cancer

3.88   Beth has slowly progressing ascites due to liver failure associated with metastatic ovarian carcinoma. She is uncomfortable from the pressure and asks what can be done. Which of the following supportive measures is *most appropriate* to manage her discomfort?
  a.   fluid and sodium restriction
  b.   diuretic therapy
  c.   paracentesis
  d.   all of the above

3.89   Ascites is a presenting symptom in what percentage of women with ovarian cancer?
  a.   10%
  b.   30%
  c.   50%
  d.   70%

3.90   Approximately what percentage of women with ovarian carcinoma eventually develop ascites?
  a.   90%
  b.   80%
  c.   60%
  d.   30%

3.91   From a physiological point of view, which of the following best describes how peritoneal ascites occurs?
  a.   tumor seeding of the peritoneum resulting in obstruction of the diaphragmatic and/or abdominal lymphatics
  b.   thoracic duct obstruction and dilation
  c.   excess intraperitoneal fluid production
  d.   all of the above

3.92   Which of the following chemotherapy agents is known to cause fluid retention that may manifest as abdominal ascites, as a pleural effusion, or as a combination?
  a.   mitoxantrone
  b.   megestrol acetate
  c.   docetaxel
  d.   paclitaxel

3.93 Andrea has ovarian cancer and complains of abdominal fullness. In this patient the presence of shifting dullness would be indicative of which of the following?
    a. abdominal carcinomatosis
    b. liver enlargement
    c. ascites
    d. all of the above

3.94 Malignant peritoneal effusion (ascites) is caused by which of the following?
    a. obstruction of diaphragmatic lymphatics
    b. tumor seeding of the peritoneum
    c. humoral factors that cause increased capillary leakage of proteins
    d. all of the above

3.95 Your patient with ascites has had a peritoneal tap and removal of 1–2 liters repeatedly in the past and is calling now with a request for another tap because the fluid has come back and he is uncomfortable. Your response is based on knowledge of which of the following?
    a. Sclerosis with instillation of chemotherapy is the most effective treatment
    b. Draining the peritoneum only makes fluid accumulate faster.
    c. Repeated paracentesis can lead to severe protein depletion.
    d. Peritoneal tap can lead to tumor seeding.

ALTERATIONS IN ELIMINATION

Incontinence

3.96 Urinary incontinence following transurethral resection of the prostate is related to which of the following?
    a. damage to the muscle controlling the striated urethral sphincter
    b. damage to the cavernous nerve
    c. prolonged urethral catheterization
    d. all of the above

3.97 A patient's prostate cancer has recurred, and he is receiving radiation to a portal including the prostate, periprostatatic tissue, and pelvic lymph nodes. Possible complications of radiation to this area include *all but* which of the following?
    a. constipation and bowel narrowing
    b. urinary incontinence
    c. lower extremity edema
    d. cystitis

3.98 Laser therapy is an option for small superficial bladder tumors. The advantages of this procedure include *all but* which of the following?
    a. An indwelling catheter is necessary for only a short time period.
    b. Dissemination of disease in the bladder is less likely compared to fulguration.
    c. It can be performed under local anesthesia.
    d. The risk for bladder perforation is minimal.

3.99 Complications of the continent urinary diversion include:
a. urinary leakage
b. difficult catheterization
c. ascending infection
d. a and b

3.100 Mr. Benson presents with some pain and frequency of urination. During a rectal palpation, the examiner detects a diffuse enlargement of the prostate. There seems to be no mass, however. With no other information, one might infer that Mr. Benson is *most likely* to have:
a. nephritis
b. cancer of the prostate
c. cancer of the bladder
d. benign prostatic hypertrophy

3.101 Your patient is being prepped for a radical prostatectomy and is concerned about urinary incontinence. Your best advice to him would be which of the following?
a. Urinary incontinence is a major problem in only about 50% of patients.
b. Stress incontinence occurs in about 25% of patients but is manageable.
c. 92% of patients achieve urinary control following radical prostatectomy.
d. He should talk to his doctor.

3.102 Following TURP your patient experiences dribbling and stress incontinence. He asks you what his treatment options are. The most appropriate response would include which of the following?
a. Surgery, because the goal is urethral compression
b. Kegal exercises to strengthen the pelvic floor muscles
c. alpha-adrenergic agonists drugs to increase sphincter resistance
d. all of the above

Constipation

3.103 A patient is receiving cyclophosphamide, doxorubicin, and vincristine for lung cancer. He also is receiving opioid analgesics for pain. He normally has a bowel movement every day. He reports that he has not had a bowel movement in 3 days but does not feel the urge and has not been eating normally. Appropriate nursing assessment and management include which of the following?
a. He has not had a normal routine so it is a good idea to increase fiber and fluids and call if there is no bowel movement in 24 hours.
b. He should take a laxative, such as milk of magnesia, and call if he has no bowel movement in 48 hours.
c. Elderly patients often have a decrease in colonic transit time, and with time he will have results.
d. He should take a laxative and a suppository and call if there are no results in 24 hours.

3.104 Which of the following chemotherapeutic agents is *least likely* to cause constipation?
a. vinorelbine
b. vincristine
c. vinblastine
d. carmustine

3.105   A patient is receiving vinorelbine and complains of colicky abdominal pain and abdominal distention. Physiologically the patient's symptoms are *most likely* caused by:
a.   the effect of the vinorelbine on the GI mucosa
b.   decreased colonic transit time with vinorelbine
c.   diminished afferent and efferent pathways from the sacral cord
d.   cramping and gas pains, which are common with vinorelbine

3.106   Twenty four hours after taking a laxative, a patient calls and complains of nausea and inability to pass gas. He has not had a bowel movement in 4 days. The most appropriate approach to this situation includes which of the following?
a.   The patient needs to have an enema.
b.   A stool softener and a laxative should be recommended.
c.   The patient should have a physical exam and a flat plate of the abdomen because he could be obstipated.
d.   An oil retention enema and milk of magnesia should be given and repeated if there are no results in 24 hours.

3.107   Opioids affect the gastrointestinal (GI) tract, contributing to constipation by which of the following mechanisms?
a.   activation of opioid receptors in the GI tract and the central nervous system (CNS)
b.   increased water absorption due to increased transit time
c.   insensitivity to rectal distention
d.   all of the above

3.108   Which of the following statements regarding vincristine-induced constipation is *not* true?
a.   Vincristine may damage the myenteric plexus of the colon.
b.   Vincristine is more likely to cause constipation than is vinblastine.
c.   Bowel effects usually occur with peripheral nerve dysfunction.
d.   Severe constipation may occur in up to 35% of patients.

3.109   Which of the following is *not* commonly associated with increased risk for constipation?
a.   vincristine
b.   vinorelbine
c.   vindesine
d.   etoposide

3.110   Chemotherapy-related constipation is associated with which of the following?
a.   colicky abdominal pain
b.   peripheral nerve dysfunction
c.   decreased colonic transit time
d.   reduced rectal emptying due to spinal cord compression

3.111   Opioid-induced constipation is best managed by which of the following approaches?
a.   increase fiber to 3–4 grams per day
b.   increase fluid intake to eight 8-ounce glasses of fluid per day
c.   1 senokot tablet + 100 mg tablet of colace per 30 mg tablet of MS Contin
d.   all of the above

Diarrhea

3.112 Radiation-induced enteritis can cause significant diarrhea. Which of the following interventions is *not* appropriate management of this problem?
    a. a liquid diet high in milk and milk products
    b. Sandostatin given subcutaneously
    c. anticholinergics
    d. paragoric elixir

3.113 Physiologically the etiology of chemotherapy-induced diarrhea involves which of the following?
    a. shortening or denuding of the intestinal villa
    b. the destruction of the actively dividing epithelial cells
    c. microvilli flattening and reducing the absorbtive surface
    d. all of the above

3.114 A patient is receiving 5-fluorouracil and leucovorin weekly for 4 weeks. He reports abdominal cramping, rectal urgency, and diarrhea that wake him at night time. On questioning, he reports four diarrhea stools on each of the past 3 days, each with a volume of about 1 cup. Appropriate nursing action would include:
    a. Encourage him to take loperamide with each loose stool and to push fluids and delay treatment for 1 week.
    b. Diarrhea is expected with 5-fluorouracil, and he should receive his chemotherapy with instructions to take loperamide with each loose stool.
    c. Myelosuppression is the dose-limiting toxicity of 5-fluorouracil, so if the counts are good, he should receive treatment.
    d. Assess the patient for dehydration including orthostatic blood pressures.

3.115 A patient receiving chemotherapy complains of severe diarrhea for 6 days and agrees to come to the outpatient clinic to be evaluated. Appropriate nursing action would include:
    a. Monitor the patient for orthostatic hypotension, lethargy, and weakness.
    b. Monitor fluids and electrolytes.
    c. Notify the physician for fluid replacement and evaluation.
    d. all of the above

3.116 5-Fluorouracil is commonly given with leucovorin to treat GI malignancies. This combination of drugs results in which of the following?
    a. manipulation of the metabolism of the 5-fluorouracil
    b. potentiate the effect of 5-fluorouracil
    c. decrease diarrhea occurrence
    d. a and b

3.117 Which of the following chemotherapy agents is *least likely* to cause diarrhea?
    a. bleomycin
    b. irinotecan
    c. docetaxel
    d. methotrexate

3.118 A patient reports diarrhea 2 weeks after paclitaxel therapy. He had a fever 5 days after his treatment and was placed on antibiotics empirically. He states that he feels well, but he has no appetite and the diarrhea is not slowing down. Appropriate nursing action includes which of the following?
   a. Encourage the patient to take antidiarrheal agents and to push fluids.
   b. Monitor the fluids and electrolytes and give results to the physician.
   c. Send a stool culture for *Clostridium difficile*.
   d. b and c

3.119 In general, antidiarrheal agents should *not* be given to patients as treatment for diarrhea that might be caused by an infectious agent. What is the rationale for this?
   a. The antidiarrheal agent would slow the passage of stool.
   b. The antidiarrheal agent increases the exposure of the mucosa to the infectious agent.
   c. The risk of systemic absorption is increased.
   d. all of the above

3.120 The *most common* injury to the large bowel that occurs following radiotherapy is:
   a. increased bowel motility
   b. proctosigmoiditis
   c. abdominal cramping
   d. loose, watery stools

3.121 Mr. Brown has had a bone marrow transplant and suffers from chronic diarrhea. A cause for his diarrhea is *most likely* which of the following?
   a. viral infection
   b. GVHD
   c. herpes simplex
   d. varicella zoster

Bowel Obstruction

3.122 Which of the following clinical manifestations are *most likely* to exist in patients with a cancer of the sigmoid colon?
   a. anemia and a vague, dull, persistent pain in the upper right quadrant
   b. abdominal pain and melena
   c. sensations of incomplete evacuation and tenesmus
   d. bright red bleeding through the rectum

3.123 Physical examination and diagnostic studies of a patient with cancer of the right colon are *most likely* to find which of the following?
   a. a palpable mass
   b. polyps in the rectum
   c. anemia
   d. high levels of carcinoembryonic antigen (CEA)

3.124 During Ms. Harris's rectal examination for her complaints of abdominal distention and pain, you detect a stony, hard mass in the cul-de-sac. What does this indicate?
   a. Ms. Harris has small amounts of intra-abdominal fluid forming a "puddle sign" on the pelvic floor.
   b. Ms. Harris has pancreatic or hepatic lesions pressing on the pelvic floor.
   c. Ms. Harris has a carcinoma that has metastasized to the pelvic floor.
   d. Ms. Harris has metastasis at Virchow's node.

3.125 Which of the following is contraindicated for a patient with constipation due to structural blockage by a tumor?
a. increase fiber in the diet to greater than 6 grams per day
b. administer magnesium citrate or GoLYTELY as needed
c. soap suds enemas
d. all of the above

3.126 Alfred is newly diagnosed with a bowel obstruction secondary to an abdominal mass. The physician is proposing the patient begin total parenteral nutrition (TPN) as soon as possible. Which of the following is *not* appropriate rationale for TPN in this case?
a. TPN will probably be needed for the rest of his life.
b. TPN will be used throughout surgery, radiation, and chemotherapy.
c. TPN will provide nutrients for 2–3 months.
d. TPN is the best chance for the patient to maintain nutrition during treatment.

3.127 Your patient has a bowel obstruction complicated by intractable hiccups. Which of the following medications for hiccups is contraindicated?
a. metoclopramide
b. chlorpromazine
c. cisapride
d. amitriptyline

3.128 Biliary vomiting is indicative of which of the following?
a. intermittent bowel obstruction
b. obstruction in the upper part of the abdomen
c. obstruction in the lower ileus
d. progressive constipation

3.129 Susan has end-stage cancer with a bowel obstruction and is currently in hospice care. Which of the following would be an appropriate intervention to minimize her discomfort?
a. placement of a nasogastric tube to manage nausea and vomiting
b. enemas every other day to promote evacuation
c. avoiding the use of opioids, because they will only make it worse
d. octreotide acetate to minimize secretions

Ostomies, Urinary Diversions

3.130 Mr. James is scheduled for a radical cystectomy with urinary diversion. He is especially concerned about the possibility of being impotent following surgery. Your comments and counsel are based on which of the following?
a. Because the surgery involves removal of the bladder, attached peritoneum, the prostate, and seminal vesicles, impotence is nearly always unavoidable.
b. It is possible that the nerves crucial to achieving penile erection may be spared and he should be encouraged to talk to his surgeon.
c. Refer him to an enterostomal therapist for information about a penile prosthesis and placement of the urinary diversion.
d. all of the above

3.131   Which of the following procedures is the surgeon *most likely* to perform when a lesion involves the middle and left transverse colon?
a.   a right hemicolectomy that includes the related lymphatic and circulatory channels
b.   a one-stage procedure involving resection of the lesion and a primary anastomosis
c.   a two-stage procedure involving a temporary colostomy or ileostomy
d.   a three-stage procedure involving a diverting colostomy, a resection of the tumor, and takedown of the colostomy

3.132   For proximal and midrectal adenocarcinomas, the treatment technique of choice is:
a.   low anterior resection, preserving external anal sphincter control
b.   abdominoperineal resection with a temporary colostomy
c.   laser therapy to the tumor bed through a colonoscope or flexible sigmoidoscope
d.   prophylactic oophorectomy

3.133   The primary complications of a cystectomy and urinary diversion are related primarily to *all but* which of the following?
a.   stoma construction and placement
b.   wound dehiscence
c.   long-term kidney damage
d.   stoma stenosis

3.134   A continent urinary diversion is a surgical method substituting for the functions of the lower urinary tract. Which of the following is *not* a correct description of this procedure?
a.   A continent urinary diversion provides control of voiding.
b.   One-way valves prevent urinary reflux.
c.   An intra-abdominal pouch is created for storage of urine.
d.   All continent urinary diversions are constructed from terminal ileum.

3.135   Following a radical cystectomy, the nurse is instructed to irrigate the pouch regularly to maintain patency. The patient expresses dismay, stating that he does not feel that he can learn to do this. The nurse's best response is which of the following?
a.   "Has your doctor told you it will be necessary for you to irrigate the pouch?"
b.   "Most of the time, the mucus becomes very thin and easy to pass."
c.   "Mucus production will decrease over time and irrigation will become unnecessary."
d.   "Irrigation is necessary to prevent urinary reflux."

3.136   Mr. Makela has an ileal conduit placed following cystectomy for advanced bladder cancer. Which of the following would be considered normal?
a.   a delay of urinary output for 4–5 hours after surgery
b.   protrusion of the stoma 3 inches above the skin surface
c.   a stoma that is dark red in color and slightly edematous
d.   a small amount of leakage from the appliance

3.137   If the urine passing from a stoma is cloudy, it may be that:
a.   the patient is dehydrated
b.   the stoma was formed from intestinal tissue
c.   a leak in the stoma pouch has occurred, allowing air and bacteria to enter a sterile area
d.   antispasmodics are indicated

3.138 Placement of a stoma following colorectal surgery is *least likely* to be:
   a. on smooth skin large enough in area to allow the appliance to be secured to the abdomen
   b. in a location that the patient can see without difficulty
   c. outside the borders of the rectus muscle to avert accidental dislodgment of the appliance
   d. on a site close to the transverse colon

3.139 Which of the following postoperative assessments of stoma viability is a matter of concern that should be brought to the surgeon's attention?
   a. persistent peristalsis in the bowel
   b. bleeding of the stoma when rubbed
   c. a dusky or gray stoma
   d. protrusion of the stoma

3.140 Postoperative care and teaching of the patient undergoing abdominoperineal resection (APR) for rectal cancer is *most likely* to be influenced by which of the following?
   a. the type of colostomy to be performed
   b. the patient's age, sex, and physical condition
   c. the extent of hepatic invasion
   d. the type of closure of the perineal wound to be used

Renal Dysfunction

3.141 Nephrotic syndrome is a paraneoplastic syndrome (PNS) characterized by which of the following?
   a. the presence of lesions in the renal glomerulus
   b. a secondary benign disorder resulting from a primary glomerular disease
   c. impaired renal function due to obstruction of the glomerulus by tumor products
   d. all of the above

3.142 As you take the history of a client with nephrotic syndrome, what signs and symptoms would you expect to see or hear reported?
   a. brown, foamy urine
   b. "gaunt" face and generalized weight loss with anorexia
   c. mild hypotension
   d. a and b

3.143 Multiple myeloma is associated with renal failure precipitated by numerous factors. Which of the following contributes most to renal failure in multiple myeloma?
   a. infection
   b. hypercalcemia
   c. dehydration
   d. any of the above

3.144 Several years ago, a patient was given concomitant radiation therapy and chemotherapy for cancer of the bladder. Recently, she developed cystitis. If this condition is a late effect of her cancer treatment, which agent is *least likely* to have been the responsible one involved?
   a. cyclophosphamide
   b. ifosfamide
   c. methotrexate
   d. cisplatin

3.145   Management of tenesmus, cystitis, and urethritis that may result when radiation is given to the pelvic area involves several nursing options, including all of the following *except:*

    a.   administering gastrointestinal and urinary antispasmodics

    b.   administering antibiotics if there is evidence of infection

    c.   encouraging high fluid intake by the patient

    d.   providing sitz baths if the perineal area is being irradiated

3.146   Mr. Prang is at high risk for developing hemorrhagic cystitis in response to conditioning therapy for BMT. You propose to help prevent this development with the use of:

    a.   hydration

    b.   a Foley catheter

    c.   the uroprotectant mesna

    d.   all of the above

3.147   The only consistent risk factor for kidney cancer is:

    a.   cigarette smoking

    b.   coffee

    c.   heredity

    d.   asbestos

3.148   Prolonged diarrhea without adequate management can lead to all of the following *except*:

    a.   renal failure

    b.   dehydration

    c.   circulatory collapse

    d.   nutritional malabsorption

ANSWER EXPLANATIONS

3.1   **The answer is d.** All management is directed at symptom relief and supportive care. This is best accomplished through dietary manipulation, topical anesthesia, and systemic analgesia when needed.

3.2   **The answer is c.** The most common early symptoms of esophagitis include dysphagia (difficulty swallowing), odynophagia (painful swallowing), and epigastric pain. Esophageal pain that worsens and becomes continuous and substernal indicates progressing esophagitis.

3.3   **The answer is a.** Sucralfate suspension is used to treat radiation- and chemotherapy-induced esophagitis. Some suggest that it promotes comfort and possibly healing by binding to proteinaceous exudate in exposed mucosa.

3.4   **The answer is b.** Prior or concurrent radiation may augment the severity and extent of mucosal injury. Some drugs, such as dactinomycin and doxorubicin, potentiate radiation injury to the esophagus, and others, including 5-fluorouracil, hydroxyurea, procarbazine, and vinblastine, produce an additive toxic effect with irradiation.

3.5   **The answer is d.** Esophageal fistula, stricture, hemorrhage, radiation pneumonitis, and pericarditis are all possible complications of radiotherapy for esophageal cancer. Side effects to be expected are swallowing difficulties, including burning, pain, dryness, and skin reactions.

3.6   **The answer is b.** Because carcinoma of the thyroid can rapidly invade surrounding structures, symptoms may occur that are related to compressive effects of the enlarging mass on adjacent structures. Patients may experience dyspnea or stridor when the trachea is compressed or infiltrated. Compression of the esophagus may cause dysphagia. Hoarseness can result from malignant infiltration or destruction of the laryngeal or vagus nerves.

3.7   **The answer is b.** Dysphagia and weight loss are classic symptoms of esophageal carcinoma.

3.8   **The answer is a.** Scopolamine is used to manage excessive salivation and respiratory tract secretions.

3.9   **The answer is c.** Liquids are the most difficult to manage and are tried last. Semisolids stay together as a bolus and are easier to swallow. These patients do not have a feeding tube, so they must begin a swallowing program as soon as their nasogastric tube is removed.

3.10   **The answer is d.** Cytokines have been proposed as one class of circulating anorectic agents. There is also support for an effect of serotonin and bombesin on appetite suppression, especially among individuals with carcinoid or lung cancers.

3.11   **The answer is a.** Megestrol acetate has been found to improve appetite, cause weight gain, control nausea, and improve quality of life among individuals with cancer. Dosages range from 160 to 800 mg/day.

3.12   **The answer is c.** Anorexia may occur among individuals receiving radiotherapy; regardless of the treatment site. Anorexia is probably related to the presence in the patient's system of the waste products of tissue destruction.

3.13   **The answer is d.** Anorexia or declining food intake implies alterations in food perception, taste, and smell that result from the effects of chemotherapy. Abnormalities of carbohydrate, protein, and fat metabolism are central features of anorexia. Visceral and lean body mass depletion are common, along with muscle atrophy, visceral organ atrophy, and hypoalbuminemia.

3.14   **The answer is a.** Anorexia can lead to compromised immune status as manifested by decreased macrophage mobilization, depressed lymphocyte function, and impaired phagocytosis. Hypoalbuminemia occurs, but it is not as accurate an indicator of immune status.

3.15   **The answer is d.** A loss of more than 10% of body weight within the previous 6 months or an unintentional weight loss of more than 1 kilogram per week is considered a significant risk factor. A macrobiotic diet places the patient at risk for protein malnutrition.

3.16   **The answer is a.** Although all the other answers are appropriate, anorexia and cancer cachexia are common manifestations of lung cancer, other factors are contributory.

3.17   **The answer is a.** Enteral and parenteral nutrition can lead to congestive heart failure, increased tracheal and bronchial secretions, painful edema, diarrhea, and ultimately a worse quality of life and death.

3.18   **The answer is d.** Megestrol acetate increases appetite and lean body mass and decreases the breakdown of fat reserves. Steroids, hydrazine sulfate, and dronabinol may affect appetite, but rarely result in weight gain, and are associated with significant side effects.

3.19   **The answer is c.** Anorexia-cachexia does not result from the nutritional demands of the malignancy or reduced food intake, but from multiple metabolic and physiologic abnormalities.

3.20   **The answer is a.** Mucositis is observed more often with 5-FU when combined with other mucositis-producing drugs such as methotrexate and doxorubicin and when 5-FU is given concurrently with leucovorin to augment its cytotoxicity.

3.21   **The answer is d.** Management of stomatitis in the cancer patient includes all these choices.

3.22   **The answer is d.** All three choices are risk factors that contribute to stomatitis in the cancer patient.

3.23   **The answer is c.** Gentle, frequent mouth care with soothing solutions can be helpful. Care should be taken, however, not to dislodge the plaque-like formations of mucositis and cause bleeding.

3.24   **The answer is d.** Areas of the oral cavity adjacent to metal tooth fillings are at greater risk for increased reaction due to radiation scatter from the metal fillings. Mucositis will be enhanced and prolonged in patients who have preexisting poor oral or dental hygiene, continue to smoke, use chewing tobacco, consume alcohol, and have poorly fitting dentures.

3.25   **The answer is b.** The dose-limiting side effect for 5-FU when given as an IV bolus is myelosuppression, but when the drug is given by continuous IV infusion the dose-limiting side effect is mucositis.

3.26   **The answer is c.** The incidence of oral herpes simplex virus infection in cancer patients receiving chemotherapy is approximately 50%. In the bone marrow transplantation population, the incidence approaches 90%.

3.27   **The answer is d.** Hydrogen peroxide solutions are highly effective at removing mucosal debris, but they are not recommended for long-term use because of their destructive effects on new granulation tissue and the risk of tooth decalcification with chronic exposure and the overgrowth of the white papillae of the tongue, which is an excellent growth medium for fungus.

3.28   **The answer is c.** Because the incision in surgery for a pituitary adenoma is located in the upper gingiva, oral inspection and meticulous mouth care are instituted to maintain integrity of the mucous membranes and to prevent infection. In addition, sneezing and nose-blowing are contraindicated during this period to minimize pressure on the operative site.

3.29   **The answer is d.** Gingival hypertrophy is the result of infiltration of the gums by leukemic cells. Chemotherapy will treat the underlying cause. The other measures may reduce infection and add to comfort.

3.30   **The answer is a.** Xerostomia is a transient dysfunction of the salivary gland that occurs following chemotherapy. It is a decrease in the quality and quantity of saliva.

3.31   **The answer is c.** Oral care before meals helps to freshen the mouth and stimulate appetite. Increasing fluid intake during meals and snacks helps to lubricate food and ease swallowing. Vegetable or corn oil swished in the mouth may be a cost-effective alternative for artificial lubrication. Lemon glycerin is contraindicated as a mouthwash because it dries and irritates the mucosa and can decalcify the teeth.

3.32   **The answer is b.** Specific agents for dissolving and breaking up thick saliva include papain (found in papaya) and amylase (found in pineapple). Sialogogues stimulate the secretion of endogenous saliva and include gustatory stimulants such as sugar-free lemon candy and masticatory stimulants such as sugar-free gum. Pilocarpine to increase saliva should be used with caution for those with cardiovascular disease.

3.33   **The answer is a.** Mucositis is an inflammatory response of the oral mucosa to radiation therapy. The oral cavity appears inflamed, and white patchy areas may be seen. The patient complains of a sore throat and mouth. Xerostomia is a drying of the oral mucosa that results from loss of saliva due to damage that occurs to the salivary glands subsequent to radiation therapy to the head and neck; it manifests in a thicker saliva. Trismus or jaw hypomobility may occur if the posterior mandible is included in the irradiated field.

3.34   **The answer is a.** Although some salivary function may return following the cessation of treatment, the patient should understand that salivary function will never reach the preradiated level.

3.35   **The answer is b.** Oral pilocarpine has been approved for use as a stimulant to the exocrine glands. This results in diaphoresis, salivation, lacrimation, and gastric and pancreatic secretion. Symptomatic improvements of xerostomia are found in 87% of users.

3.36   **The answer is d.** Radiotherapy to the head and neck region destroys taste buds and cells responsible of saliva secretion, resulting in xerostomia. A person who is experiencing this effect produces little saliva, and the saliva that is produced is viscid, acidic, and high in organic content. Affected individuals often complain of decreased taste perception and difficult mastication.

3.37   **The answer is d.** Unlike mucositis, which is reversible, xerostomia is often a permanent oral complication.

3.38   **The answer is b.** Saliva provides lubrication for oral tissues and protection from bacterial infections. Saliva also inhibits enamel decalcification and provides an important excretory route for blood-borne urea, uric acid, and ammonia.

3.39   **The answer is d.** Cisplatin causes delayed nausea, and a serotonin antagonist plus a steroid is the most effective treatment.

3.40   **The answer is a.** Side effects of ^{131}I include nausea and vomiting, fatigue, headache, bone marrow suppression, salivary gland inflammation, and infrequently leukemia and radiation-induced pulmonary fibrosis.

3.41   **The answer is d.** Nausea and vomiting have been effectively treated with stress-reduction and distraction methods, exercise, and oral ginger.

3.42   **The answer is d.** Although cisplatin is most commonly associated with delayed nausea, doxorubicin, cyclophosphamide, and ifosfamide can also delay nausea.

3.43   **The answer is c.** Anticipatory nausea and vomiting occur in 25% of patients as a result of classic operant conditioning from stimuli associated with chemotherapy.

3.44   **The answer is c.** Drug sequencing does not predict the degree and severity of nausea and vomiting. Characteristics that affect the occurrence of nausea and vomiting include susceptibility to motion sickness, poor previous emetic control, and being young.

3.45   **The answer is a.**

3.46   **The answer is d.** The combination of the serotonin antagonist ondansetron and dexamethasone has been found to be more efficacious than ondansetron alone.

3.47   **The answer is d.** Nausea and vomiting following chemotherapy and TBI is a consistent problem. Protracted nausea and vomiting also may be caused by GVHD, CMV esophagitis, or gastrointestinal infections.

3.48   **The answer is b.** In the earlier days of transplant, total-body irradiation was delivered in a single dose, which often resulted in lethal organ toxicity. The current standard is for several days of fractionated dosing to provide maximum effect with minimal toxicity.

3.49   **The answer is a.** Nausea, due to DMSO, is often acute but brief. The patient also experiences nausea and vomiting, chilling, cramping, and a bad taste from DMSO. Cough, dyspnea, chest tightness, decreased or increased blood pressure, and tachypnea may indicate pulmonary emboli or pulmonary overload. High fever is not usually reported.

3.50   **The answer is c.** Vomiting as a sign of increased ICP may be preceded by nausea, or it may be sudden, unexpected, and projectile. It is not related to food ingestion. Paclitaxel and carboplatin are not usually associated with the sudden onset of nausea and vomiting, especially when it has not been a problem before. Dexamethasone is an appropriate choice for either problem, but the patient's symptoms can progress quickly and he needs to be evaluated.

3.51   **The answer is c.** Younger patients are more sensitive to the extrapyramidal effects of the prochlorperizine, but this does not mean they are allergic to it. The combination of diphenhydramine and prochlorperazine can prevent EPS and dystonia.

3.52   **The answer is c.** Chemotherapy does interfere with specific metabolic and enzymatic reactions, as well as causing excitation of the true vomiting center, alteration of intestinal absorptive surface, and, indirectly, food aversions.

3.53   **The answer is d.** Terms commonly used to describe conditions that result from cancer or its treatment include hypogeusia (decreased taste sensitivity), dysgeusia (perverted taste perception), odynophagia or dysphagia (painful swallowing), and hyposmia (diminished ability to smell).

3.54   **The answer is c.** Altered taste and smell sensors, with loss of taste and olfactory cues, change the normal references that are part of appetite and intake. Changes may be caused by direct tumor invasion; cancer-induced deficiencies in zinc, copper, nickel, vitamin A, and niacin, or cancer-associated circulating factors.

3.55   **The answer is a.** Physiological increases in the recognition thresholds for sweet, sour, and salt and decreases in the recognition levels for bitter are common. These threshold changes can lead to meat and other food aversions.

3.56   **The answer is d.** Alterations in taste are reported during the second week of treatment. Doses in the 50–65 Gy range cause maximum taste loss. The most severely affected taste qualities are salt and bitter. Sweet taste is generally least affected.

3.57   **The answer is c.** Choices **a**, **b**, and **d**, along with excessive lacrimation and swelling of the cheeks or orbit, are all clinical manifestations of carcinoma of the nasal cavity and paranasal sinus.

3.58   **The answer is b.** Normal eating is possible after use of a nasogastric tube for nutrition in the immediate postoperative period. Speech is affected by the excision of the vocal cords—esophageal speech or use of a handheld artificial larynx is necessary. Hyposomia and decreased taste acuity are also noted postlaryngectomy.

3.59   **The answer is b.** A common complaint during intravenous administration of drugs such as nitrogen mustard, cisplatin, and cyclophosphamide is that they cause a metallic taste. Some individuals become so sensitized to this taste that they become nauseated in anticipation of their administration.

3.60   **The answer is d.** Although the exact mechanisms responsible for taste changes in individuals with cancer are unknown, it appears that nutritional deficiencies, among them deficiencies of vitamin A, zinc, copper, nickel, and niacin, may play a role.

3.61   **The answer is a.** Alternative and complementary therapies are gaining in popularity. Nurses and doctors need to teach patients about the harmful aspects of vitamin overdosing and the importance of moderation, given that patients will pursue alternative approaches.

3.62   **The answer is b.** Cisplatin frequently causes hypomagnesemia, which manifests as shaking. Daily magnesium supplementation is indicated during cisplatin therapy, and electrolyte levels should be monitored frequently.

3.63   **The answer is d.** Although properly constructed diets are adequate, many practitioners do not provide balanced diets. Potential hazards of macrobiotic diets include protein, calorie, iron, vitamin D, and vitamin B_{12} deficiencies. Colitis is more common with a metabolic diet.

3.64   **The answer is d.** Although the scientific information is far from complete, in general most clinicians agree that megadose vitamins are harmful because they can cause cardiac abnormalities and especially liver damage. Kidney stones and coagulation abnormalities are common with high doses of vitamins.

3.65   **The answer is d.** Aside from its usefulness as a diagnostic tool, fluid removal by paracentesis alone is of little therapeutic value. It is usually reserved until a large volume of fluid has accumulated and the patient is profoundly symptomatic because the fluid accumulates rapidly.

3.66   **The answer is b.** Platinum-based chemotherapy can cause a specific nutritional deficiency, resulting in hypomagnesemia. The deficiency is highly specific to the particular drug.

3.67   **The answer is d.** Hyperuricemia involves a release of uric acid in the plasma during the process of tumor lysis. Urate crystals may be deposited in the kidney, causing damage and perhaps renal failure.

3.68   **The answer is a.** Midarm muscle circumference (arm circumference minus triceps skinfold) is felt to be an accurate indicator of protein status that correlates with serum albumin levels when done correctly by a trained individual. It is estimated that the measurement of midarm muscle circumference in the same person can vary by as much as 5% when calculated by different individuals.

3.69   **The answer is d.** Because all muscle produces creatinine, the proportion of creatinine produced is directly proportional to the amount of muscle in the body. In individuals with cancer and in other malnourished individuals creatinine excretion is decreased as muscle protein is degraded for use as energy.

3.70   **The answer is d.** Surgery can increase energy requirements by 1.5 times the normal dietary requirements. Betty can be somewhat reassured that her cancer is not in the aerodigestive or gastrointestinal tract because she is likely to have nutritional problems resulting from the surgery only in the immediate perioperative period.

3.71   **The answer is a.** A classic triad is apparent with cancer of the head of the pancreas: progressive jaundice, profound weight loss, and pain. Jaundice, which is precipitated by common bile duct obstruction, is the presenting symptom in 80% of all cases of cancer of the head of the pancreas, and is the symptom that inevitably leads individuals to seek medical attention.

3.72   **The answer is b.** The majority of women who receive adjuvant chemotherapy for breast cancer gain weight. There is no evidence to support the idea that women with breast cancer who do not receive chemotherapy will lose weight, and there is some evidence to indicate that women who are obese may have a poorer survival rate than women who are not.

3.73   **The answer is c.** The skinfold measure, if taken in all seven sites, can produce a fairly accurate measure of body composition. However, if fewer than five of the sites are measured, the accuracy is lowered.

3.74   **The answer is c.** The percentage of Charles's weight change can be determined by subtracting his actual weight from his usual weight and dividing the result by the usual weight. This number is multiplied by 100 to get the actual percentage.

3.75   **The answer is d.** Because Charles's eating habits have changed considerably and because he is not going to be staying in the hospital for most of his treatment, both the calorie count method and the 24-hour recall method are inappropriate. Food frequency reporting is not ideal because Charles has a hard time remembering what he ate. A diet diary would provide an extended record of Charles's eating habits that would rely on his cooperation and honesty—both of which you feel you can count on.

3.76   **The answer is b.** Hemorrhage, hypovolemia, and hypotension pose the greatest threats to the individual who has just undergone surgery for cancer of the pancreas. As soon as possible after pancreatectomy, small feedings will be started with a diet that is usually bland, low in fat, and high in carbohydrates and protein. Restrictions include caffeine, alcohol, and overindulgence. The stool should be examined daily for the characteristic signs of steatorrhea: frothy, foul-smelling stool with fat particles floating in the water.

3.77   **The answer is b.** From 40 to 70% of women with breast cancer who receive adjuvant chemotherapy gain weight and some become obese.

3.78   **The answer is b.** Corticosteroids are not indicated in William's case because he is a diabetic, and both metoclopramide and THC are indicated for patients experiencing chemotherapy-induced nausea—which William is *not* experiencing. Even though diabetics taking megestrol acetate must monitor themselves closely, the drug is indicated in this case because it increases appetite, causes weight gain, and improves quality of life.

3.79   **The answer is d.** Treatment-induced nutritional problems are often successfully handled by medication and self-care actions. Cancer-associated nutritional problems are best resolved by successful treatment of the malignancy.

3.80   **The answer is a.** Early nutritional intervention, while the tumor burden is still small, has the best chance to alter patient outcomes.

3.81   **The answer is b.** Cancer-induced sepsis initiates an increase of energy needs, which may or may not bring about an increase of appetite, but which would *not* contribute to loss of appetite. All of the rest of these factors—bombesin, cytokines, and psychological distress—could produce a loss of appetite.

3.82   **The answer is a.** Charles is suffering from primary cachexia. Secondary cachexia is caused by mechanical effects of the tumor or treatment—unlikely in David's case because he is suffering from lung cancer. Simple starvation and marasmus are not indicated when hepatic glucose production is at normal levels.

3.83   **The answer is c.** In cachexia, body fat can drop as much as 85% and skeletal muscle can drop as much as 75%.

3.84   **The answer is c.** The endocrine PNSs are the most frequently occurring PNSs and the most well-defined in terms of their etiology.

3.85   **The answer is c.** Inanition is progressive deterioration with muscle wasting and energy loss. Cachexia is a general term meaning ill health. It can occur in nonneoplastic diseases but is characterized by anorexia, weight loss, skeletal muscle atrophy, and asthenia.

3.86   **The answer is a.** Cancer cachexia is characterized by anorexia, weight loss, skeletal muscle atrophy, and asthenia (loss of strength). Marasmus is simple starvation with protein-calorie malnutrition.

3.87   **The answer is a.** Malignant peritoneal effusion (ascites) is most common in patients with ovarian cancer. Ascites is found at presentation in 33% of these patients, and over 60% will develop ascites at some time before death.

3.88   **The answer is d.** Ascites can become severe in advanced disease. Palliative measures to control ascites include fluid and sodium restriction, diuretic therapy, paracentesis, and albumin administation.

3.89   **The answer is b.** See answer to 3.87.

3.90   **The answer is c.** Over 60% of women will develop ascites at some time before death. The appearance of ascites in patients with advanced disease is prognostically grim, and palliation is usually all that can be offered. Life expectancy is a few months.

3.91   **The answer is d.** The most common cause of ascitic fluid buildup is tumor seeding the peritoneum, resulting in obstruction of the diaphragmatic and/or abdominal lymphatics. Excess intraperitoneal fluid production may also be a factor contributing to ascites.

3.92   **The answer is c.** A side effect of docetaxel is fluid retention. The incidence is related to the cumulative dose, which can be disabling and worsens with higher doses. Fluid retention is exhibited peripherally as abdominal ascites, as a pleural effusion, or as a combination.

3.93   **The answer is c.** The clinical test for ascites is to assess for shifting dullness to ascertain the presence of fluid.

3.94   **The answer is d.** The most common cause of ascitic fluid buildup is tumor seeding of the peritoneum, resulting in obstruction of the diaphragmatic and abdominal lymphatics. The tumor itself may elaborate humoral factors that cause increased capillary leakage of proteins and fluids into the peritoneum.

3.95   **The answer is c.** Removal of 2–3 liters of fluid and repeated paracentesis taps can lead to severe protein depletion, postural hypotension, and electrolyte abnormalities. Although sclerosing therapy is effective in treating pleural effusions, it is less successful with ascites.

3.96   **The answer is d.** After radical prostatectomy, 92% of patients achieve urinary control, 8% experience stress incontinence, and 6% wear one or fewer incontinence pads per day. Approximately 1% of men are incontinent after a TURP.

3.97   **The answer is a.** Radiation therapy side effects include impotence, urinary incontinence, bone marrow depression, lower extremity edema, cystitis, urethral strictures, diarrhea, proctitis, and rectal bleeding. Diarrhea can be problematic, as a part of the colon and rectum lie within the pelvic field.

3.98 **The answer is a.** Out-patient photodynamic therapy, laser therapy, can be done while the patient is under local anesthesia through a small cystoscope, without causing bleeding or the stimulation of the obturator nerve. An indwelling catheter is not necessary following the procedure.

3.99 **The answer is d.** Late complications usually involve problems with continence or catheterization, such as urinary leakage at the stoma or through the urethra, difficult catheterization, electrolyte abnormalities, pyelonephritis, hydronephrosis, and stone formation. The idea with the continent urinary diversions is that there would be less infection.

3.100 **The answer is d.** The normal prostate on palpation is usually a rounded structure about 4 cm in diameter that feels firm. Cancer of the prostate typically appears as a stony, hard nodule, whereas benign hypertrophy usually results in a diffuse enlargement of the prostate without masses.

3.101 **The answer is c.** After radical prostatectomy, 92% of patients achieve urinary control, 8% experience stress incontinence, and 6% wear one or fewer incontinence pads per day. Approximately 1% of men are incontinent after a TURP.

3.102 **The answer is d.** Sphincter incompetence presents as dribbling and stress incontinence. Treatment includes alpha-adrenergic agonist drugs and surgery. The drugs increase sphincter resistance. The goal of surgery is urethral compression.

3.103 **The answer is d.** If a bowel movement does not occur every other day, a laxative must be taken. His risk factors are high for constipation and it should be stressed to the patient never to wait more than three days without a bowel movement before calling the physician.

3.104 **The answer is d.** Vincristine, vinblastine, and vinorelbine are the most common chemotherapy agents to cause constipation.

3.105 **The answer is c.** Rectal emptying is specifically diminished because nonfunctional afferent and efferent pathways from the sacral cord are interrupted.

3.106 **The answer is c.** The fact that he is nauseated and not passing gas means he could be obstipated and needs to be evaluated immediately.

3.107 **The answer is d.** Opioids affect the bowel by activation of specific opioid receptors in both the GI tract and the central nervous system. Increased tone and nonpropulsive motility in the ileum and colon results in increased transit time and water absorption. Morphine-induced insensitivity to rectal distention further contributes to constipation.

3.108 **The answer is c.** Bowel effects of the vinca alkaloids may be unaccompanied by peripheral nerve dysfunction.

3.109 **The answer is d.** Vincristine, vinorelbine, and vindesine are all associated with constipation. Etoposide is not predisposed to cause constipation.

3.110 **The answer is a.** Chemotherapy agents cause constipation as a result of autonomic nerve dysfunction manifested as colicky abdominal pain. Rectal emptying is diminished because nonfunctional afferent and efferent pathways from the sacral cord are interrupted.

3.111 **The answer is d.** Combining the softening action with the peristaltic stimulant effect lessens constipation.

3.112 **The answer is a.** Management of severe diarrhea in patients with radiation-induced enteritis include all of these choices *except* a liquid diet high in milk products.

3.113 **The answer is d.** When these cells are destroyed, atrophy of the intestinal mucosa and shortening of the intestinal villa with flattening and reduction of the absorptive surface results in a "slick gut." Thus the intestinal contents move rapidly through the gut, reducing absorption of nutrients.

3.114 **The answer is d.** Patients may experience abdominal cramps and rectal urgency with 5-fluorouracil which can evolve into nocturnal diarrhea or fecal incontinence leading to lethargy, weakness, orthostatic hypotension, and fluid/electrolyte imbalance.

3.115 **The answer is d.** Nocturnal diarrhea or fecal incontinence leads to lethargy, weakness, orthostatic hypotension, and fluid/electrolyte imbalance. Without adequate management, prolonged diarrhea will cause dehydration, nutritional malabsorption, and circulatory collapse.

3.116 **The answer is d.** The leucovorin potentiates the antitumor effect of the 5-fluorouracil but it also increases the diarrhea.

3.117 **The answer is a.** Bleomycin can cause some mucositis, but not like the others which cause mucositis plus potentially severe diarrhea.

3.118 **The answer is d.** Performing a stool culture, giving fluids, monitoring the electrolytes, and reporting results to the physician are all appropriate. Giving antidiarrheal agents to a patient who has recently had antibiotics is not.

3.119 **The answer is d.** Stool cultures need to be obtained initially to rule out an infectious process so appropriate antibiotics can be implemented. *Clostridium difficile* has been reported in patients receiving chemotherapy who have had prior antibiotic exposure.

3.120 **The answer is b.** The most common injury to the large bowel that occurs after radiotherapy is proctosigmoiditis. Another commonly encountered side effect is increased bowel motility, which creates abdominal cramping and loose, watery stools.

3.121 **The answer is b.** After allogeneic BMT, diarrhea is a prominent manifestation of intestinal involvement with GVHD.

3.122 **The answer is b.** Cancers of the sigmoid colon are most often manifested by abdominal pain and melena. The manifestations in choice **a** are those of a tumor of the right colon; manifestations in choices **c** and **d** are those of rectal cancer.

3.123 **The answer is a.** Because the transverse colon is the most anterior and movable part of the colon, tumors here are more accessible to detection by palpation. Other possible symptoms that might have been determined by inspection, auscultation, palpation, and percussion of the abdomen include distention of the abdomen, enlarged and visible abdominal veins, occult blood in the stool, and enlarged lymph nodes or organs (especially the liver). Diagnostic examination by fiberoptic colonoscopy confirms the presence of the tumor. Anemia is more likely to occur with cancer of the right colon. Polyps in the rectum may be present and may indicate the patient was at high risk for colorectal cancer. CEA, although useful in evaluating the efficacy of treatment, is of limited value in the detection of colon cancer.

3.124 **The answer is c.** On palpation during a rectal exam, the examiner may feel a a stony, hard mass in the cul-de-sac. The shelf indicates a carcinoma that has metastasized to the pelvic floor, initiating obstruction and pain, and therefore is a sign of advanced malignancy.

3.125 **The answer is d.** High-fiber diets are contraindicated in patients whose constipation results from structural blockage of the bowel, because increasing bulky intraluminal contents may increase the obstruction. Do not give GoLYTELY with bowel obstruction because of a high risk of perforation. Soap suds enemas are contraindicated because of the risk of acute colitis.

3.126 **The answer is a.** TPN is appropriate only for short-term nutritional support.

3.127 **The answer is a.** Metoclopramide is particularly useful in hiccups due to gastric stasis or distention and gastroespohageal reflux; however, it is contraindicated in patients with bowel obstruction.

3.128 **The answer is b.** Biliary vomiting is almost odorless and indicates an obstruction in the upper part of the abdomen. The presence of foul-smelling, fecaloid vomiting can be the first sign of an ileal or colonic obstruction.

3.129 **The answer is d.** A gastrostomy tube or a PEG would be chosen over a nasogastric tube, which is uncomfortable. Enemas are contraindicated and lead to cramping pain. Opioids are important, since over 90% of patients have continuous abdominal pain.

3.130 **The answer is d.** A radical cystectomy with urinary diversion, particularly if accompanied by a lymphadenectomy, can affect many aspects of sexual functioning. Erectile impotence that results after radical cystectomy may be helped by the insertion of a penile prosthesis. When the nerves crucial to the mechanisms of penile erection are spared, erectile potency has been preserved.

3.131 **The answer is b.** When a malignant lesion involves the middle and left transverse colon, the standard procedure involves resection of the lesion and a primary anastomosis. The two- and three-step procedures are riskier and less often performed. A right hemicolectomy is performed on the cecum or ascending colon.

3.132 **The answer is a.** For proximal and midrectal adenocarcinomas, the treatment technique of choice is low anterior resection. This preserves external anal sphincter control, thus eliminating the need for a permanent colostomy. Abdominoperineal resection is usually used for poorly differentiated adenocarcinoma and more advanced disease. Laser therapy to the tumor bed through a colonoscope or flexible sigmoidoscope is used for smaller tumors of the colon and rectum, and prophylactic oophorectomy is recommended for only some women diagnosed with adenocarcinoma of the colon and rectum.

3.133 **The answer is b.** Wound dehiscence is not primarily related to cystectomy. Complications are related to stoma construction and placement and to the possibility of long-term kidney damage. Other complications include stomal stenosis.

3.134 **The answer is d.** There are several types of continent urinary diversions. They differ largely in the portion of intestine used to create the pouch.

3.135 **The answer is c.** Continent urinary reservoirs and bladder substitutes produce much mucus. They should be irrigated regularly in the early postoperative period to prevent mucus accumulation. Mucus production will decrease over time, and irrigation will become unnecessary.

3.136 **The answer is c.** A urinary diversion should produce urine from the time of surgery, and flow should be more or less continuous. The stoma should protrude $1/2$–$3/4$ inches above the skin to allow the urine to drain into the aperture of an appliance. Leakage from the appliance is abnormal and could lead to skin breakdown. The stoma itself should be deep pink to dark red in color.

3.137 **The answer is b.** The intestine normally produces mucus, and mucus will almost always be present in diversions using segments of the bowel, causing the urine to appear cloudy. Excessive mucus may clog the urinary appliance outlet, and if this occurs, an appliance with a larger outlet may be used.

3.138 **The answer is c.** Preoperative selection and marking of a stoma site is critical to postoperative management. The stoma site should be located within the borders of the rectus muscle. Bringing the bowel through this muscle sheath prevents later complications of peristomal hernia and prolapse. To determine the ideal location of the stoma, the patient's abdomen is observed in sitting, standing, bending, and lying positions.

3.139 **The answer is c.** An important postoperative nursing function is assessment of stoma viability to identify early signs of compromised circulation to the stoma. A stoma that is dusky, gray, or black indicates an inadequate blood supply and is documented and brought to the surgeons's attention. A stoma with necroses sloughs and generally leads to stomal stenosis. The postoperative occurrences in choices **a**, **b**, and **d** all are normal.

3.140 **The answer is d.** Because APR requires a combined surgical approach through the abdomen and perineum, a major complication of APR is the occurrence of perineal and abdominal wound infections. The type of closure employed—primary closure, partial closure with an incisional drain, or leaving the wound open and packing it—determines the necessary postoperative care and teaching.

3.141 **The answer is d.** Nephrotic syndrome is impaired renal function resulting in massive proteinuria due to obstruction. It is caused by the presence of paraneoplastic lesions in the renal glomerulus and is a secondary benign disorder resulting from a primary glomerular disease.

3.142 **The answer is a.** Signs and symptoms of nephrotic syndrome include massive proteinuria and brown, foamy urine, as well as facial and peripheral edema, which may progress to anasarca or edema of all body tissues. The combined water and electrolyte retention may cause mild to moderate hypertension, not hypotension.

3.143 **The answer is d.** Infection, hypercalcemia, and dehydration are all possible contributing factors to the renal failure associated with multiple myeloma.

3.144 **The answer is c.** Nephritis and cystitis are the major long-term renal toxicities that result from cancer treatment. Damage to the nephrons and bladder has been documented in patients treated with cyclophosphamide, ifosfamide, and cisplatin.

3.145 **The answer is d.** Sitz baths are contraindicated if the perineal area is being irradiated.

3.146 **The answer is d.** Prevention of hemorrhagic cystitis is the key to success including aggressive use of hydration, use of a Foley catheter, and administration of the uroprotectant mesna.

3.147 **The answer is a.** The only risk factor that has been linked persistently to kidney cancer by both cohort studies and epidemiological studies is cigarette smoking. The links to occupational exposures (lead, asbestos) and genetics are less frequent.

3.148 **The answer is a.** The degree and duration of diarrhea depend on the agent, dose, nadir, and frequency of chemotherapy administration. Patients may experience abdominal cramps and rectal urgency with 5FU-leucovorin therapy, which can evolve into nocturnal diarrhea or fecal incontinence, leading to lethargy, weakness, orthostatic hypotension, and fluid/electrolyte imbalance. Without adequate management, prolonged diarrhea causes dehydration, nutritional malabsorption, and circulatory collapse. Renal failure does not result from untreated diarrhea.

STUDY NOTES

STUDY NOTES

C H A P T E R **4**

CARDIOPULMONARY FUNCTION

ALTERATIONS IN VENTILATION

Anatomical or Surgical Alterations

4.1   A patient has recently returned from the operating room with a tracheotomy. He has a high-humidity oxygen collar with orders to suction the trachea every 2 hours as needed. The need for the continuous-high-humidity collar is best explained by which of the following?
   a.   The collar provides necessary oxygen to the lungs.
   b.   The collar provides humidity to the air normally supplied by the nose.
   c.   The collar protects the airway.
   d.   The collar provides humidified air to a permanently altered airway.

4.2   Which of the following is *not* a problem postoperatively for the patient who has had a laryngectomy?
   a.   wound dehiscence
   b.   flap failure
   c.   aspiration
   d.   stomal infection

4.3   The primary purpose of a laryngectomy tube postoperatively is which of the following?
   a.   to prevent tracheal trauma
   b.   to prevent tracheal closure
   c.   to maintain adequate stomal size
   d.   a and c

4.4   Individuals with advanced esophageal cancer are considered at high risk for the development of:
   a.   other gastrointestinal cancers
   b.   superior vena cava syndrome
   c.   aspiration pneumonia
   d.   xerostomia

149

4.5   You are asked to demonstrate proper suctioning of a tracheostomy for a group of student nurses. Points you will be sure to make during the demonstration include:
a.   "Limit suctioning to 10 seconds or less at 120 mm Hg or less."
b.   "Hyperoxygenation is advised before and after suctioning."
c.   "Hyperinflation of the lungs is advised both before and after the procedure to prevent suction-induced hypoxemia and subsequent arrhythmias."
d.   all of the above

4.6   Stan has a well-differentiated tumor on his true vocal folds that seems to be growing fairly slowly. Stan's tumor is most likely to be a _____ tumor.
a.   subglottic
b.   supraglottic
c.   glottic
d.   either a or c

4.7   Most small cell lung cancer tumors:
a.   are not associated with necrosis
b.   are responsible for 55% of all lung cancers
c.   are centrally located, developing around a main bronchus, and eventually compressing the bronchi externally
d.   have a longer doubling time than that of any other lung cancer type

4.8   In the presence of a known bone tumor, symptoms such as hemoptysis, cough, fever, weight loss, and malaise may indicate:
a.   pulmonary metastases
b.   pernicious anemia
c.   radiotherapy toxicity
d.   infection

4.9   After surgery, a patient develops aspiration pneumonia. Which of the following symptoms may have caused this?
a.   difficulty in swallowing
b.   mechanical obstruction from cancer
c.   excessive sedation
d.   all of the above

4.10   Mrs. Alexander has been diagnosed with local-regional lung cancer. You are told she has a central, rather than peripheral, tumor. What kinds of symptoms will Mrs. Alexander be *most likely* to have?
a.   symptoms due to extrathoracic involvement
b.   chest pain
c.   symptoms associated with airway obstruction
d.   weakness, anorexia, and cachexia

Pulmonary Toxicity Related to Cancer Therapy

4.11 Ms. Daniels, who had an allogeneic BMT, develops certain pulmonary complications. You are mindful that, because of prolonged periods of immunosuppression caused by her medication, she is at greater risk for developing:
a. interstitial pneumonia
b. CMV pneumonia
c. idiopathic pneumonia
d. RSV pneumonia

4.12 Davis has received prior irradiation to his chest; therefore, his doctor would be particularly cautious prescribing which of the following?
a. bleomycin
b. cytarabine
c. mitomycin C
d. all of the above

4.13 Your patient with disseminated testicular cancer has just completed bleomycin, etoposide, cisplatin (BEP) treatment and is scheduled for surgery to remove a residual retroperitoneal mass. Which of the following is appropriate to emphasize in your teaching of this patient?
a. Bleomycin-induced pulmonary toxicity is a potential side effect.
b. This treatment is designed to be curative.
c. This treatment is not curative but will significantly increase his survival.
d. a and b

4.14 Which of the following describes the features of chemotherapy-induced pulmonary toxicity?
a. The site of damage is the endothelial cells of the lungs.
b. There is an inflammatory-type reaction.
c. It is a drug-induced pneumonitis.
d. all of the above

4.15 The most sensitive pulmonary function test to detect pulmonary toxicity before the onset of clinical symptoms is:
a. the carbon monoxide diffusion capacity measurement
b. pulmonary blood gases
c. CO_2 binding capacity
d. a chest x-ray

4.16 The best method to establish a histopathological diagnosis of pulmonary toxicity is:
a. a sputum specimen
b. fiberoptic bronchoscopy
c. thoracotomy
d. needle biopsy

4.17 The earliest symptom of pulmonary toxicity is:
a. bilateral basilar rales
b. hypoxia with hypocapnia
c. productive cough
d. hyperthermia

4.18 Risk factors for pneumothorax with placement of a central line in the bone marrow transplant patient includes *all but* which of the following?
 a. high-dose steroids
 b. total body irradiation
 c. recent weight loss
 d. bedrest

4.19 Pulmonary edema due to fluid overload can occur in the first few days following marrow or blood cell transplant. Which of the following factors increases the risk of pulmonary edema in this population?
 a. previous anthracycline therapy
 b. previous cyclophosphamide therapy
 c. total body irradiation (TBI)
 d. all of the above

4.20 The mortality of marrow transplant patients with pneumonitis who require intubation and mechanical ventilation is:
 a. 15%
 b. 30%
 c. 60%
 d. >90%

4.21 Which of the following is the most definitive test for determining total lung functioning in the patient with radiation-induced pulmonary fibrosis?
 a. chest x-ray
 b. CT scan
 c. diffusion capacity
 d. pulmonary function tests

4.22 Which of the following best explains the mechanism for bleomycin-induced pulmonary fibrosis?
 a. pressure necrosis
 b. allergic reaction with scarring
 c. formation of free radicals and lipid peroxidation
 d. damage to type III pneumocytes

Anemia

4.23 You learn that one of the probable causes for Mark's fatigue is bone marrow suppression that is at the level of classic anemia. Mark is receiving transfusions to treat the anemia. Which is *most likely* to occur as a result?
 a. Mark's hemoglobin will improve but his hematocrit will not, resulting in an improvement in the anemic condition but not the fatigue.
 b. Mark's hemoglobin and hematocrit will improve, resulting in an improvement in both the anemic condition and the fatigue.
 c. Mark's hematocrit will improve but his hemoglobin will not, resulting in an improvement in the anemic condition but not the fatigue.
 d. Mark's hematocrit will remain the same and his hemoglobin will improve, resulting in an improvement in both his fatigue and his anemia.

4.24   You have a patient, Karen, who is experiencing some symptoms of anemia and chronic cancer-related fatigue. You ask your colleague, who has studied a great deal of outside information on the topic, what is likely to happen. He tells to you to expect that her anemic symptoms will be treated:
    a.   with similar expected results for both the anemia and the fatigue
    b.   with better expected results for both the anemia and the fatigue
    c.   with worse expected results for both the anemia and the fatigue
    d.   with no expectations

4.25   Your patient suffers from borderline anemia and is about to receive 5-FU and mitomycin for treatment of colon cancer. Your teaching plan is based on which of the following facts regarding anemia?
    a.   It rarely occurs because the bone marrow recovers so quickly.
    b.   It is treated prophylactically with the administration of platelets if their count falls too low.
    c.   It can be treated with erythropoietin injections 1–3 times a week.
    d.   a and c

4.26   Anemia can occur as a remote effect of neoplastic disease. This is caused by:
    a.   tearing of interstitial tissue with subsequent slow but long-term blood loss
    b.   tumor product impairment of bone marrow function
    c.   red cell metabolism
    d.   b and c

4.27   Anemia of chronic disease is characterized by which of the following?
    a.   erythroid hypoplasia of the bone marrow
    b.   increase in reticulocytes
    c.   hyperferremia
    d.   increased serum erythropoietin

4.28   Which of the following chemotherapeutic agents causes anemia by inhibiting the maturation of the erythroid lineage cells in the bone marrow?
    a.   cyclophosphamide
    b.   nitrogen mustard
    c.   cisplatin
    d.   carboplatin

4.29   A 72-year-old patient with lung cancer complains of extreme fatigue. He is not very active, but with a hemoglobin of 7.7 g/100 ml the decision is made to bring him in to the out-patient infusion center to be transfused with 3 units of packed red blood cells. The primary problem associated with a low hemoglobin and the reason to transfuse is which of the following?
    a.   risk for hemorrhage
    b.   risk for angina
    c.   risk for stroke
    d.   risk for hypovolemia

4.30   Your patient complains of extreme fatigue, headache, irritability, and dizziness. You suspect he is suffering from which of the following disorders?
    a.   iron deficiency
    b.   hypercalcemia
    c.   anemia
    d.   low magnesium

4.31   As a treatment for anemia, erythropoietin is meant to do what?
a.   replenish and stimulate iron stores
b.   increase reticulocytosis
c.   increase erythropoiesis
d.   decrease reticulocytosis

4.32   Anemia of chronic illness is associated with which of the following?
a.   erythroid hypoplaisa of the bone marrow
b.   a decrease in reticulocytosis
c.   hypoferremia
d.   all of the above

4.33   Which of the following chemotherapeutic agents is known to cause anemia because of its effect on the erythroid cell line?
a.   cisplatin
b.   mitomycin
c.   nitrogen mustard
d.   cyclophosphamide

Pleural Effusions

4.34   Mr. Allen has lung cancer and complains that he cannot catch his breath. He is scheduled to have a chest x-ray to determine the etiology of his shortness of breath and dyspnea. Which of the following statements would be accurate counsel for this patient?
a.   His symptoms are probably due to the side effects of radiation and chemotherapy.
b.   The chest x-ray will probably show that the tumor has grown, and he should think about palliative care.
c.   Dyspnea in the person with lung cancer is often associated with pleural effusions, all of which are considered to be malignant.
d.   If a pleural effusion is found, it is possible to manage the problem with a procedure called pleurodesis.

4.35   Janis frequently experiences dyspnea due to recurrent pleural effusions. Her doctor has suggested that she have a more permanent device placed into her pleural space to make it easier to drain the fluid from her lung. Which of the following is an accurate description of this device?
a.   A pleuroperitoneal shunt can be inserted to divert fluid from the chest cavity to the abdomen.
b.   A pleural port can be implanted underneath the skin just below the ribs, with the catheter resting in the pleural space. The port is accessed with a 19-gauge Huber point needle whenever she complains of difficulty breathing.
c.   A small-bore catheter may be placed into the pleural space and allowed to drain through a one-way valve by gravity drainage.
d.   all of the above

4.36   Thoracentesis involves fluid removal from:
a.   the pericardial sac
b.   the pleural cavity
c.   the abdominal cavity
d.   the spinal column

4.37   The first and most common means of obliteration of the pleural cavity in a patient with chronic, recurrent malignant pleural effusions is:
   a.   pleuroperitoneal shunt
   b.   pleural stripping
   c.   sclerosis
   d.   local radiation

4.38   Which of the following chemotherapy agents is known to cause fluid retention that may manifest as abdominal ascites, as a pleural effusion, or as a combination?
   a.   mitoxantrone
   b.   megestrol acetate
   c.   docetaxel
   d.   paclitaxel

4.39   Cytarabine and mitomycin C can cause diffuse alveolar damage, resulting in which of the following pulmonary disorders?
   a.   pneumonia
   b.   capillary leak syndrome
   c.   obliteration of alveoli
   d.   pleural effusion

4.40   Mr. Eliot, 64 and a smoker for 47 years, has an undifferentiated neoplasm arising in the proximal right bronchus. On examination of Mr. Eliot, you hear a dullness on percussion. What might this indicate?
   a.   tumor in the main bronchus
   b.   bagpipe sign
   c.   bronchophony
   d.   pleural effusion

4.41   Your patient is immediate post-op following a right hepatectomy. He is most at risk for which of the following non–liver-related complications?
   a.   pneumonia and pleural effusion
   b.   deep-vein thrombosis
   c.   hemorrhage
   d.   subphrenic abscess

4.42   What percentage of pleural effusions are malignant?
   a.   100%
   b.   75%
   c.   50%
   d.   <25%

4.43   Which of the following tumor-related pathologies is *not* known to cause pleural effusion?
   a.   disseminated intravascular coagulopathy
   b.   superior vena cava syndrome (SVCS)
   c.   postobstructive pneumonitis
   d.   pericardial constriction

4.44   Which of the following differentiates a malignant pleural effusion from a nonmalignant pleural effusion?
   a.   Malignant effusions are almost always grossly bloody.
   b.   Malignant effusions are almost always an exudate.
   c.   Nonmalignant effusions are almost always a transudate.
   d.   all of the above

4.45   Which of the following is the most commonly reported symptom of pleural effusion?
   a.   fever
   b.   sharp pleuritic chest pain
   c.   dry irritating cough
   d.   dyspnea

ALTERATIONS IN CIRCULATION

Lymphedema

4.46   Which of the following is *not* considered a risk factor for lymphedema?
   a.   axillary irradiation
   b.   infection
   c.   weight lifting
   d.   breast reconstruction

4.47   Which of the following conditions is benign and iatrogenic in origin and is usually secondary to radical cancer surgery?
   a.   pericardial effusion
   b.   lymphedema
   c.   pleural effusion
   d.   anasarca

4.48   Although the incidence of lymphedema has decreased because breast surgeries have become less radical, the percentage of women who experience lymphedema following a modified radical mastectomy is approximately:
   a.   2–5%
   b.   5–10%
   c.   10–12%
   d.   12–15%

4.49   A woman who is about to have a modified radical mastectomy for diffuse multicentric breast cancer states, "Having a lymph node dissection is all right with me. I want all the cancer cells taken out if they are there." The most appropriate nursing response would be:
   a.   The axillary dissection could cause lymphedema depending on the number of nodes removed.
   b.   The purpose of the lymph node dissection is staging; it is not a therapeutic procedure.
   c.   Because her disease is all over the breast, it is a good idea that she is having a more extensive dissection under her arm.
   d.   If any nodes are left behind, radiation can always be used.

4.50   A woman is more at risk for lymphedema if she has which of the following risk factors?
    a.   obesity
    b.   inflammation or infection
    c.   radiation therapy
    d.   all of the above

4.51   A woman with a history of modified radical mastectomy with axillary dissection and radiation therapy completed chemotherapy 6 months ago and calls concerned about slight swelling and redness in her affected arm. On questioning her, you learn that she has recently been to Europe. What is the appropriate nursing action and why?
    a.   She should keep the arm elevated. Slight swelling is common following exposure to compression changes in an airplane. Wear a sleeve.
    b.   The swelling is probably due to the flight and the fact that she probably carried a suitcase. The redness is a problem. She should be on antibiotics, so she should see her doctor as soon as possible.
    c.   Keep the arm elevated. If it is not better in a week, call back.
    d.   She needs a diuretic and an antibiotic, so she should see her doctor.

4.52   The physiological reason for lymphedema is best explained by which of the following?
    a.   An increased resistance to venous flow occurs.
    b.   A disturbance in oncotic pressure occurs because of protein accumulation.
    c.   Lymphatic obstruction causes backflow of fluid.
    d.   a and b

4.53   The mainstay of symptomatic lymphedema treatment is:
    a.   redirection of fluid
    b.   manual lymphatic drainage (MLD)
    c.   stimulation of the dermal lymphatomes
    d.   all of the above

4.54   Complex decongestive physiotherapy for the management of lymphedema involves all but which of the following?
    a.   deep massage
    b.   compression garments
    c.   exercises
    d.   bandaging

4.55   The overall incidence of lymphedema in breast cancer is:
    a.   <10%
    b.   20%
    c.   30%
    d.   50%

Cardiovascular Toxicity Related to Cancer Therapy

4.56   In tissues that are relatively radioresistant, such as the liver or heart, high doses of radiation are most likely to damage:
    a.   parenchyma
    b.   vascular tissue
    c.   mucous membranes
    d.   rapidly dividing cells

4.57   Althea has received both extensive mediastinal radiation and chemotherapy. Toxic effects to monitor for include:
        a.   pericarditis and hemodynamic compromise
        b.   chest pain, edema, and cardiac tamponade
        c.   coronary artery disease and cardiomyopathy
        d.   all of the above

4.58   Chronic cardiotoxic effects can occur months after treatment with certain chemotherapeutic agents. Patients are routinely monitored for:
        a.   nonproductive cough, dyspnea, pedal edema
        b.   biventricular CHF
        c.   low-voltage QRS complex
        d.   all of the above

4.59   An individual is admitted with congestive heart failure. Medical records indicate a history of acute leukemia, which was treated 10 years ago with anthracyclines. The most likely late effect of this treatment is:
        a.   angina
        b.   pulmonary fibrosis
        c.   pericarditis
        d.   cardiomyopathy

4.60   Cardiotoxicity associated with doxorubicin can be minimized by the administration of which of the following cardioproctective agents?
        a.   calcium gluconate
        b.   digitalis
        c.   amifostine
        d.   dexrazoxane (Zinecard)

4.61   Which of the following is considered to be a significant risk factor for cardiotoxicity?
        a.   an ejection fraction of 45% or less at rest
        b.   anthracycline cumulative dose of 300 mg/m^2
        c.   combination of doxorubicin and paclitaxel chemotherapy
        d.   total body irradiation

4.62   Which of the following is not considered to be a significant risk factor for cardiac tamponade:
        a.   lung cancer
        b.   radiation to the pericardium
        c.   pericardial fluid accumulation of 300 cc
        d.   increased catecholamine production

4.63   In a blood cell transplant patient who receives cyclophosphamide, the most critical risk factor for cardiac toxicity is:
        a.   dose
        b.   prior anthracycline therapy
        c.   bolus versus continuous infusion
        d.   mediastinal radiation

4.64 Delayed radiation injury to the heart can manifest as which of the following?
a. pericardial disease
b. myocardial disease
c. coronary heart disease
d. all of the above

4.65 The mechanism of cardiac damage following anthracycline therapy includes *all but* which of the following?
a. overexpression of genes encoding for cardiac muscle protein
b. binding to membranes rich in cardiolipin
c. formation of free radicals
d. inhibited expression of genes encoding for cardiac muscle protein

4.66 The mechanism of cardiac damage from radiation therapy primarily involves which of the following?
a. microvascular thrombosis
b. rupture of the endothelial cells
c. swelling of the cells of the myocardial capillaries
d. all of the above

Fluid and Electrolyte Imbalances

4.67 What side effects may a patient experience as a direct result of pheresis?
a. Fever—especially localized fever—from rapid movement and return of large volumes of blood to the body
b. Hypercalcemia from high volumes of IV calcium gluconate
c. Hypovolemia, especially for patients with a history of cardiac problems
d. a and c

4.68 A patient receiving mitomycin and 5-FU develops a 15-lb weight gain, decreased hemoglobin, thrombocytopenia, ascites, encephalopathy, and elevated bilirubin and SGOT lab values. You recognize these as classic symptoms of:
a. liver failure
b. severe dehydration
c. veno-occlusive disease
d. intractable ascites

4.69 Control of extracellular calcium levels within a narrow range is achieved through the action of several agents, including all of the following *except:*
a. parathyroid hormone (PTH), which controls renal regulation of calcium
b. 1,25-dihydroxyvitamin D, which controls intestinal calcium absorption
c. calcitonin
d. glucocorticoids, which control osteoclast activity

4.70 How does the body typically respond to elevated levels of extracellular calcium?
a. by reducing PTH secretion
b. by increasing bone resorption
c. by increasing renal synthesis of 1,25-dihydroxyvitamin D
d. by decreasing urinary calcium excretion

4.71   The location and frequency of bone remodeling activity is controlled by several factors, including all of the following *except:*
a.   local factors such as prostaglandins, regulatory proteins, and constituents of the organic matrix
b.   mechanical factors such as weight bearing
c.   skeletal calcium, which couples bone resorption and bone formation
d.   osteotropic hormones, especially PTH and 1,25-dihydroxyvitamin D

4.72   Third spacing is:
a.   the normal fluid distribution in the extracellular and intravascular compartments
b.   an excess of interstitial fluid accumulation
c.   fluid retention in sites that normally have very little or no fluid
d.   lack of normal osmotic pressures

4.73   Choose the statement that most accurately describes the degree of subjective symptoms produced by malignant pericardial and pleural effusions.
a.   Symptoms tend to be related more to the rate of fluid accumulation than to the volume collected.
b.   Symptoms tend to be related more to the volume of fluid collected than to the rate of the collection.
c.   Symptoms are related more to the underlying disease and length of time the patient has been diagnosed with cancer.
d.   Symptoms correspond directly to whether the metastatic disease is from microscopic seeding of the cavities or from local extension.

4.74   Acute renal failure secondary to tumor lysis syndrome (TLS) is primarily due to:
a.   hyperuricemia and hyperkalemia
b.   hyperkalemia and hyperphosphatemia
c.   hyperuricemia and hyperphosphatemia
d.   hyperuricemia and hypokalemia

4.75   The cardiac conduction abnormalities related to tumor lysis syndrome (TLS) are due to:
a.   intracellular hypokalemia
b.   extracellular hyperkalemia
c.   intracelular hypercalcemia
d.   extracellular hypercalcemia

4.76   In a patient whose calcium is 11.8 mg/dl and serum albumin is 2.5 g/dl, a formula is needed to determine the total serum calcium. Why is this formula necessary?
a.   When a patient has less serum albumin to bind with calcium, a greater portion of the total serum calcium must be ionized.
b.   Ionized calcium and calcium bound to albumin are inversely related.
c.   Albumin binds calcium, precipitating hypocalcemia.
d.   Low albumin levels drive calcium to abnormally high levels.

Thrombotic Events

4.77 Vaginal cancer is generally treated with surgery and radiation. Complications following treatment include *all but* which of the following?
   a. venous thrombosis and vaginal engorgement
   b. vaginal fibrosis and scarring
   c. constriction in blood supply
   d. loss of vaginal elasticity

4.78 Mr. Archer has had an implanted port for 4 weeks and recently complained of pain in his right neck and shoulder, just above the catheter insertion site. On examination, you notice slight swelling over the neck, face, shoulder, and arm. He also complains that his arm is cold at times and there is some tingling in his arm and shoulder. What is the most appropriate action to take?
   a. These symptoms are normal following port placement and should resolve in 2–3 weeks. Have him return to the clinic in a week if he is not better.
   b. Flush the line with heparin to make sure it is not clotted.
   c. Notify the physician to examine the patient. A venogram will probably demonstrate a venous thrombosis.
   d. Notify the physician to obtain an order for urokinase. The patient probably has a fibrin sheath formation around the tip of the catheter.

4.79 Thromboembolism (TE) is most frequently seen with which of the following?
   a. small cell lung cancer
   b. non–small cell lung cancer
   c. mucin-secreting bladder carcinoma
   d. mucin-secreting adenocarcinoma of the GI tract

4.80 The etiology of thromboembolism is:
   a. the tumor secretion of cytokines, such as interleukin-1 (IL-1), affecting red cell metabolism
   b. the ability of tumor cells to affect systemic activation of coagulation and cause platelet dysfunction
   c. chronic hemorrhage
   d. bone marrow failure

4.81 Tumor cells may remotely precipitate paraneoplastic thromboembolism by:
   a. activation of the coagulation pathway
   b. damage to the endothelial lining of blood vessels
   c. protein-calorie malnutrition
   d. a and b

4.82 The prognosis for a patient with colorectal cancer is probably poorest if which of the following exists?
   a. venous and lymph node invasion
   b. high blood pressure
   c. location of the tumor above the peritoneal reflection
   d. squamous cell involvement

4.83   Mrs. Mura has chronic myeloma and has recently begun to complain of blurred vision, headache, drowsiness, and occasional confusion. These symptoms may be caused by which of the following?
    a. a high concentration of proteins that increases serum viscosity
    b. chronic effects of steroid use
    c. hyperviscosity syndrome
    d. a and c

4.84   On inspection, you note that Ms. Harris exhibits edema and a bluish tint to the face and that her neck veins seem too prominent. What might be causing these symptoms?
    a. blockage of the inferior vena cava
    b. nodular umbilicus
    c. distention
    d. intra-abdominal fluid

4.85   The incidence of thromboembolic disease is estimated to occur in what percentage of patients with cancer?
    a. 1–10%
    b. 10–20%
    c. 20–30%
    d. >30%

4.86   Cancers most likely to be associated with thromboembolism include *all but* which of the following?
    a. lung cancer
    b. colon cancer
    c. pancreatic cancer
    d. melanoma

4.87   Thromboembolic disease that is refractory to anticoagulation therapy is often indicative of underlying cancer.
    a. true
    b. false

4.88   Tissue plasminogen activator (t-PA) is an effective thrombolytic agent in the treatment of catheter-related thrombosis. *All but* which of the following statements regarding this medication are true?
    a. It must be given as a continuous infusion.
    b. There is less likelihood of hemorrhage compared to urokinase.
    c. Clot lysis is faster compared to urokinase.
    d. There is less likelihood of hemorrhage with t-PA.

4.89   The major complication related to thrombocythemia includes which of the following?
    a. bleeding
    b. thrombosis
    c. pulmonary embolism
    d. all of the above

ANSWER EXPLANATIONS

4.1 **The answer is b.** Patients with a tracheotomy have lost the functions of the nose in warming, moistening, and filtering the air when breathing. A tracheotomy is not permanent.

4.2 **The answer is c.** Patients who have a laryngectomy no longer have communication between the mouth and throat so aspiration is not physically possible.

4.3 **The answer is d.** The tube will help prevent trauma to the tracheal mucosa due to suctioning and, most important, will maintain an adequate stoma size. Because the laryngectomy stoma is permanent, the tube may be removed and cleaned without fear of stomal closure.

4.4 **The answer is c.** When an esophageal tumor gets so large that it causes saliva, food, and liquids to spill over into the lungs, affected individuals are at high risk for the development of aspiration pneumonia. Because of this potential, pulmonary hygiene and aspiration precautions should be a focus of nursing care for the person with esophageal cancer.

4.5 **The answer is d.** Some points to remember regarding suctioning a tracheostomy include limiting suctioning to 10 seconds or less at 120 mm Hg or less. Hyperoxygenation and hyperinflation of the lungs are advised both before and after the procedure to prevent suction-induced hypoxemia and subsequent arrhythmias.

4.6 **The answer is c.** The glottic area includes the true vocal folds and the anterior and posterior glottic commissures. Tumors in this area tend to be well-differentiated, grow slowly, and metastasize late. Lesions that lie superior to a horizontal plane passing through the floor of the ventricles and including the epiglottis, aryepiglottic folds, arytenoids, and ventricular bands (false cords) are classified as supraglottic.

4.7 **The answer is c.** Most SCLC tumors are centrally located, developing around a main bronchus as a whitish-gray growth that invades surrounding structures, eventually compressing the bronchi externally. Necrosis is frequently seen, and SCLC is responsible for 25% of all lung cancers, not 55%. Its doubling time is shorter, not longer, than that of any other lung cancer type.

4.8 **The answer is a.** Metastatic spread in bone cancer occurs primarily to the lungs by the hematogenous route. Symptoms of pulmonary metastases include weight loss, malaise, hemoptysis, cough, chest pain, and fever.

4.9 **The answer is d.** Aspiration pneumonia in the surgical oncology patient may be caused by difficulty in swallowing, mechanical obstruction from the cancer, or excessive sedation.

4.10 **The answer is c.** Central tumors are more likely to cause symptoms associated with airway obstruction, such as wheezing, stridor, dyspnea, atelectasis, and pneumonia. Chest pain is associated with peripheral tumors, which cause chest pain in as many as 50% of patients. Weakness, anorexia, and cachexia are systemic symptoms.

4.11 **The answer is b.** CMV pneumonia is the leading cause of infectious pneumonia after BMT. The incidence of CMV pneumonia may be higher in allograft versus autograph recipients, specifically because of prolonged periods of immunosuppression caused by medication.

4.12 **The answer is d.** Agents associated with pulmonary toxicity include, among others, bleomycin, cytarabine, mitomycin C, cyclophosphamide, carmustine, and methotrexate. Prior irradiation to the chest enhances risk for toxicity.

4.13 **The answer is d.** Men who received bleomycin at a cumulative dose of greater than 200 mg/m^2 are at greater risk of pulmonary edema with subsequent respiratory failure. Treatment is curative.

4.14. **The answer is d.** Pulmonary toxicity usually is irreversible and progressive as a result of chemotherapy administration. The initial site of damage seems to be the endothelial cells, with an inflammatory-type reaction resulting in drug-induced pneumonitis.

4.15 **The answer is a.** The most sensitive pulmonary function test is the carbon monoxide diffusion capacity measurement that becomes abnormal before the onset of clinical symptoms.

4.16 **The answer is b.** The best method to establish a histopathological diagnosis is to obtain involved tissues by means of an open-lung biopsy or a fiberoptic bronchoscopy.

4.17 **The answer is a.** Pulmonary toxicity usually presents clinically as dyspnea, unproductive cough, bilateral basilar rales, and tachypnea.

4.18 **The answer is d.** Predisposing factors for pneumothorax include high-dose steroids, total body irradiation, and poor nutrition with recent weight loss.

4.19 **The answer is d.** Pulmonary edema can be seen in the first few days following marrow or blood cell transplant and is the result of fluid overload. Previous exposure to anthracyclines and the use of cyclophosphamide and TBI during conditioning can exacerbate this complication.

4.20 **The answer is d.**

4.21 **The answer is c.** Lung scarring is seen on chest x-ray, CT scan may provide definitive imaging for diagnosis, and pulmonary function tests (PFTs) may suggest reduced tidal volume; however, PFTs do not demonstrate significant changes when small volumes of lung are irradiated. Diffusion capacity may be the best measure of total lung function, because this test is least likely to be affected by compensatory changes in unirradiated portions of the lung.

4.22 **The answer is c.** The mechanisms of bleomycin injury include formation of free radicals and lipid peroxidation of phospholipid membranes. Subsequently, interstitial edema and damage to type 1 pneumocytes occurs.

4.23 **The answer is b.** Mark's hematocrit and hemoglobin values are expected to improve, resulting in an improvement in both the anemic condition and, in a case like this, the fatigue.

4.24 **The answer is d.** Studies focused on reversing severe anemia caused by bone marrow suppression may not generalize to most patients receiving cancer treatments. Karen's much less severe anemia could be caused by many different factors and may be treated in a number of different ways, all of which may or may not improve the condition and her fatigue.

4.25 **The answer is d.** Chemotherapy-induced anemia occurs rarely because the bone marrow begins to recover before the number of circulating RBCs decreases significantly. Erythropoietin can be administered to correct anemia induced by chemotherapy. The most common side effect from the erythropoietin is hypertension, and the prophylactic administration of platelets (if their count falls below 20,000 mm^3) is for potential bleeding—*not* the anemia.

4.26 **The answer is d.** Anemia as a remote effect of neoplastic disease is caused by tumor product impairment of bone marrow function and/or red cell metabolism.

4.27 **The answer is a.** Anemia of chronic disease is associated with erythroid hypoplasia of the bone marrow. This results in a slight decrease in reticulocytosis, hypoferremia, and a decrease in serum erythropoietin.

4.28   **The answer is c.** Cyclophosphamide and nitrogen mustard are alkylators and quite toxic but generally do not cause significant anemia. Carboplatin is platelet sparing.

4.29   **The answer is b.** Anemia manifests as pallor, hypotension, headaches, irritability, and fatigue. Tachycardia and tachypnea may be present due to the hypoxic effects on the heart.

4.30   **The answer is c.** Anemia manifests as pallor, hypotension, headaches, irritability, and fatigue.

4.31   **The answer is c.** Erythropoietin is a growth factor for erythroid progenitor cells that promotes proliferation and maintains their survival.

4.32   **The answer is d.** Anemia of chronic disease is associated with erythroid hypoplasia of the bone marrow. This results in a slight decrease in reticulocytosis, hypoferremia, and a decrease in serum erythropoietin.

4.33   **The answer is a.** Actions of certain chemotherapeutic agents, such as cisplatin, may inhibit the maturation of the erythroid lineage cells in the bone marrow.

4.34   **The answer is d.** Not all pleural effusions are malignant and etiology should be established before palliative treatment is initiated. When pleural effusions reaccumulate, as is often the case, pleurodesis is the recommended therapy.

4.35   **The answer is d.** Pleural fluid removal through an implanted port and interpleural catheter can be performed by the nurse on an outpatient basis. New technology using small-bore needles may permit management of malignant pleural effusions on an outpatient basis. These radiologically placed small-bore catheters are connected to a plastic bag with a one-way valve system for gravity drainage. In cases of recurrent effusion, a pleuroperitoneal shunt can be inserted to divert fluid from the chest cavity to the abdomen.

4.36   **The answer is b.** Relief of pleural effusion symptoms such as dyspnea, cough, and dull, aching chest pain is a short-term treatment goal that is usually achieved when the pleural fluid is mechanically drained. Thoracentesis involves pleural fluid removal by needle aspiration through the chest wall. Fluid tends to reaccumulate when it is not possible to control the underlying cancer. Long-range treatment goals are directed toward the obliteration of the pleural space so that pleural fluid cannot reaccumulate.

4.37   **The answer is c.** Sclerosis with chemical agents is the most common method used to obliterate the pleural space in patients with malignant pleural effusions. Chemical sclerosing does not prolong the patient's life but may enhance quality of life by relieving symptoms and reducing the time a patient spends in the hospital. Shunts and stripping are surgical methods that become options after other approaches have been tried and the pleural effusion remains uncontrolled. Although external beam radiation may be used as local treatment for mediastinal tumors, hemithoracic radiation is not recommended as a first-line management of malignant pleural effusions because of the hazard of pulmonary fibrosis.

4.38   **The answer is c.** A side effect of docetaxel is fluid retention. The incidence is related to the cumulative dose, which can be disabling and worsens with higher doses. Fluid retention is exhibited peripherally as abdominal ascites, as a pleural effusion, or as a combination.

4.39   **The answer is b.** A capillary leak syndrome, involving primarily the lung, occurs 2–21 days after the first dose of cytarabine, resulting in pulmonary edema and respiratory failure. Mitomycin C damage to the lung presents as diffuse alveolar damage with capillary leak and pulmonary edema.

4.40   **The answer is d.** Dullness on percussion indicates either pleural effusion or a consolidated lung. Lung cancer is the most common cause of hemorrhagic pleural effusion in middle-aged and elderly male smokers. Mr. Eliot has smoked since he was 17.

4.41   **The answer is a.** Pleural effusion is common following liver resection and is most often seen after right hepatectomy.

4.42   **The answer is c.**

4.43   **The answer is a.** Tumor-related pathologies that can cause pleural effusion include SVCS, endobronchial obstruction with atelectasis, postobstructive pneumonitis, and pericardial constriction.

4.44   **The answer is d.**

4.45   **The answer is d.** Dyspnea caused by the accumulating effusion is the most commonly reported symptom. Sharp pleuritic chest pain may or may not be accompanied by a pleural rub. Other symptoms include fever; dry, irritating cough; and hypoxia.

4.46   **The answer is d.** The most common causes of chronic or late lymphedema are infection and tumor recurrence or tumor enlargement in the axilla. Heat, strenuous exercise, or lifting objects weighing more than 5–10 pounds contribute to lymphedema.

4.47   **The answer is b.** Lymphedema is a benign, iatrogenic problem caused by radical cancer surgery. Arm lymphedema often developed after the most common treatment for all types of breast cancer in the past: radical mastectomy with axillary node dissection followed by radiation. It now occurs much less frequently. Lymphedema of the leg may develop after groin dissection that is performed for the treatment of metastatic disease from primary tumors. Mechanical interruption (surgical technique) and radiation often produce lymphatic obstruction, the most common cause of lymphedema.

4.48   **The answer is b.**

4.49   **The answer is b.** A lymph node dissection stages disease. It is not a therapeutic procedure.

4.50   **The answer is d.** Factors that contribute to the development of lymphedema are obesity, insufficient muscle contraction, inflammation, trauma, formation of fibrosclerotic tissue within the lymph vessel, and scarring secondary to radiation therapy or infection.

4.51   **The answer is b.**

4.52   **The answer is d.** Lymphatic obstruction is a factor, but it is an anatomic reason for lymphedema, not a physiological one.

4.53   **The answer is d.** The mainstay of symptomatic lymphedema treatment is MLD performed by a physical therapist trained in lymphedema management. It is light stimulation of the dermal lymphatomes and the lymphatic vessels to redirect the protein-rich fluid and is not to be confused with deep massage.

4.54   **The answer is a.** Complex decongestive physiotherapy consists of skin care, manual lymphatic drainage, bandaging, exercises, and wearing a compression garment.

4.55   **The answer is b.** The extent of the surgery including axillary dissection is a primary factor in the occurrence of lymphedema.

4.56   **The answer is b.** Many of the acute reactions to high doses of radiation occur as the result of indirect effects on the stromal components (especially the vasculature) that support the parenchyma of irradiated tissues and organs. This explains the damage that can occur to organs in which parenchymal tissue is relatively radioresistant.

4.57   **The answer is d.** Toxic effects include acute and chronic pericarditis, along with a spectrum of symptoms ranging from cough and chest pain to edema, paradoxical pulse, cardiac tamponade, and hemodynamic compromise. Coronary artery disease and cardiomyopathy are also seen following extensive mediastinal radiation.

4.58   **The answer is d.** Chronic cardiotoxic effects include a nonproductive cough, dyspnea, and pedal edema and involve irreversible cardiomyopathy presenting as a classic biventricular CHF with a characteristic low-voltage QRS complex.

4.59   **The answer is d.** One of the most serious side effects of anthracyclines is cardiac toxicity, which typically presents as cardiomyopathy with clinical signs of congestive heart failure. Recent evidence, however, indicates that structural damage can occur in the absence of clinical signs and that cardiac failure may occur many years after completion of therapy.

4.60   **The answer is d.** Zinecard interferes with the intracellular process responsible for anthracycline-induced cardiomyopathy.

4.61   **The answer is a.** Further doses of chemotherapy are not recommended if the ejection fraction drops to 45% or less at rest or deteriorates more than 5% from baseline.

4.62   **The answer is d.** Catecholamine production results in an increase in heart rate, which is a compensatory mechanism.

4.63   **The answer is a.** The dose of cyclophosphamide is a major factor in the development of cardiac toxicity. The contribution of prior anthracycline therapy or mediastinal radiation therapy is unclear.

4.64   **The answer is d.**

4.65   **The answer is a.** The mechanism of cardiac damage following anthracycline therapy includes inhibited expression of genes encoding for cardiac muscle protein, binding to membranes rich in cardiolipin, and the formation of free radicals.

4.66   **The answer is d.** Cardiac damage following radiation primarily involves the endothelial cells of the myocardial capillaries. The injury causes swelling, microvascular thrombosis, or rupture.

4.67   **The answer is c.** Chilling can occur because of the large volume of blood being returned to the patient. A large volume of the anticoagulant sodium citrate can cause hypocalcemia. IV calcium gluconate may be needed if the hypocalcemia becomes severe. Hypovolemia may be a problem, especially for patients with a history of cardiac problems. Thrombocytopenia is problematic with some types of equipment.

4.68   **The answer is c.** Signs of chemotherapy-induced VOD have been described as (1) unexplained thrombocytopenia refractory to platelets, (2) sudden weight gain, (3) sudden decrease in hemoglobin, (4) increase in liver enzymes, (5) intractable ascites, and (6) encephalopathy.

4.69 **The answer is d.** Glucocorticoids, including prednisone and hydrocortisone, are used to treat hypercalcemia. They are not part of the body's normal homeostatic mechanism that regulates serum calcium. PTH and 1,25-dihydroxyvitamin D exert their effects by controlling movement of calcium across bone, kidney, and small intestine. PTH's action on the kidney occurs through the formulation and action of NcAMP, which acts as a second messenger influencing calcium transport.

4.70 **The answer is a.** The body's homeostatic response to increased calcium loads involves suppression of PTH, which decreases bone resorption and inhibits intestinal calcium absorption. This inhibitory effect occurs as a result of decreased renal synthesis of 1,25-dihydroxyvitamin D and increased urinary calcium excretion. The calcium load is cleared principally by the kidney.

4.71 **The answer is c.** Bone remodeling, the process of bone formation and resorption, involves three types of bone cells: osteoblasts, osteocytes, and osteoclasts. Incitement of bone remodeling is thought to be directed at the osteocyte. Bone remodeling is said to be coupled; bone resorption is coupled with bone formation. Uncoupling refers to the failure of bone formation to follow the resorption process. Bone remodeling activity is influenced by mechanical factors such as weight bearing, by the activity of osteotropic hormones, and by local factors such as prostaglandins, regulatory proteins, and constituents of the organic matrix.

4.72 **The answer is c.** The distribution pattern of body water is termed *fluid spacing. First spacing* describes a normal distribution of fluid in both the extracellular and the intracellular compartments. *Second spacing* refers to an excess accumulation of interstitial fluid (edema), and *third spacing* is fluid retention in sites that normally have no fluid or a minimum of fluid (effusion).

4.73 **The answer is a.** Common presenting signs and symptoms of malignant effusions are distressing to most patients. The degree of subjective symptoms produced by a pleural effusion depends less on the amount of fluid involved than on the rapidity with which it accumulates. If fluid accumulation is gradual, the heart and lungs can accommodate, but rapid accumulation can trigger an oncologic emergency.

4.74 **The answer is c.** Acute renal failure secondary to TLS is primarily due to hyperuricemia and hyperphosphatemia.

4.75 **The answer is b.** When cell lysis occurs, potassium is released from the intracellular compartment to the extracellular compartment and serum potassium levels increase, depressing cardiac function.

4.76 **The answer is a.** Ionized calcium and calcium bound to albumin are in equilibrium. Therefore, when a patient has less serum albumin to bind with calcium, a greater portion of the total serum calcium portion must be ionized. Conversely, when serum albumin is high, less calcium is in the ionized form.

4.77 **The answer is a.** For women receiving radiation therapy to the vagina, vaginal fibrosis and scarring with a loss of blood supply and elasticity is a major adverse effect.

4.78 **The answer is c.** Signs and symptoms of a venous thrombosis are related to impaired blood flow and include: edema of the neck, face, shoulder, or arm; prominent superficial veins; neck pain; tingling of the neck, shoulder, or arm; and skin color or temperature changes. A venogram with contrast media is used to assess for a venous thrombosis.

4.79   **The answer is d.** The type of cancer most often implicated in incidence of TE is mucin-secreting adenocarcinoma of the GI tract. Other malignancies primarily associated with TE include SCLC, NSCLC, and colon and pancreatic cancers. To a lesser extent, TE-associated cancers include breast, prostate, ovarian, and bladder carcinomas.

4.80   **The answer is b.** The etiology of thromboembolism is the ability of tumor cells to affect systemic activation of coagulation and cause platelet dysfunction. Anemia is caused by the other choices given: the tumor secretion of cytokines, such as interleukin-1 (IL-1), affecting red cell metabolism; chronic hemorrhage; and bone marrow failure.

4.81   **The answer is d.** Tumor cells may remotely precipitate paraneoplastic TE by activation of the coagulation pathway, damage to the endothelial lining of blood vessels, or platelet activation. Choice **c**—protein-calorie malnutrition—is involved in the etiology of anemia of malignancy.

4.82   **The answer is a.** Poor prognosis has been associated with obstructing or perforating carcinomas, occurrence in young people, location of the tumor below the peritoneal reflection, lymph node involvement, venous invasion, hepatic metastasis, and invasion of the bowel wall.

4.83   **The answer is d.** The patient's symptoms could be caused by hyperviscosity syndrome, a rare occurrence in myeloma patients caused by a high concentration of proteins that increases the serum viscosity.

4.84   **The answer is a.** Venous distention is caused by blockage of the inferior vena cava, which can occur from spread of cancer. With this condition, there is edema of the eyelids, a bluish face and lips, prominent neck veins, and pitting edema of the arms and large veins over the upper portions of the chest and shoulders.

4.85   **The answer is a.**

4.86   **The answer is d.** Mucin-secreting adenocarcinomas of the gastrointestinal tract are most often associated with a thromboembolism (TE). The malignancies primarily associated with TE include small cell lung cancer; non–small cell lung cancer; and colon and pancreas and, to a lesser extent, breast, prostate, ovarian, and bladder carcinomas.

4.87   **The answer is a.** Several prospective studies have confirmed a relationship between recurrent, episodic idiopathic deep-vein thrombosis and the subsequent development of malignancy.

4.88   **The answer is a.** t-PA is administered as a bolus infusion.

4.89   **The answer is d.** Thrombocythemia and thrombocytosis are a result of overproduction of platelets. The major complications related to an increased platelet count are bleeding and thrombosis. Thrombosis may result in symptoms associated with venous thrombosis pulmonary embolism, transient cerebral ischemia, myocardial infarction and angina.

STUDY NOTES

CHAPTER 5

ONCOLOGIC EMERGENCIES

METABOLIC

Disseminated Intravascular Coagulation

5.1   The symptoms of disseminated intravascular coagulation (DIC) seem paradoxical because:
a.   both platelet function and platelet numbers are implicated in DIC
b.   patients may experience fever at the same time their bodies are hypothermic
c.   DIC may be both the cause and effect of malignancy
d.   thrombosis and hemorrhage may occur simultaneously

5.2   Therapy for disseminated intravascular coagulation (DIC) often involves the administration of several substances. Which of the following is *not* a common treatment for DIC?
a.   heparin
b.   epsilon-amino caproic acid (EACA or Amicar)
c.   vitamin K
d.   platelet replacement

5.3   Patients with cancer may have bleeding, despite normal platelet counts and coagulation factors. An example of this problem is bleeding caused by:
a.   platelet sequestration
b.   disseminated intravascular coagulation (DIC)
c.   decreased platelet adhesiveness
d.   hypocoagulability

5.4   Which of the following statements best describes the physiologic characteristics of disseminated intravascular coagulation (DIC)?
a.   All clotting factors are prolonged.
b.   In contrast to what would be expected, the INR, PT, and PTT are elevated.
c.   The platelet count is decreased, the plasma fibrinogen is low due to consumption of fibrinogen by the clotting cascade, and the prothrombin time is prolonged.
d.   There is an absence of coagulation, and therefore there is widespread hemorrhage.

5.5   The most common cause of DIC is:
   a.   thrombopoiesis
   b.   infection
   c.   tumor products
   d.   anaphylaxis

5.6   The major and only definitive treatment for DIC is:
   a.   aggressive antibiotic therapy
   b.   treatment of the underlying cancer
   c.   administration of platelets and fresh frozen plasma
   d.   reversing the clotting cascade by the administration of heparin

5.7   Which of the following is *not* considered an early sign of disseminated intravascular coagulation?
   a.   petechiae
   b.   purpura
   c.   acral cyanosis
   d.   hemoptysis

Syndrome of Inappropriate Antidiuretic Hormone Secretion (SIADH)

5.8   Which of the following is *not* true of paraneoplastic syndromes (PNSs)?
   a.   Most PNSs appear in the middle stages of the disease course.
   b.   PNSs rarely occur with childhood malignancies.
   c.   The existence of a PNS frequently predicts a poor prognosis with regard to the malignancy.
   d.   Response of the PNS to therapy frequently correlates with tumor response.

5.9   Mr. Bradford, a patient with small cell lung cancer (SCLC), develops anorexia, weakness, and fatigue. At first, these are attributed to the cancer itself. As his condition worsens, though, Mr. Bradford's wife, who is caring for him through a hospice arrangement, calls you in tears, reporting that he has suddenly become combative. You tell her that he must have a serum chemistry as soon as possible because you suspect:
   a.   hypercalcemia
   b.   hyponatremia
   c.   pACTH syndrome
   d.   end-stage cancer

5.10   The incidence of SIADH in small cell lung cancer is:
   a.   2–5%
   b.   9–14%
   c.   25–35%
   d.   35–50%

5.11   Which of the following is indicative of SIADH?
   a.   increased plasma sodium and decreased urine output
   b.   hyponatremia with high serum osmolality and high urine osmolality
   c.   hypernatremia with high serum osmolality and high urine ismolality
   d.   hyponatremia with low serum osmolality, high urine sodium, and high urine osmolality

5.12 The problem with ectopic ADH secretion as a paraneoplastic syndrome in cancer compared to normal antidiuretic hormone secretion is which of the following?
a. Ectopic ADH is not regulated.
b. Ectopic ADH acts on cardiac tissue.
c. Ectopic ADH does not respond to dehydration.
d. Ectopic ADH is not related to mental status changes.

5.13 Mr. Lindy has a history of small cell lung cancer and returns for his 6-month checkup. He has felt well except for some nausea, weakness, and at times confusion, headache, and lethargy. His lab values reveal hypokalemia, hyponatremia, low BUN, and low creatinine. His clinical symptoms are suspicious for which of the following?
a. metastatic disease to the brain
b. metastatic disease to the liver
c. syndrome of inappropriate antidiuretic hormone secretion
d. adrenal insufficiency

5.14 Which of the following is *not* considered a therapeutic approach to the management of SIADH?
a. water restriction to less than 1000 mL/day
b. water load test
c. hypertonic saline infusions
d. demeclocycline

Septic Shock

5.15 Which of the following variables does *not* influence the incidence of sepsis?
a. concurrent radiotherapy and chemotherapy
b. length of myelosuppressive therapy
c. absolute granulocyte count less than 500/mm^3
d. duration of granulocytopenia

5.16 The consequence of infection with gram-negative organisms that can quickly lead to death is:
a. dehydration
b. gastrointestinal bleeding
c. endotoxic shock
d. anaphylaxis

5.17 *Pneumocystis carinii* is potentially fatal and requires treatment with:
a. foscarnet
b. ganciclovir
c. trimethoprim-sulfamethoxazole
d. an aminoglycoside

5.18 The signs of overt shock are not present in the early phase of shock. The early phase of shock is characterized by which of the following hemodynamic patterns?
a. vasodilation
b. normal to decreased cardiac output
c. mild hypotension
d. a and c

5.19 The physiologic process responsible for the clinical picture observed in late shock is:
a. hypoxemia
b. vasoconstriction
c. hypotension
d. vasodilation

5.20 Once treatment has been initiated, the nurse needs to be aware of the complications of shock, which include:
a. disseminated intravascular coagulation
b. hepatic abnormalities
c. below-normal temperature
d. a and b

5.21 Granulocytopenia is the single most important risk factor for sepsis in individuals with cancer. Which of the following is a common cause of granulocytopenia?
a. leukemia
b. chemotherapy
c. total body irradiation
d. all of the above

5.22 Septic shock ultimately causes death due to which of the following?
a. fever
b. coagulopathy
c. tissue ischemia
d. hypotension

Acute Tumor Lysis Syndrome

5.23 Acute tumor lysis syndrome (ATLS) is a complication of cancer therapy that occurs most commonly in patients with tumors that have a high proliferation index and are highly sensitive to chemotherapy. ATLS is *least likely* to be seen in which of the following cases?
a. colon cancer
b. lymphoma
c. acute myelogenous leukemia
d. non-Hodgkin's lymphoma

5.24 NHL patients with big, bulky, high-grade disease are at high risk for acute tumor lysis syndrome. One important aspect of the nursing care for such patients is:
a. looking for signs of motor incoordination and cognitive deficits
b. monitoring urine output for signs of renal failure
c. discontinuing vinca alkaloid treatment if signs of severe jaw pain occur
d. providing oral or intravenous agents that keep blood and urine acidic

5.25 Mr. James has chronic myelogenous leukemia in blastic transformation. He is considered to have a high tumor burden and has evidence of lymphadenopathy and spenomegaly. Which of the following laboratory tests indicates that he is experiencing ATLS?
a. acute hyperuricemia
b. hypokalemia
c. hypercalcemia
d. all of the above

5.26 The primary physiologic complication of ATLS is:
 a. tumor cell obstruction of microvasculature causing disseminated intravascular coagulation
 b. liver failure caused by a veno-occlusive disease
 c. uric acid crystallization in the renal tubules causing obstruction and acute renal failure
 d. tumor lysis causing release of tissue which produces pulmonary emboli

5.27 The most effective means of preventing ATLS includes which of the following?
 a. sodium bicarbonate and vigorous hydration
 b. heparinization
 c. maintaining a urine pH of less than 7
 d. all of the above

5.28 In tumor lysis syndrome, there is a release of a large amount of phosphorus into the blood and a proportional decrease in what other serum electrolyte?
 a. magnesium
 b. calcium
 c. potassium
 d. sodium

5.29 Which of the following is a key element in the prevention of tumor lysis syndrome?
 a. aggressive hydration
 b. diuresis
 c. allopurinol
 d. all of the above

5.30 Mr. Clay has lymphoma and received chemotherapy 4 days ago. He has been doing well but comes in complaining of fatigue, dizziness, and a "fluttering" feeling in his chest. Chemistries reveal potassium, 6 mEq/L; creatinine, 2.7 mg/dl; and calcium, 6 mg/dl. Your assessment is which of the following?
 a. He is dehydrated and needs fluids.
 b. He could have a life-threatening arrhythmia and should be admitted.
 c. He is probably anemic and needs blood.
 d. He is losing calcium and needs magnesium.

Anaphylaxis

5.31 A patient who received monoclonal antibody therapy 3 weeks ago presents with serum sickness that is characterized by which of the following?
 a. urticaria
 b. arthralgia
 c. generalized adenopathy
 d. all of the above

5.32 Measures to prevent a hypersensitivity reaction to a monoclonal antibody include *all but* which of the following?
 a. Speed up the infusion to decrease the amount of time the infusion takes.
 b. Administer an antihistamine prior to beginning the infusion.
 c. Administer a steroid the evening prior and morning of the infusion.
 d. Administer epinephrine 1:1000 as directed.

5.33   Mrs. Howe has just arrived for her first treatment with Herceptin, a monoclonal antibody. As you plan her teaching about her medication, you are careful to include which of the following?
   a. She should report any difficulty breathing, chills, or cough because her medication could cause an anaphylactic reaction.
   b. If she does have a reaction, the medication will be stopped temporarily and restarted after her symptoms subside.
   c. Diphenhydramine and acetaminophen are often given before the first infusion to minimize the allergic reaction.
   d. all of the above

5.34   Alex has an infection of his vascular access device and is beginning vancomycin therapy. Twenty minutes into a 60-minute infusion, you notice that his face and upper torso are flushed and he is wheezing slightly. Appropriate nursing action includes:
   a. Stop the infusion, he is having an allergic reaction.
   b. Administer decadron and benadryl immediately.
   c. Slow the infusion and administer morphine.
   d. This is not an antigen antibody reaction; slow the infusion to 90 minutes.

5.35   Allison is receiving a loading dose of Herceptin therapy. The infusion is to be administered over 90 minutes. Shortly after the infusion begins, she complains of hives, rash, and itching all over. She has a fever of 102°F and chills. Appropriate nursing action includes:
   a. Stop the infusion, administer steroids, and monitor vital signs.
   b. Stop the infusion, monitor vital signs and administer diphenhydramine and benadryl. Resume the infusion.
   c. Slow the infusion and administer morphine for the chills.
   d. Stop the infusion, administer epinephrine, and monitor vital signs.

5.36   Which of the following drugs is *not* commonly associated with a hypersensitivity reaction?
   a. paclitaxel
   b. cytarabine
   c. L-asparaginase
   d. docetaxel

5.37   Of the patients who experience a hypersensitivity reaction to paclitaxel, what percentage experience symptoms within 10 minutes of initiating the drug, after only a few milligrams had been infused?
   a. 20%
   b. 40%
   c. 60%
   d. 80%

Hypercalcemia

5.38   Which of the following types of malignancies is *least likely* to be associated with hypercalcemia?
   a. lung cancer
   b. breast cancer
   c. multiple myeloma
   d. colon cancer

5.39   Among the common early symptoms in hypercalcemic patients are all of the following *except*:
    a.   nausea and vomiting
    b.   diarrhea
    c.   hypertension
    d.   polyuria

5.40   The most important initial treatment for hypercalcemia is:
    a.   improving renal calcium excretion
    b.   treating the primary tumor
    c.   inhibiting osteoclast function
    d.   inhibiting bone resorption

5.41   The pathophysiology of hypercalcemia involves a combination of two factors—bone resorption and:
    a.   decreased renal calcium clearance
    b.   increased osteoclast activity
    c.   increased glomerular function
    d.   decreased availability of ionized calcium

5.42   Factors that are produced by tumors have been implicated in malignancy-associated hypercalcemia. Probably the most important of these humoral circulating factors is:
    a.   prostaglandin
    b.   PTH-like factor
    c.   bisphosphonate
    d.   osteoclast-activating factor

5.43   A patient is found to have a large tumor mass associated with high levels of PTH-related protein but normal levels of 1,25-dihydroxyvitamin D and normal intestinal absorption rates. Bone absorption is found to exceed bone formation. The most likely diagnosis is:
    a.   primary hyperparathyroidism
    b.   multiple myeloma
    c.   humoral hypercalcemia of malignancy (HHM)
    d.   Hodgkin's disease

5.44   Which of the following statements about the association between breast cancer and hypercalcemia is correct?
    a.   Bone resorption in breast cancer patients is probably due to cancer cells directly rather than to PGE mediation.
    b.   Tumor flare is thought to be the result of PGE inhibition by breast cancer cells.
    c.   Not all patients with metastases develop hypercalcemia, although most breast cancer patients with hypercalcemia have widespread skeletal metastases.
    d.   Hypercalcemia in breast cancer patients is usually responsive to prostaglandin inhibitors.

5.45   The symptoms of hypercalcemia in cancer patients are best described as:
    a.   similar to those of acute renal failure
    b.   easily identified but difficult to treat
    c.   distinct from those of end-stage disease
    d.   numerous, vague, and nonspecific

5.46 A patient develops confusion, disorientation, and hallucinations with an elevated serum calcium and occasional bradycardia. Therapeutic interventions might include which of the following?
   a. saline diuresis
   b. intravenous pamidronate
   c. aggressive cancer therapy
   d. all of the above

STRUCTURAL

Cardiac Tamponade

5.47 Malignant pericardial effusions:
   a. are extremely rare
   b. are easily detected by tachycardia, low blood pressure, and shortness of breath
   c. occur in 50% of all patients with cancer, especially the hematologic malignancies
   d. are not easily detected by routine tests and are found in 8–20% of autopsies.

5.48 The patient who is experiencing a pericardial effusion shows signs and symptoms that include:
   a. chest pain, confusion, nausea, and vomiting
   b. confusion, nausea, vomiting, and hypertension
   c. hypertension, bradycardia, and increased cardiac output
   d. decreased cardiac output, dyspnea, cough, and chest pain

5.49 Which of the following tumor types is *not commonly* associated with pericardial effusion and tamponade?
   a. lung cancer
   b. gastrointestinal carcinoma
   c. breast cancer
   d. leukemia

5.50 Mrs. Anderson has metastatic breast cancer and was doing well until recently when she started to complain of difficulty sleeping, anxiety, a cough, and some difficulty catching her breath. In addition, she has needed to sleep in a more upright, forward-leaning position. Which of the following most accurately describes what is probably causing her symptoms?
   a. She is most likely experiencing liver ascites, which is making lying down difficult for her. Call the doctor to see if the patient needs an antianxiety agent.
   b. Difficulty sleeping is common in cancer patients. She obviously needs something more effective to help her sleep.
   c. She is probably experiencing a slight peritoneal effusion which is causing her some anxiety and difficulty breathing. Notify the doctor because the patient needs a chest x-ray.
   d. Her symptoms are classic for pericardial effusion, and unless emergency measures are instituted to relieve the pressure she could progress to cardiac tamponade.

5.51 Which of the following statements about cardiac tamponade is *false*?
  a. An echocardiogram is the most precise method for visualization of a malignant pericardial effusion.
  b. Hypotension is an early and common objective symptom for cardiac tamponade.
  c. Pericardiocentesis is both therapeutic and diagnostic.
  d. The clinical picture in cardiac tamponade is caused by a buildup of pressure around the heart.

5.52 Cardiac tamponade results from an excess accumulation of fluid in the:
  a. pleural space
  b. pericardial sac
  c. pulsus paradoxus
  d. ventricular space

5.53 Which of the following tumor types is *not* commonly associated with pericardial effusions?
  a. lung cancer
  b. breast cancer
  c. prostate cancer
  d. lymphoma

Spinal Cord Compression

5.54 You will soon begin work in a clinic that specializes in the detection and treatment of spinal cord tumors. You are aware that the most common presenting symptom of a spinal cord tumor is:
  a. weakness
  b. cold, numbness, and tingling
  c. pain
  d. uncoordinated ataxic gait

5.55 Spinal cord compression occurs by which of the following mechanisms?
  a. direct extension of the tumor into the epidural space
  b. vertebral collapse
  c. displacement of bone into the epidural space
  d. all of the above

5.56 Mrs. Johnson has complained of back pain for 6 months and now presents with weakness. Which of the following helps to explain her symptoms?
  a. Pain is rarely a symptom of spinal cord tumors.
  b. Weakness is a classic symptom of spinal cord tumors.
  c. Back pain and weakness are likely caused by her chronic steroid use.
  d. a and b

5.57 Mark is being discharged from the hospital. His prostate cancer involves some bone metastasis. Which of the following developments is likely to indicate a need for radiation therapy?
  a. worsening back pain
  b. weakness of the lower extremities
  c. sensory deficits
  d. all of the above

5.58   A woman with breast cancer and known bone metastasis is currently on pamidronate. Her primary complaint is weakness in both arms. She has back pain, but it is unchanged from the previous week. The most logical explanation for her symptoms and the correct nursing action is which of the following?

a.   Weakness in arms and legs is common with pamidronate, and she should increase her use of the arms to avoid losing muscle strength.

b.   She has known bony metastasis that is no worse; the pamidronate will help the bone to heal, so it is appropriate to monitor her symptoms.

c.   If she has bony disease in her spine, she should have an emergency MRI to rule out thoracic cord compression.

d.   She should be encouraged not to cough, strain, or lift heavy objects because she could have osteoporosis and is at risk for disc disease.

Superior Vena Cava Syndrome

5.59   A man with a history of lung cancer calls his doctor to report the following symptoms: headache, swollen face and neck, and shoulders and chest are covered with a lacy venous pattern. Which of the following best identifies what he is describing?

a.   telangiectasia and complications of prior radiation therapy

b.   possible pneumothorax

c.   possible local recurrence with brain metastasis

d.   possible superior vena cava obstruction

5.60   Mrs. Ruthe recently had a Port-a-cath placed for long-term chemotherapy administration, and her doctor advised her to take Coumadin 1 mg a day for as long as she has the port. She is inquiring why she needs the Coumadin. The most appropriate response is which of the following?

a.   People with cancer are more prone to clotting disorders, and she is at increased risk for blood clots in her legs.

b.   Coumadin is used in place of the heparin flushes to maintain port patency.

c.   She needs the Coumadin for only about a week until she is completely healed and then she can stop it.

d.   The Coumadin is necessary to prevent clot formation around the port and possible venous thrombosis.

5.61   Which of the following is *not* characteristic of a superior vena cava syndrome (SVCS)?

a.   As the superior vena cava is compressed, there is reduced venous return to the right atrium.

b.   An increase in venous pressure causes venous hypertension.

c.   Late symptoms include cough and dyspnea.

d.   Initial symptoms include hoarseness and edema in the face, neck, and arms.

5.62   What is the most likely initial treatment of choice for quickly progressing superior vena cava syndrome (SVCS)?

a.   radiation therapy

b.   chemotherapy

c.   surgical resection

d.   administration of anticoagulants

5.63 Surgical management of chronic SVCS generally includes which of the following procedures?
   a. The portion of the vena cava that is being compressed is repositioned surgically following resection of the tumor.
   b. A bypass graft or stent is placed into the superior vena cava to dilate and expand the narrowed lumen of the vessel.
   c. A bypass graft is fashioned to redirect blood flow around the obstruction.
   d. b and c

5.64 Which of the following cancers is responsible for more than 70% of all cases of SVCS?
   a. breast cancer
   b. lung cancer
   c. Hodgkin's disease
   d. Kaposi's sarcoma

5.65 Which of the following is a primary cause of SVCS?
   a. external compression by primary tumor
   b. direct invasion by tumor
   c. thrombus formation within the vessel
   d. all of the above

Increased Intracranial Pressure

5.66 The most common acute-onset sign of malignant cerebral edema is:
   a. headache
   b. nausea/vomiting
   c. seizure
   d. disorientation

5.67 In most instances of CNS tumors, the first, earliest, and most sensitive indicator of dysfunction is a change in:
   a. level of consciousness
   b. cognitive ability
   c. motor and sensory function
   d. all of the above

5.68 After tumor resection, a patient suffers postoperative cerebral edema. This most likely results from:
   a. surgical manipulation of the surrounding brain tissue
   b. changes in regional blood flow
   c. brain injury caused by excessive retraction
   d. any of the above

5.69 Jeffrey's intracranial pressure (ICP) is acutely elevated. In acute situations like his, the drug of choice is:
   a. mannitol
   b. a corticosteroid
   c. vincristine
   d. vinblastine

5.70   Which of the following statements regarding metastatic brain tumors is *not* accurate?
   a.   Metastatic brain tumors are the most common type of brain tumor.
   b.   The incidence of metastatic brain tumors is decreasing due to advances in cancer care.
   c.   Tumors in the lung are the most likely of all solid tumors to metastasize to the brain.
   d.   Radiation therapy is the primary mode of treatment and is palliative.

5.71   In balancing intracranial pressure, the mechanism that specifically maintains a normal ICP despite fluctuations in arterial pressure and venous drainage is:
   a.   autoregulation
   b.   compensation
   c.   CSF displacement
   d.   cerebral blood flow

ANSWER EXPLANATIONS

5.1   **The answer is d.** DIC always results from an underlying disease process that triggers abnormal activation of thrombin formation. Thrombin is both a powerful coagulant and an agent of fibrinolysis. Thus small clots may be formed in the microcirculation of many organs at the same time that clots and clotting factors are being consumed. The result is hemorrhage as the body is unable to respond to vascular or tissue injury.

5.2   **The answer is c.** Vitamin K might be administered to a patient experiencing hypocoagulability, but not the hypercoagulability caused by DIC. All the other therapies may provide short-term relief of DIC symptoms. Treatment of the underlying malignancy is vital in treating the patient with DIC, inasmuch as the tumor is the ultimate stimulus.

5.3   **The answer is c.** Choices **b** and **d** are coagulation abnormalities; choice **a** is a quantitative abnormality. Qualitative abnormalities, such as choice **c**, refer principally to alterations in platelet function, which may include a decreased procoagulant activity of platelets, decreased platelet adhesiveness and decreased aggregation in response to ADP, thrombocytosis associated with myeloproliferative disorders, and the coating of platelets by fibrin degradation products as a result of the increased activation of coagulation factors.

5.4   **The answer is c.** DIC represents the most common serious hypercoagulable state in individuals with cancer. Tests generally done to help support the diagnosis of DIC include prothrombin time, platelet count, and the plasma fibrinogen level; all are reduced.

5.5   **The answer is b.** The most common cause of DIC is infection. It is believed that bacterial endotoxins, which are released from gram-negative bacteremia, activate the Hageman factor. This factor can initiate coagulation as well as stimulate fibrinolysis.

5.6   **The answer is b.** Treatment of the underlying malignancy is vital in the patient with a hypercoagulability abnormality, because the tumor is the ultimate stimulus. All other therapy, although effective on a short-term basis, provides only an interval of symptomatic relief.

5.7   **The answer is d.** Early signs of DIC include petechiae, purpura, hemorrhagic bullae, acral cyanosis, and frank gangrene. Late signs of DIC are overt hemorrhage involving multiple, unrelated sites such as hemoptysis, intraperitoneal hemorrhage, and intracranial bleeding; all are life-threatening events for the patient with DIC.

5.8   **The answer is a.** Most PNSs appear in the later stages of the disease course. It is true that PNSs rarely occur with childhood malignancies with the exception of Wilms' tumor and neuroblastoma. The existence of a PNS frequently predicts a poor prognosis for the malignancy. Finally, response of the PNS to therapy frequently correlates with tumor response.

5.9   **The answer is b.** Mr. Bradford most likely has hyponatremia secondary to SIAD. SIAD is primarily associated with small cell lung cancer. Water intoxication accounts for the signs and symptoms seen with SIAD. The early symptoms, such as nausea, weakness, anorexia, and fatigue, can be easily attributed to the cancer. However, as the hyponatremia worsens, symptoms may progress to include altered mental status, confusion, and combativeness.

5.10   **The answer is b.** SIADH is primarily associated with small cell lung cancer. Most of these patients (80%) may have some aspects of SIADH without clinical evidence of the syndrome. Only about 9–14% of patients with small cell lung cancer have SIADH.

5.11   **The answer is d.** The syndrome of secretion of inappropriate antidiuretic hormone (SIADH) results from ADH secretion by the tumor. The symptoms include hyponatremia and low serum osmolality, characterized by mental status changes, lethargy, seizures, and confusion.

5.12   **The answer is a.** Although structurally identical to normal ADH, ectopic ADH is not regulated. Atrial natriuretic peptide (ANP), a hormone arising from cardiac atrial tissue, has been identified as the cause of hyponatremia. Water intoxication accounts for the symptomatology of SIADH.

5.13   **The answer is c.** Serum chemistries frequently show low BUN, creatinine, albumin, and uric acid; this is a dilutional effect in hyponatremia associated with SIADH. SIADH occurs commonly in patients with SCLC and initially presents as nausea, weakness, confusion, and lethargy.

5.14   **The answer is b.** The water load test is a diagnostic study for SIADH, and not a therapeutic approach. Fluids are restricted to less than 1000 ml/day. Hypertonic saline is given IV with furosemide to expedite water loss. Demeclocycline is an antibiotic used to treat chronic SIADH. It stimulates diuresis by impairing the effect of AVP on the renal tubule.

5.15   **The answer is a.** There is a direct relationship between the number of circulating PMNs and the incidence of infection. When the granulocyte count is less than 500/mm^3, risk of infection is significant. As the length of therapy and the duration of granulocytopenia increase, so does the incidence of sepsis. Although concurrent radiotherapy and chemotherapy might increase the degree of myelosuppression, the incidence of sepsis is not increased.

5.16   **The answer is c.** The most significant consequence of gram-negative infection is the potential for endotoxic or systemic shock. The release of endotoxins initiates a cascade of events that, unless interrupted, will rapidly lead to death for the neutropenic patient.

5.17   **The answer is c.** *P. carinii* is a protozoan that causes infection in children with primary immunodeficiency disorders, persons with AIDS, and those with cancer who are undergoing immunosuppressive therapy. Untreated, *P. carinii* is fatal, and even with therapy mortality is high. The treatment of choice is trimethoprim-sulfamethoxazole.

5.18   **The answer is d.** Septic shock evolves through two phases that, although not always distinct, are characterized by different hemodynamic patterns. The early phase consists of vasodilation, decreased peripheral vascular resistance, normal to increased cardiac output, and mild hypotension.

5.19   **The answer is b.** The late phase of septic shock is characterized by a profound reduction in cardiac output, increased peripheral vascular resistance, oliguria, and metabolic acidosis. These factors create a cycle of vasoconstriction, ischemia, and vasodilation that results in irreversible damage to the heart, vascular system, kidneys, liver, and vasomotor center of the brain.

5.20   **The answer is d.** Once treatment has been initiated, nurses closely monitor for complications of shock, including disseminated intravascular coagulation, renal failure, GI bleeding, and hepatic abnormalities.

5.21   **The answer is d.** Granulocytopenia occurs secondary to leukemia, bone marrow infiltration, total body irradiation, and cytotoxic chemotherapy.

5.22   **The answer is c.** The clinical picture of septic shock illustrates the cumulative effects of coagulopathy, hypotension, hypoperfusion, and ultimately tissue ischemia involving virtually every organ system in the body.

5.23   **The answer is a.** ATLS is most commonly seen in patients with high-grade lymphoma, acute myelogenous leukemia, chronic myelogenous leukemia, and non-Hodgkin's lymphoma.

5.24   **The answer is b.** Acute tumor lysis syndrome generally occurs when the patient is initially treated. Tumor cells spill their contents into the general circulation, causing a metabolic disturbance. Renal failure and death may occur. The treatment of choice is prevention, including hydration, sodium bicarbonate, and intravenous or oral allopurinol to prevent hyperuricemia nephropathy include decreased urine output and increased lethargy.

5.25   **The answer is a.** ATLS is most often characterized by the development of acute hyperuricemia, hyperkalemia, hyperphosphatasemia, and hypocalcemia with or without acute renal failure.

5.26   **The answer is c.** Uric acid crystallization in the renal tubules causing obstruction, decreased glomerular filtration, and/or acute renal failure is a major complication of ATLS.

5.27   **The answer is a.** ATLS can be prevented by prophylactic alkalinization of urine—maintaining the urine pH at a level greater than 7—with the use of sodium bicarbonate and vigorous hydration.

5.28   **The answer is b.** In TLS, there is an inverse relationship between phosphorus and calcium, whereby if one mineral increases, the other decreases in the same proportion.

5.29   **The answer is d.** Aggressive hydration is needed, to at least 3 liters of fluid per day with adequate urinary output and using diuretics to prevent renal tubular damage. Allopurinol inhibits the enzyme xanthine oxidase and prevents the formation of uric acid, which in turn prevents uric acid nephropathy.

5.30   **The answer is b.** An increase in phosphate, potassium, uric acid, BUN, and creatinine or a 25% decrease in calcium within 4 days of chemotherapy is indicative of TLS and places the patient at risk for life-threatening arrhythmias.

5.31   **The answer is d.** Mab therapy can cause a serum sickness that may occur 2–4 weeks after therapy and results from circulating immune complexes.

5.32   **The answer is a.** Anaphylactoid reactions have most commonly occurred with Mab therapy. Most of these reactions occurred with Mabs in their early development and in administration to patients with lymphoma or leukemia or when Mabs were administered by rapid infusion.

5.33   **The answer is d.** Acute side effects that occur during Mab infusion are most commonly fever, chills, malaise, myalgia, nausea, and vomiting. Dyspnea, cough, and chest pain can occur during a Mab infusion and may be related to the rate of infusion. The symptoms often resolve if the rate is slowed.

5.34   **The answer is d.** Vancomycin causes release of histamine from the mast cells, which causes vasodilation and the appearance of an allergic reaction. The red neck or red man syndrome is common with vancomycin and improves with slowing to a 90-minute infusion.

5.35   **The answer is b.** Fever, chills, and rash are common with the first infusion and respond to acetaminophen and diphenhydramine. Stop the infusion temporarily when hives, rash, pruritus, and fever are present. Notify physician and monitor vital signs. Resume the infusion and monitor the patient.

5.36   **The answer is b.** Hypersensitivity reactions (HSRs) due to cytarabine are rare and seen only within the past few years where the doses used are 10–15 times normal. HSRs are frequent enough with paclitaxel, docetaxel, and asparaginase therapy to be a treatment-limiting toxicity.

5.37   **The answer is d.** Most (80%) of the patients who have an HSR develop the reaction within 10 minutes of initiating the drug. The remainder of those who develop a reaction (20%) do so during their second infusion.

5.38   **The answer is d.** Patients with lung and breast cancer account for the highest percentage of malignancy-induced hypercalcemia. However, multiple myeloma, which is relatively rare, is the underlying cause in 10% of malignancy-associated hypercalcemia cases.

5.39   **The answer is b.** Constipation, and *not* diarrhea, is more likely to be observed during the early stages of hypercalcemia. Elevated extracellular calcium levels depress smooth muscle contractility, leading to delayed gastric emptying and decreased gastrointestinal motility.

5.40   **The answer is a.** Before excessive bone resorption can be treated, impaired renal calcium excretion must be improved, usually by correcting dehydration and removing factors that may exacerbate hypercalcemia, including thiazide diuretics. Oral or intravenous hydration with normal saline may be required.

5.41   **The answer is a.** Hypercalcemia is characterized by excess extracellular calcium. This condition results from bone resorption—the release of skeletal calcium into serum—and from the failure of the kidneys to clear extracellular calcium. As calcium levels rise, symptoms of hypercalcemia appear.

5.42   **The answer is b.** Malignancy-associated hypercalcemia is a complex metabolic complication in which bone resorption exceeds both bone formation and the kidney's ability to excrete extracellular calcium. Humoral circulating factors include a PTH-like factor, transforming growth factors (TGF-alpha), and 1,25-dihydroxyvitamin D. Hypercalcemia that develops in patients with solid tumors but without bone metastases is thought to be caused by PTH-like factor.

5.43   **The answer is c.** In humoral hypercalcemia of malignancy (HHM), patients secrete high levels of PTH-related protein but have normal levels of 1,25-dihydroxyvitamin D and normal intestinal absorption rates. Osteoblastic and osteoclastic activities are "uncoupled" so that bone resorption exceeds bone formation. Hypercalcemia and hypercalciuria thus occur.

5.44   **The answer is c.** Bone resorption in breast cancer patients is probably the result of PGE-mediated osteolysis, rather than direct bone resorption. Tumor flare is thought to indicate the release of PGE by a hormonally responsive tumor. Hypercalcemia in breast cancer patients is generally unresponsive to prostaglandin inhibitors.

5.45   **The answer is d.** Hypercalcemia symptoms are numerous, vague, and nonspecific, and because many cancer patients with hypercalcemia have large tumor burdens and will die in 3–6 months, symptoms of hypercalcemia may be confused with those of end-stage disease.

5.46   **The answer is d.** Paraneoplastic hypercalcemia often presents as confusion, disorientation, and hallucinations with bradycardia. Treatment of hypercalcemia includes vigorous hydration and pamidronate.

5.47   **The answer is d.** Malignant pericardial effusions are not easily detected by routine tests and are found in 8–20% of autopsies. Only 30% of affected patients are symptomatic. Since pericardial effusion is not easily detected by routine tests, it is often not discovered while the patient is alive.

5.48   **The answer is d.** Pericardial effusion interferes with cardiac function because the fluid burden occupies space and reduces the volume of the heart in diastole. Systemic circulatory effects of decreased cardiac output and impaired venous return lead to generalized congestion. The body tries to compensate in several ways: tachycardia, an increase in systemic and pulmonary venous pressure, and increased ejection fraction.

5.49   **The answer is b.** Gastrointestinal cancer rarely results in pericardial effusion and tamponade probably because of its natural pattern of metastases to the liver and surrounding organs.

5.50   **The answer is d.** Subjective symptoms of pericardial effusion most commonly include dyspnea and cough. The person with cardiac tamponade positions himself or herself in an upright, forward-leaning stance for maximum relief and has anxiety.

5.51   **The answer is b.** Hypotension occurs, but in only about one-third of patients who have cardiac tamponade.

5.52   **The answer is b.** Cardiac tamponade results from an excess accumulation of fluid in the pericardial sac (pericardial effusion). The fluid collection causes an increase in pressure around the heart, resulting in diminished flow of blood to the ventricles.

5.53   **The answer is c.** Several tumor types are associated with the development of pericardial effusion including lung, breast, lymphoma, and leukemia. Other tumor types include malignant melanoma, gastric, ovarian, kidney, pancreas, and head and neck cancers.

5.54   **The answer is c.** Pain is the most common presenting symptom of a spinal cord tumor. Weakness is the most readily identified objective finding and may follow the appearance of sensory symptoms. Specific sensory deficits depend on where the tumor is on a cross section of the spine. A lateral tumor affects pain and temperature, causing cold, numbness, and tingling. Anterior tumors lead to weakness and an uncoordinated ataxic gait.

5.55   **The answer is d.** Spinal cord compression occurs either by direct extension of the tumor into the epidural space or by vertebral collapse and displacement of bone into the epidural space. It can also occur by direct extension through the intervertebral foramina.

5.56   **The answer is b.** Weakness is the most readily identified objective finding for spinal cord tumor. Choice **a** cannot be correct because pain is the most common presenting symptom of a spinal cord tumor. There is no evidence to support choice **c**.

5.57   **The answer is d.** All patients with bone metastasis are at risk for spinal cord compression. Worsening back pain, weakness of the lower extremities, or sensory deficits require immediate medical attention—usually radiation therapy to control tumor impingement on the spinal cord.

5.58   **The answer is c.** Imminent spinal cord compression should be suspected in individuals who have known bone metastases, progressive back pain associated with weakness, paresthesias, bowel or bladder dysfunction, or gait disturbances.

5.59   **The answer is d.** Obstruction of the superior vena cava is a common complication of lung cancer. The clinical picture includes edema of both eyelids, arms, and hands; the face is a dusky blue color; the lips are deeply cyanotic; and the shoulders, chest, and upper abdomen are covered with a lacy collateral venous pattern.

5.60   **The answer is d.** Catheter-induced SVCS, most often the result of thrombosis, is treated with fibrinolytic therapy, such as urokinase. Prevention involves using Coumadin 1 mg daily.

5.61   **The answer is c.** Initial symptoms of SVCS include cough; dyspnea; stridor; hoarseness; edema in the face, neck, and arms; and neck and chest vein distention.

5.62   **The answer is a.** Fractionated irradiation of the mediastinum is the treatment of choice. Doses of 300–400 cGy/day are administered initially followed by 200 cGy doses to achieve a cumulative dose of 3,000–3,500 cGy to the obstructing tumor site.

5.63   **The answer is d.** One of two approaches, superior vena cava bypass graft or stent placement, may be performed for the patient with a good prognosis who has chronic or recurrent SVCS for whom other treatment options have been exhausted. The graft creates a new vessel that circumvents the obstruction; the stent is inserted into the superior vena cava to dilate and expand its narrowed lumen.

5.64   **The answer is b.** Lung cancer is responsible for 70% of all cases of SVCS. Small cell carcinoma of the lung is the most common histologic type, followed by squamous cell carcinoma of the lung.

5.65   **The answer is d.** SVCS may be caused by external compression by primary or metastatic cancer, direct invasion by tumor, or thrombus formation within the vessel

5.66   **The answer is c.** Malignant cerebral edema produces diffuse signs and symptoms reflecting its more global effects on brain functioning, as opposed to the focal signs and symptoms caused by direct destruction of tissue by tumor. Subtle early changes in the patient's status are vague and usually are observed only by someone who knows the patient well. Seizure is the most common acute-onset sign. Headache, another common early symptom, is caused by distortion and traction of pain-sensitive structures by the edema.

5.67   **The answer is a.** In most instances the first, earliest, and most sensitive indicator of dysfunction is a change in the level of consciousness. Mental status and cognitive ability, as well as motor and sensory function and cranial nerve function, are assessed.

5.68   **The answer is d.** Postoperative cerebral edema results from the surgical manipulation of the surrounding brain tissue, changes in regional blood flow, or brain injury caused by excessive retraction.

5.69   **The answer is a.** In situations in which ICP is acutely elevated, corticosteroids alone are insufficient and osmotic diuretics (hyperosmolar agents), usually mannitol, are required.

5.70   **The answer is a.** Gliomas are the most common primary brain tumor in adults.

5.71   **The answer is a.** In balancing intracranial pressure, autoregulation is the mechanism that specifically maintains a normal ICP, despite fluctuations in arterial pressure and venous drainage.

STUDY NOTES

STUDY NOTES

CHAPTER 6

SCIENTIFIC BASIS FOR PRACTICE

CARCINOGENESIS

6.1 A patient asks, "What are cancer-suppressor genes?" As part of your answer, you explain that cancer-suppressor genes code for proteins that _____ growth-promoting factors.
   a. enhance
   b. fuel
   c. inactivate
   d. duplicate

6.2 The *p53* gene is:
   a. a potent oncogene
   b. the most frequently mutated gene in human cancer
   c. the "guardian of the oncogene"
   d. protected from DNA viruses

6.3 In clonal selection:
   a. mutation in the genome of a cell may confer a survival advantage on that cell
   b. a cell becomes weaker with each mutation
   c. oncogenes are destroyed
   d. telomeres develop, which are completely duplicated during cell division

6.4 A patient asks you to describe the "types of things that cause cancer." Because of her interest in "types" of causes, you might begin by explaining that cancer is *ordinarily* classified as being caused by a combination of factors that include:
   a. biological, viral, physical, or chemical
   b. occupational, viral, dietary, or familial
   c. chemical, viral, physical, or familial
   d. viral, chemical, familial, occupational, or lifestyle

6.5   Mr. Henderson's cancer is said to have been induced by familial carcinogenesis. From this, you can assume that in his case certain genes:
   a.   caused cancer by functioning to excess
   b.   caused cancer by their absence
   c.   acted as growth promoters
   d.   lost their ability to prevent malignant growth by their loss of homozygosity

6.6   One encouraging aspect of research into tumor-associated viruses is the discovery of:
   a.   their direct tumor causation
   b.   their promise for prevention through development of vaccines from animal forms of the viruses
   c.   their promise for prevention through inactivation
   d.   similar viruses in animals that have been eliminated by vaccines made from attenuated viruses

6.7   Which of the following is *not* true of carcinogenesis and chemoprevention?
   a.   Chemoprevention is the most promising form of host modification, using nutrients or pharmacological agents to inhibit or reverse carcinogenesis.
   b.   Proto-oncogenes are most likely involved in initiation and promotion of cancer.
   c.   Chemoprevention has the potential for both secondary and tertiary prevention, but by definition, it cannot be useful in primary prevention.
   d.   Agents that inhibit carcinogenesis generally are classified by the point in the process at which they are effective.

6.8   The *ras* oncogenes:
   a.   have a screening usefulness of about 45%
   b.   function early in the process of carcinogenesis
   c.   are a late event
   d.   are not effective as targets for early detection

6.9   Ms. Harris has hepatocellular carcinoma, which is apparently viral. The *most likely* assumption, then, is that she was exposed somehow to:
   a.   HTLV-1
   b.   ATL
   c.   HCC
   d.   HBV

6.10 Fat and fiber are two dietary factors that appear to be correlated with the occurrence of colorectal cancer. It is thought that they operate by affecting, in opposite ways, the:
   a.   conversion of ionized bile salts into insoluble compounds
   b.   rate of uptake of calcium by the GI tract
   c.   breakdown of carcinogenic compounds by digestive enzymes
   d.   exposure of the GI tract to promoters of carcinogenesis

SPECIFIC CANCERS

Pathophysiology

6.11   Ms. Jantzen will soon begin induction therapy for acute myelogenous leukemia. As her oncology nurse, you explain that the goal of therapy is to cause severe bone marrow hypoplasia, using:
    a.   busulfan and hydroxyurea
    b.   cytosine arabinoside and daunorubicin
    c.   vincristine, prednisone, L-asparaginase, and daunorubicin
    d.   chlorambucil and cyclophosphamide

6.12   Which of the following statements about lymphomas is correct?
    a.   Non-Hodgkin's lymphoma (NHL) is distinguished from Hodgkin's disease (HD) primarily on the basis of its different clinical manifestations.
    b.   Lymphomas are preeminently a malignancy of the lymphocyte.
    c.   There seems to be a single malignancy for all stages in the developmental sequence from primitive to mature lymphocyte.
    d.   In general, B-lymphocyte malignancies are more aggressive than T-lymphocyte malignancies.

6.13   The most common form of skin cancer is:
    a.   basal cell carcinoma (BCC)
    b.   squamous cell carcinoma (SCC)
    c.   malignant melanoma
    d.   superficial spreading melanoma (SSM)

6.14   Ms. Smith, who has acute myelogenous leukemia, is in complete remission after two courses of induction therapy. She is beginning post-remission therapy, in which she will receive very high doses of the same drugs used for induction therapy. She asks, "What's the point of this? I'm so sick of treatment. I'm in remission, aren't I?" You explain that this type of post-remission therapy is:
    a.   consolidation therapy to prevent leukemic recurrence related to minimal residual disease
    b.   intensification therapy to treat substantial toxicities, including extended myelosuppression and cerebellar dysfunction
    c.   maintenance therapy, which is used to help prevent a recurrence in some specific cases
    d.   CNS prophylaxis to prevent leukemic recurrence related to minimal residual disease

6.15   You are the new oncology nurse in a large hospital. On your first day you meet Mr. Jackson. His physician neglects to tell you what type of leukemia Mr. Jackson has, but he says to you, "He still has the Philadelphia chromosome, so we don't exactly have a cure yet." From this you are able to discern that Mr. Jackson has:
    a.   acute lymphocytic leukemia
    b.   acute myelogenous leukemia
    c.   chronic lymphocytic leukemia
    d.   chronic myelogenous leukemia

6.16 The most common site of metastasis for tumors of the bone is the:
a. GI tract
b. central nervous system
c. liver
d. lungs

6.17 All of the following are common metastatic sites for breast cancer *except* the:
a. brain
b. liver
c. bone
d. gastrointestinal tract

6.18 The glioblastoma multiforme (GBM):
a. is most common in individuals who are between 30 and 50 years of age
b. has less necrosis than anaplastic astrocytoma
c. is the most common adult primary brain tumor
d. a and c

6.19 Which of the following conditions is commonly associated with colorectal carcinoma?
a. appendicitis or gallbladder disease
b. hemorrhoids
c. anal condylomata acuminata
d. chronic ulcerative colitis

6.20 During the initial workup, Mr. Smith, who has testicular cancer, complains of low back pain that has been present for about 1 month. This may indicate:
a. metastatic disease to the lumbar spine
b. that the cancer has spread to the prostate
c. that the cancer has spread into the retroperitoneal lymph nodes
d. a and c

6.21 Multiple myeloma is a cancer of which of the following cell types?
a. B lymphocyte
b. plasma cell
c. monoclonal lymphocyte
d. a and b

Diagnostic Measures

6.22 You are preparing for an initial meeting with Mr. Jennings, who is about to undergo diagnostic screening for a suspected abdominal cancer. In describing this process, you intend to tell him that major goals of the diagnostic evaluation may be to establish, among other things, the:
a. tissue type of the malignancy
b. primary type of the malignancy
c. extent of disease within the body
d. all of the above

6.23 Mr. Phillips has liver cancer. The preferred procedure for imaging the abdomen is usually:
a. ultrasonography
b. CT scan
c. thermography
d. x-ray

6.24   Mrs. Plyman is about to undergo ultrasonography to evaluate a possible pelvic tumor. She asks you for information on the procedure. Which of the following statements will *not* be part of your education plan?
   a.   Ultrasonography can be used to discriminate masses.
   b.   The procedure is most applicable in detecting tumors within the pelvis, retroperitoneum, and peritoneum.
   c.   It is an excellent means of visualizing through bone or air, especially in comparison with radiography or CT scans.
   d.   Ultrasonography is noninvasive, directing reflecting echoes of high-frequency sound waves into specific tissues.

6.25   Mrs. Plyman says, "I don't like the idea of ultrasonography. Why can't I be examined using MRI?" Your best explanation is:
   a.   MRI is most helpful in detecting and staging cancer in the central nervous system, spine, head and neck, and musculoskeletal system.
   b.   MRI is more dangerous than ultrasonography because it uses radio-labeled monoclonal antibodies to visualize microscopic sites of metastasis.
   c.   MRI exposes patients to ionizing radiation and therefore is not safer than ultrasonography, although both are easily used within safe limits.
   d.   There is no way to enhance MRI imaging, as there is with ultrasonography.

6.26   Mrs. Ellis has stage II breast cancer and is receiving adjuvant doxorubicin and cyclophosphamide. She has no symptoms of bone involvement but asks that a bone scan and a Ca 15-3 tumor marker be done. The most appropriate response would be which of the following?
   a.   A bone scan would not be useful because Mrs. Ellis has no symptoms.
   b.   CA-15-3 is used to monitor metastatic disease, and not as an early detection test.
   c.   Both tests should have been done prior to surgery.
   d.   a and b

6.27   Mrs. Wilson is about to have a sputum cytology study. She asked the nurse to "explain this type of test. I already had a chest x-ray. Why isn't that enough?" The best answer is to explain that sputum cytology:
   a.   is probably the most helpful diagnostic study for lung cancer
   b.   can be particularly helpful in evaluating mediastinal lymph nodes
   c.   has a diagnostic yield of up to 80% for small peripheral tumors
   d.   has a diagnostic yield of up to 80% for central tumors

6.28   The diagnosis of either HD or NHL usually is established by:
   a.   cytologic examination of the Reed-Sternberg cells
   b.   CT and MRI scans of the nodular tissue
   c.   lymph node biopsy
   d.   exploratory laparotomy

6.29   The preferred initial surgical procedure for suspected cutaneous melanoma (CM) is:
   a.   excisional biopsy
   b.   incisional biopsy
   c.   wide excision
   d.   curettage and electrodesiccation

6.30 Which of the following procedures is considered the standard approach for definitive pathological diagnosis of testicular cancer?
   a. biopsy
   b. fine-needle biopsy
   c. transcrotal approach orchiectomy
   d. inguinal orchiectomy

6.31 All of the following are commonly used in the diagnosis/staging of cervical cancer *except:*
   a. Pap smear
   b. colposcopy
   c. biopsy
   d. laparoscopy

6.32 Adenocarcinomas:
   a. constitute 30% of all lung cancers and are more common in males than in females
   b. arise from the basal cells of the bronchial epithelium and usually present as masses in large bronchi
   c. are the most common lung cancer in males, in females, and in nonsmokers, accounting for 40% of all tumors
   d. are the least common type of lung cancer, representing approximately 10–15%

6.33 A sarcoma is a malignant tumor of the connective tissue, whereas a carcinoma is a malignant tumor arising from which of the following tissues?
   a. epithelium
   b. endothelial
   c. mesenchymal
   d. hematopoietic

6.34 Approximately what percentage of people diagnosed with cancer are diagnosed with a tumor of unknown origin?
   a. 20–25%
   b. 15–20%
   c. 10–15%
   d. 5–10%

6.35 The primary objective of classification and staging of malignant tumors is to do which of the following?
   a. to provide the information necessary for treatment planning
   b. to identify individuals who might be candidates for research studies
   c. to provide prognostic information
   d. all of the above

Classification

Tumor Classification

6.36 Mr. Mayle's clinical exam reveals evidence of an extensive primary tumor with fixation to a deeper structure, bone invasion, and lymph nodes of a similar nature. The lesion is operable but not resectable, and gross disease is left behind. There is some chance of survival. How would you classify Mr. Mayle's cancer?
   a. Stage IV, T4, N3, M+
   b. Stage I, T1, NO, MO
   c. Stage II, T2, N1, MO
   d. Stage III, T4, N2, MO

6.37 A benign tumor:
   a. is well circumscribed or encapsulated and appears orderly
   b. is not made up of cells similar to those of its parent tissue
   c. invades the organs from which it originated and is made up of cells that vary greatly in size and shape
   d. a and b

6.38 Malignant tumors arising in glandular epithelial tissues are known as:
   a. sarcomas
   b. osteosarcomas
   c. transitional cell carcinomas
   d. adenocarcinomas

6.39 CIN III (cervical intraepithelial neoplasia stage III) is characterized by neoplastic changes involving up to full thickness of the epithelium with no areas of stromal invasion or metastases. CIN III is also known as:
   a. preclinical invasive carcinoma
   b. carcinoma in situ
   c. adenocarcinoma
   d. verrucous carcinoma

6.40 Two patients have been diagnosed with bronchogenic cancer. You know that this does not mean that both patients will necessarily have a similar symptomatology or course of treatment because bronchogenic cancers are grouped into two broad categories:
   a. small cell lung cancer (SCLC) and the non–small cell lung cancers (NSCLC)
   b. adenocarcinoma and large cell carcinoma
   c. heterogeneous and histological
   d. hyperplasia and carcinoma in situ

Staging

6.41 In the TNM staging system:
   a. cTNM indicates that assessment has been obtained clinically
   b. cTNM indicates whether carcinogenesis has occurred
   c. rTNM indicates that remission of the cancer is occurring
   d. aTNM indicates that the cancer has been detected on first assessment

6.42 Stage groupings involve:
   a. combining the various classification elements of tumor site, regional lymph node involvement, and the presence or absence of metastasis
   b. two main staging periods: pretreatment and posttreatment
   c. two main staging periods: clinical diagnostic staging and pretreatment staging
   d. a and b

6.43 After a course of treatment, Ms. Trent's treatment response is evaluated. This reevaluation or restaging:
   a. makes possible the redesignation of a more appropriate stage to be referenced throughout the remaining course of the illness, replacing the stage ascribed at the time of diagnosis
   b. focuses attention on the disease parameters that were positive at diagnosis
   c. determines whether the patient is eligible to participate in a clinical trial
   d. a and b

6.44 In determining the survival rate for persons with cancer of the renal pelvis, the most important factor seems to be:
   a. the stage of the tumor
   b. whether or not radiotherapy was used in treatment
   c. whether or not the tumor is hormone sensitive
   d. the age and physical condition of the patient at diagnosis

6.45 The AJCC staging system for lung cancer uses:
   a. eight stages, each of which is distinct relative to treatment and 5-year survival statistics
   b. the TNM letters
   c. the simple two-stage system
   d. two defining terms—limited-stage disease and extensive-stage disease—to stage lung cancers

6.46 Which of the following statements about the staging of Hodgkin's disease is correct?
   a. Stage II malignancy is determined by a positive bone marrow biopsy.
   b. Stage determination is important because it influences what treatment option will be used.
   c. Stage II presentation is usually indicative of a more aggressive HD type.
   d. HD rarely presents as stage II.

6.47 Accurate staging of a patient with Hodgkin's disease is *least likely* to include which of the following procedures?
   a. a chest radiograph
   b. an exploratory laparotomy
   c. blood chemistries, including liver and kidney function tests
   d. a complete blood count

6.48 The phase of cutaneous melanoma tumor growth that is characterized by focal deep penetration of atypical melanocytes into the dermis and subcutaneous tissue is the:
   a. radial phase
   b. vertical growth phase
   c. nodular phase
   d. acral lentiginous phase

Grading

6.49   Treatment of advanced intermediate/high-grade non-Hodgkin's lymphoma (NHL) is *most likely* to involve:
    a. invasive surgery
    b. high doses of topical radiation
    c. combination chemotherapy
    d. cyclophosphamide combined with radiation

6.50   A liver tumor may be suspected if laboratory tests reveal elevated levels of:
    a. gastrin
    b. cholesterol
    c. alpha-fetoprotein
    d. amylase

6.51   A primary tumor is one that is histologically confirmed to arise from a specific site of tumorigenesis, whereas a secondary tumor refers to:
    a. a tumor that arises in another site after the primary tumor has been discovered
    b. a tumor of unknown origin
    c. a metastatic tumor resembling the primary tumor histologically
    d. a second primary cancer that is histologically different from the primary tumor

6.52   Grading a malignant neoplasm is a method of classification based on histopathological characteristics of the tissue. Which would *not* be considered to be a primary objective of grading?
    a. establishing the aggressiveness or degree of malignancy of tumor cells
    b. providing prognostic information for all cancers
    c. quantifying information to assist in treatment planning
    d. determining the stage of disease of selected cancers

6.53   Mr. Fleischman's cancer is given an AJCC classification of G2. This means his cancer is:
    a. undifferentiated
    b. well differentiated
    c. poorly differentiated
    d. moderately well differentiated

6.54   Histopathological type refers to:
    a. a qualitative assignment given to a lesion at a site other than the orginal site that is of the *same* cell type as the original; this is used to determine metastatic tumors
    b. a quantitative assessment of the extent to which the tumor resembles the tissue of origin
    c. a qualitative assessment whereby a neoplasm is categorized in terms of the tissue or cell type from which it has originated
    d. a qualitative assignment that indicates that a lesion at a site other than the original site is of a *different* cell type than the original tumor; this is used to indicate a second primary cancer

6.55   The *least* threatening prostate cancers are those that:
    a. feature large tumor volume
    b. have a Gleason grade of 3–5
    c. originate in the peripheral zone
    d. are indolent

6.56 The primary application of flow cytometry analysis in solid tumors is to do which of the following?
    a. determine DNA content (ploidy)
    b. determine the percentage of cells synthesizing DNA (the S-phase fraction)
    c. measure tumor markers
    d. a and b

Prognosis

6.57 In determining the progression of bladder cancer, the *most important* feature is the:
    a. degree of hematuria present
    b. presence of bladder neck obstruction
    c. depth of penetration into the bladder wall
    d. presence of pain in the suprapubic region

6.58 Carry asks you to explain the relationship among tumor size, node involvement, and prognosis. Which of the following statements is *most accurate*?
    a. Smaller tumors with positive node involvement have the best prognosis.
    b. Larger tumors with negative node involvement have the best prognosis.
    c. Smaller tumors with negative node involvement have the worst prognosis.
    d. Larger tumors with positive node involvement have the worst prognosis.

6.59 The prognosis for a patient with HD is *most closely* related to:
    a. elevated lactic dehydrogenase level
    b. histologic type
    c. abdominal lymph node involvement
    d. stage at presentation

6.60 Which of the following patients with prostate cancer is *most likely* to be given "watchful waiting" as a treatment choice?
    a. Frank, who is 37, recently married, and still hopes to have children
    b. Harold, who is 76 and enjoying an active retirement with his wife
    c. Byron, who is 56 and has poorly differentiated localized disease
    d. Phil, who is 40 and has a high-grade tumor

6.61 Of the following factors related to cutaneous melanoma prognosis, the one *most closely* correlated with decreased survival rates in patients with stage I CM is:
    a. anatomic level of tumor invasion
    b. tumor location
    c. Clark level
    d. tumor thickness

6.62 Alpha-fetoprotein (AFP) and human chorionic gonadotropin (BHCG) are measured primarily for which of the following reasons?
    a. staging of testicular cancer
    b. documenting disease recurrence
    c. monitoring response to treatment
    d. all of the above

6.63   Mr. James has been told by his physician that he has a seminoma of the testis that is high grade—meaning it has a high tumor cell doubling time. Mr. James is confused about what this means in terms of his prognosis. Your explanation would include which of the following?
   a. High-grade tumors generally carry a poor prognosis.
   b. Tumors with a high tumor cell doubling time typically become resistant to chemotherapy.
   c. A high tumor cell doubling time means the disease has probably metastasized.
   d. A high tumor cell doubling time means he has a favorable prognosis.

6.64   In oncology, the tendency is to use the term *cure* to refer to:
   a. groups of cancer patients
   b. an individual who has a normal recovery with a return to health
   c. an individual who no longer exhibits symptoms, gains lost weight, and resumes normal activity
   d. all of the above, but in differing circumstances

6.65   The prognosis for a patient with colorectal cancer is probably poorest if which of the following exists?
   a. venous and lymph node invasion
   b. high blood pressure
   c. location of the tumor above the peritoneal reflection
   d. squamous cell involvement

MAJOR TREATMENT MODALITIES

Surgery

6.66   Mr. Vance just had surgery and needs both radiation and chemotherapy. Why would these both be given after surgery?
   a. Sometimes it is difficult for the surgeon to assess before surgery whether invasion has occurred and excision is the best choice.
   b. Most likely, the tumor was found to be invading nearby tissues that could not be surgically resected, and micrometastasis is a potential problem.
   c. Radiotherapy before surgery is appropriate only as a first-line means of defense; the surgery was a second-line treatment that was unsuccessful, so a more aggressive third line—combination therapy—is now being employed.
   d. b and c

6.67   You have recently become part of a new, interdisciplinary oncological team. You are aware that situations lending themselves best to surgical treatment include such factors as:
   a. slow-growing tumors that consist of cells with prolonged cell cycles
   b. an ability to achieve resection of the entire tumor mass as well as a margin of safety of normal, healthy tissue surrounding the tumor
   c. embedded tumors
   d. a and b

6.68   The following patients have been recently diagnosed: Mr. Alexander has a superficial skin cancer; Ms. Jeffries has a musculoskeletal encapsulated tumor; Mrs. Myers's tumor is embedded deep within the abdomen and pelvis; Mr. Mitchell's tumor has invaded tissues and organs in multiple directions. Which of the following are true?
  a.   Mr. Mitchell's and Ms. Jeffries's cancers need immediate resection.
  b.   Mrs. Myers's tumor should be treated with radiation, and Mr. Alexander's should be treated only with a topical antineoplastic agent; neither will benefit from surgery at this point.
  c.   Mr. Alexander and Ms. Jeffries will most likely benefit from surgical resection.
  d.   None of the above offer the best treatment options.

6.69   Which of the following is *not* an example of palliative surgery?
  a.   Joshua's leg, which has a sarcoma, is amputated because it is nonfunctioning and painful.
  b.   Mary Ellen receives breast reconstruction following mastectomy.
  c.   Mike undergoes removal of an ulcerative lesion that is a likely source of infection.
  d.   Shante has undergone resection of her primary tumor to prevent obstruction.

6.70   Within a week of surgery for esophageal cancer, contrast studies are likely to be done to check for:
  a.   local edema
  b.   any signs of residual tumor
  c.   anastomotic leaks
  d.   swallowing ability

6.71   All of the following are possible contraindications to hepatic resection for liver cancer *except:*
  a.   jaundice
  b.   severe cirrhosis
  c.   chemotherapy failure
  d.   ascites

6.72   In women, radical cystectomy includes removal of the:
  a.   bladder, urethra, uterus, ovaries, fallopian tubes, and the anterior wall of the vagina
  b.   bladder, urethra, and anterior wall of the vagina only
  c.   bladder and urethra only
  d.   bladder only

6.73   Mr. Keller has NSCLC that is in stage I; Ms. Harris's is a stage II. Mr. DeBalivere has stage IIIA, Mrs. Jensen has stage IV, and Ms. Jording has stage IIIB NSCLC. Who will benefit most from surgical resection?
  a.   Mr. Keller and Ms. Harris
  b.   Mr. DeBalivere and Ms. Jording
  c.   Ms. Jording and Mrs. Jensen
  d.   Mr. Keller only

6.74   Tomorrow morning, Steven, an oncology nursing candidate, will observe a pneumonectomy for the first time. You know he is prepared when he tells you that pneumonectomy is:
  a.   never performed if a tumor cannot be completely excised by lobectomy as well
  b.   performed for primary lung cancer confined to a single lobe of the lung
  c.   chosen when the tumor involves the proximal bronchus, is widespread throughout the lung, or is fixed to the hilum
  d.   used when the tumor is confined to the bronchus or pulmonary artery and there is no evidence of metastasis

6.75 A new patient, Charles, undergoes transurethral resection of the prostate (TURP). He asks if this will cure the disease. You explain that:
   a. TURP is sometimes found to cure prostate cancer, but the chances diminish with patient age and tumor involvement
   b. TURP is used to treat symptoms of bladder outlet obstruction
   c. TURP provides pathological evidence that a cancer, previously unsuspected, is present
   d. b and c

Radiation

6.76 An important advantage of megavoltage equipment over conventional or orthovoltage equipment used in radiotherapy is that it:
   a. is more effective in treating surface lesions
   b. reduces absorption of radiation by bone
   c. delivers radioisotopes to the site of the tumor
   d. limits release of dangerous heavy ions and negative pi-mesons

6.77 Subjective systemic reactions to radiation, including fatigue, anorexia, and nausea are *most often* caused by:
   a. acute exposure of the organism to doses of radiation in a matter of minutes rather than hours or days
   b. chronic exposure of the whole body to low doses of radiation
   c. acute, site-specific reactions that occur at the cellular and molecular levels
   d. the release of toxic wastes into the bloodstream resulting from tumor destruction

6.78 The possibility of contamination of equipment, dressings, and linens is greatest when radioactive isotopes are delivered as:
   a. implants
   b. colloids or solutions
   c. moulds
   d. ovoids separated by a spacer

6.79 Compounds that assist in maximizing the tumor cell kill achieved with radiation while minimizing injury to normal tissues are called:
   a. radioantagonists
   b. radiosensitizers
   c. oxygen-enhancement ratios
   d. linear energy transfer

6.80 Nurses are often involved with managing the side effects that result from radiotherapy. To minimize the degree of the symptoms experienced, the nurse should schedule to see most patients:
   a. immediately after the first fractionated dose
   b. on completion of the scheduled 5-week course
   c. at the end of the first week
   d. 10–14 days after treatment has begun

6.81 Simulators are used in treatment planning for radiotherapy to localize a tumor and to:
   a. define the volume to be treated with radiotherapy
   b. remove a section of a tumor for a laboratory evaluation
   c. reduce the size of a tumor prior to surgical resection
   d. prepare a histopathologic profile of a tumor

6.82   Radiation effects take place primarily at the level of:
a.   cells
b.   tissues
c.   organs
d.   the whole body

6.83   One of the primary goals of dose fractionation is to:
a.   redistribute cell age within the cell cycle, making normal cells less radiosensitive
b.   allow tumor cells to repopulate, making them more vulnerable to the late consequences that occur if new growth was inhibited
c.   deliver a dose sufficient to prevent tumor cells from being repaired while allowing normal cells to recover before the next dose is given
d.   provide time between treatments for normal cells to reoxygenate, thus making them less radiosensitive

6.84   The late effects of radiation that are often seen 6 months or more after radiotherapy are the result of:
a.   cell damage in which mitotic activity is temporarily altered in some way
b.   acute damage that occurs to tissues and organs outside the treatment field
c.   the organism's attempt to repair the damage inflicted by ionizing radiation
d.   acute, site-specific reactions to treatment

6.85   The use of radiotherapy in the treatment of gastric cancer is limited by the:
a.   radiosensitivity of the tumor
b.   close proximity of the liver, kidneys, and spinal cord
c.   severity of the side effects experienced
d.   size of the tumor mass

6.86   Hank received prostatic brachytherapy with implantation of seeds of iodine-125. Which of the following is *not* included as part of your patient education plan for Hank and his family?
a.   Hank must remain hospitalized until the source that emits gamma radiation has completely decayed so that he is not a source of radiation to those around him.
b.   Hank's hospitalization will last until decay of the source is reduced to 30 millicuries or less.
c.   A condom should be worn during intercourse for 2 months after implantation.
d.   a and c

Biotherapy

6.87   Which of the following substances is *not* a cytokine?
a.   α-interferon
b.   interleukin-2
c.   levamisole
d.   tumor necrosis factor (TNF)

6.88   The drug regimen *least likely* to cause fatigue is:
a.   high daily schedules of interferon
b.   interleukins given in long-term outpatient regimens
c.   Mab or CSF therapy
d.   none of the above (all cause fatigue)

6.89 Which of the following patients is *most likely* to have an anaphylactoid reaction in response to therapy?
   a. Eddie, who is undergoing Mab therapy
   b. Ginny, who is undergoing interleukin therapy
   c. Meredith, who is taking IL-2
   d. a and b

6.90 Biologic response modifiers are:
   a. agents that restore, augment, or modulate host antitumor immune mechanisms
   b. cells or cellular products that have direct antitumor effects
   c. biological agents that have other biological antitumor effects
   d. all of the above

6.91 Among the therapeutic cellular activities of interferons (IFNs) are all of the following *except:*
   a. antiviral activity—protecting a virally infected cell attack by another virus
   b. immunomodulatory activity—interacting with T-lymphocytes that stimulate the cellular immune response
   c. antiproliferative activity—directly inhibiting DNA and protein synthesis in tumor cells
   d. immunoregulatory activity—mediating the proliferation and activation of hematopoietic factors

6.92 IFN therapy has been most effective in the treatment of what kinds of malignancies?
   a. solid tumors, especially colon and cervical cancers
   b. basal cell and other skin carcinomas
   c. hematologic diseases, including hairy cell leukemia
   d. metastatic foci when a low tumor burden exists

6.93 Most of the toxicities that occur with the administration of the various types of IFN appear to be related to:
   a. dose
   b. route of administration
   c. schedule
   d. IFN type

6.94 Ms. Nichols has just received intravesical bacillus Calmette-Guerin. The nurse should instruct her to:
   a. regard fever and cough as normal during treatment
   b. disinfect the toilet with bleach twice daily for 6 days
   c. retain the drug in her bladder for 2 hours
   d. all of the above

Antineoplastic Agents

6.95 The metabolic activation and inactivation or catabolism of drugs is carried out primarily by the:
   a. liver
   b. spleen
   c. gastrointestinal system
   d. kidneys

6.96   Chemotherapy drug resistance occurs primarily because the cancer cell has the ability to do which of the following?
    a.   increase the number of target enzymes
    b.   repair DNA lesions
    c.   modify target enzymes so as to interfere with binding to antagonistic drugs
    d.   all of the above

6.97   Which of the following nursing measures are useful to promote safe administration of oral antineoplastic agents?
    a.   administering oral methotrexate after radiation therapy
    b.   avoiding overdose by dispensing only one course of oral chemotherapy at a time
    c.   giving the patient a written schedule of when to take leucovorin following high-dose methotrexate
    d.   b and c

6.98   Which of the following statements regarding administration of a vesicant antineoplastic agent is *incorrect?*
    a.   An extravasation can occur despite an adequate blood return.
    b.   If a vein takes a nonvesicant without any problem, the vesicant will infuse without difficulty.
    c.   The risk of infiltration of any IV increases over time.
    d.   When administering a vesicant agent, it is wiser to administer any antiemetic or antianxiolytic agent *after* the vesicant.

6.99   Mrs. Collins has breast cancer and is about to begin docetaxel. She has taken her decadron as premedication. As you check her lab tests, you notice her liver function test results are elevated. Which of the following statements is important regarding your course of action?
    a.   The docetaxel should be delayed until liver function improves.
    b.   Docetaxel is eliminated by the kidney, so liver function is not important.
    c.   The docetaxel dose may need to be reduced because of elevated liver function results.
    d.   The steroid often causes an elevation of liver functions and can be ignored.

6.100   The rationale for the use of preoperative chemotherapy in patients with osteogenic sarcoma includes *all but* which of the following aspects?
    a.   It treats micrometastases.
    b.   It decreases the size of the primary tumor, possibly facilitating limb salvage surgery.
    c.   It enhances the effect of postoperative radiation.
    d.   It evaluates the effectiveness of the chemotherapy.

6.101   When telling Jeanne about cyclophosphamide, methotrexate, and 5-fluorouracil, you are careful to give her instructions regarding which of the following potential side effects?
    a.   severe thrombocytopenia and bleeding
    b.   symptoms of bladder infection as early signs of hemorrhagic cystitis
    c.   transient peripheral neuropathies
    d.   all of the above

6.102   Richard has advanced disseminated disease and receives an orchiectomy. Which treatment is the most likely choice for cytoreduction and potential cure?
    a.   a platinum-based regimen to follow up the orchiectomy
    b.   cisplatin, etoposide, and bleomycin
    c.   radiation plus chemotherapy
    d.   radiation alone

6.103   Although 5-fluorouracil is the cytotoxic agent of choice for colorectal cancer, it is most commonly administered in combination with:
a.   floxuridine (FUDR)
b.   CPT-11
c.   leucovorin
d.   none of the above

6.104   Mrs. Otis has been diagnosed with multiple myeloma and will begin therapy with melphalan and prednisone. You will monitor Mrs. Otis closely for adverse drug effects such as:
a.   decreased BUN and creatinine
b.   hypercalcemia and bone pain
c.   bone marrow–suppressive effects
d.   all of the above

Bone Marrow Transplant

6.105   In future allogeneic transplantations, the use of bone marrow may be replaced by the use of:
a.   blood cells
b.   chemotherapy
c.   irradiation
d.   syngeneic transplants

6.106   It is determined that Ms. Daniels, who had an allogeneic bone marrow transplant, will most likely need pharmacologic intervention as prophylaxis or treatment of graft versus host disease. What is the first-line therapy?
a.   methotrexate
b.   cyclosporine
c.   PUVA
d.   a cyclosporine and methotrexate combination

6.107   After transplantation, Ms. Daniels is monitored for complications. Naturally, you will monitor her for possible relapse and any related complications. Besides relapse, what reaction is the most common life-threatening complication experienced by BMT patients in response to preparative regimen–related toxicity?
a.   renal complication
b.   veno-occlusive disease
c.   congestive heart failure
d.   interstitial pneumonia

6.108   If Ms. Daniels were to acquire chronic GVHD as a late complication of BMT, which factor is *most likely* to be a causative risk factor?
a.   mismatched donor and recipient
b.   male-to-female transplant
c.   age under 18
d.   failure to receive methotrexate and cyclosporine as chronic GVHD prophylaxis in CML

6.109   Four patients with whom you have been working have asked about the possibility of marrow transplantation. The only patient for whom BMT may be a treatment choice is:
a.   Sibyl, who does not have SCIDS
b.   Derek, who has sickle cell anemia
c.   Francis, who has an HLA-matched sibling
d.   Molly, whose mother may be a match

6.110 Mr. Jackson is admitted for marrow infusion. He will receive allogeneic BMT and is about to undergo total-body irradiation. You tell him that TBI:
   a. offers optimal tumor cell kill but without penetrating the CNS
   b. is given before marrow infusion to prevent graft rejection by the patient's own immune system
   c. is usually given in single doses to reduce toxicities
   d. should not be given as a booster in any form to patients with bulky disease because of the risk of major organ toxicity

6.111 Blood cell transplant (BCT) involves:
   a. obtaining and infusing an unspecified number of true PPSCs
   b. infusion with committed progenitor cells
   c. infusion without precursor cells
   d. all of the above

6.112 A patient is first considered for bone marrow transplant. However, the physician selects blood cell transplantation as the treatment of choice, using peripheral PPSCs and progenitor cells obtained from peripheral blood. This procedure:
   a. delays recovery of neutrophils and platelets when progenitor cells are used
   b. enables neutrophils and platelets to recover rapidly
   c. involves collecting committed progenitors that are not as far along the differentiation pathway as the PPSCs harvested from the bone marrow
   d. b and c

6.113 Mrs. Adams has diseased marrow as a result of leukemia. Her physician plans a bone marrow transplant and chooses autologous rather than allogeneic BMT. Mrs. Adams tells you, "I've never heard of using a person's own bone marrow cells. Why would anyone do that when I'm the one with the disease?" You explain that autologous bone marrow transplantation:
   a. eliminates the risk of GVHD and other toxicities, such as myelosuppression
   b. is less toxic, although there is an increased risk of veno-occlusive disease
   c. reduces the risk of tumor contamination seen in allogeneic BMTs
   d. reduces the risk of the GVL effect (GVL effect can increase the risk of relapse)

IMMUNOLOGY

6.114 The macrophage:
   a. manufactures interleukin-3, -4, and -6 and alpha- and gamma-interferon to aid in its ultimate function of target cell wall damage
   b. is a glycoprotein product that initiates effector defense functions
   c. is a primary initiator to an inflammatory immune response
   d. a and c

6.115 How do most biologic response modifiers (BRMs) work?
   a. They control the growth of cells.
   b. They modulate the immune system.
   c. They control the maturation of cells.
   d. They target tumor cells through an antibody-antigen response.

6.116 Diseases such as Kaposi's sarcoma that are common in AIDS are referred to as *opportunistic*. This is because they:
   a. affect any or all organs and tissues in the body
   b. normally occur in a benign state in most individuals
   c. occur in patients with preexisting immunodeficiency
   d. affect only HIV-infected individuals who have other diseases

6.117 Which of the following best describes what cytokines do?
   a. They bind to surface receptors of target cells and act as regulators of cell growth or as mediators of defense functions.
   b. They are capable of nonspecific tumor cell killing.
   c. They are sedentary cells located in the spleen.
   d. They facilitate the attachment of an NK cell and other cytotoxic cells.

6.118 Which of the following is *not* included in a teaching plan for a patient beginning levamisole?
   a. The main action of levamisole is to restore the immune system.
   b. The purpose of the drug is to cause mitotic arrest of colon cancer cells.
   c. Patients should avoid drinking alcohol while taking levamisole.
   d. Side effects include nausea, skin rash, and flu-like syndrome.

6.119 The scientific basis for using immunotherapy to treat cutaneous melanoma (CM) is based on which of the following observations?
   a. Patients with CM treated with chemotherapy generally do not respond.
   b. Patients with CM generally have a negative skin test and a poor immune response.
   c. Patients with CM experience more spontaneous remissions than do persons with other adult tumors.
   d. Patients with lymphocytic infiltrates at the tumor site have a worse prognosis.

6.120 Each of the following is an important function of the body's immune system *except*:
   a. protecting the body against injury from foreign substances
   b. preserving the body's internal environment
   c. preventing the growth of aberrant cells that might develop into neoplasms
   d. providing support and nourishment to the body's genetic machinery

6.121 The body is generally able to respond to a nonself invader cell more quickly and powerfully the second time it encounters such as cell than it did the first time, even if months have passed between invasions. Which of the following cells is *most closely* related to this ability?
   a. PMN granulocytes
   b. memory B lymphocytes
   c. NK cells
   d. mononuclear phagocytes

6.122 Antibody is the final product in the differentiation of:
   a. B lymphocytes
   b. helper T lymphocytes
   c. mononuclear phagocytes
   d. suppressor T lymphocytes

GENETICS

6.123   Which of the following is the *best* example of the role of genetic predisposition in the development of cancer?
   a.   The mortality rates for Japanese Americans with stomach cancer are significantly higher than those for the white American population.
   b.   As more women smoke, more women are developing lung cancer.
   c.   A study of Johns Hopkins medical students found that 55 students who later developed cancer perceived themselves as less close to their parents than did their healthy counterparts.
   d.   Familial aggregates of cancer have been found to occur.

6.124   Which of the following statements best describes the significance of the *BRCA1* gene?
   a.   It is an inherited gene that identifies women who are ensured of having breast cancer during their premenopausal years.
   b.   It is an inherited gene mutation that identifies families at significant risk for breast cancer and ovarian cancer.
   c.   It is an inherited gene mutation that identifies women likely to have breast cancer in their postmenopausal years.
   d.   It is an inherited gene that is present in over 90% of women with breast cancer.

6.125   Approximately what percentage of human cancers have a hereditary component?
   a.   15%
   b.   20%
   c.   25%
   d.   30%

6.126   Which of the following statements regarding our understanding of the genetic susceptibility in breast cancer is *not* correct?
   a.   The *BRCA1* gene is associated with increased susceptibility to both breast and ovarian cancer.
   b.   The *BRCA2* gene is associated only with an increased susceptibility to breast cancer.
   c.   The genes are estimated to be involved in 20% of breast cancer cases.
   d.   The genes are associated with breast cancer diagnosed at an early age.

6.127   Which of the following statements regarding genetic susceptibility to colon cancer is *not* correct?
   a.   Individuals who have a first-degree relative with colorectal cancer have double the risk for developing colon cancer.
   b.   Adenomatous polyps are considered to be precursors of colorectal carcinoma.
   c.   An inheritable autosomal dominant trait is found in families with a high incidence of colon cancer.
   d.   Individuals who have nonpolyposis syndrome are at a 50% risk for developing cancer of the colon.

6.128   Knudson observed that acquired retinoblastoma occurs as a single tumor, whereas children with hereditary retinoblastoma had multiple primary tumors. What does this observation suggest about retinoblastoma?
   a.   Retinoblastoma must result from a proto-oncogene left permanently in the "on" position.
   b.   All cells in the retinal tissue of an affected eye are genetically predisposed to retinoblastoma.
   c.   Retinoblastoma must be the result of recessive inheritance.
   d.   Only one copy of the retinoblastoma gene is needed for the malignancy to be expressed.

6.129   Which of the following variables appears to be the best descriptive determinant of cancer risk?
   a.   The mortality rates for Japanese Americans with stomach cancer are significantly higher than for the white American population.
   b.   As more women smoke, more women are developing lung cancer.
   c.   A study of Johns Hopkins medical students found that 55 students who later developed cancer perceived themselves as less close to their parents than did their healthy counterparts.
   d.   Familial aggregates of cancer have been found to occur.

6.130   Which of the following cancer-causing mutations is transmitted to the next generation at birth?
   a.   oncogene mutations
   b.   germ cell mutations
   c.   somatic mutations
   d.   antioncogene mutations

ANSWER EXPLANATIONS

6.1   **The answer is c.** Suppressor proteins "turn off" cell growth. Since the genes coding for these proteins have an opposite function to that of oncogenes, they are called antioncogenes; because they suppress malignant growth, they are also called cancer-suppressor genes.

6.2   **The answer is b.** The *p53* gene is one of the most important of the cancer-suppressor genes. Not only is it the most frequently mutated, but when it is not mutated, another abnormal gene blocks the *p53* protein. The protein product of *p53* is the "guardian of the genome." DNA viruses produce proteins that inactivate the *p53* protein.

6.3   **The answer is a.** In clonal selection, mutation in the genome of a cell may confer a survival advantage on that cell. The cell grows stronger, not weaker, with each mutation. The cancer cell is immortal because it seems to lack the "biological clocks" like *telomeres,* which are not completely duplicated during cell division, and thus grow progressively shorter until the chromosome can no longer replicate. In cancer, the final common path of action is through oncogenes, the growth-promoting genes: oncogenes must be mutated or relocated to be activated.

6.4   **The answer is c.** Carcinogenesis is ordinarily classified as chemical, viral, physical, or familial, even though it is likely that human carcinogenesis involves a combination of factors. Carcinogenesis can also be classified as occupational, dietary, environmental, lifestyle, and so forth.

6.5   **The answer is b.** Familial carcinogenesis is based in large part on a group of genes that, when mutated, cause cancer by their absence; that is, they seem to prevent cancer when they are functioning normally. These protective genes are the cancer-suppressor genes. The loss of the normal copy of a gene by the process of mitotic recombination is referred to as *loss of heterogeneity* or *reduction to homozygosity* because the cell becomes homozygous for the abnormal gene, thus losing its ability to prevent malignant growth.

6.6   **The answer is d.** Tumor-associated viruses probably are necessary but not sufficient for tumor causation. The discovery of cancer-causing viruses in humans shows some promise for cancer prevention in that similar viruses in animals have been eliminated by vaccines made from the attenuated (inactivated) viruses.

6.7   **The answer is c.** Chemoprevention is the most promising form of host modification, using nutrients or pharmacological agents to inhibit or reverse carcinogenesis. Proto-oncogenes are most likely involved in initiation and promotion of cancer. The theoretical disruption of carcinogenesis at several points provides the rationale for use of chemopreventive agents. Agents that inhibit carcinogenesis generally are classified by the point in the process at which they are effective. Chemoprevention has the potential for primary, secondary, and tertiary prevention.

6.8   **The answer is b.** The *ras* oncogenes appear to function early in the process of carcinogenesis and may be a good target for early detection.

6.9   **The answer is d.** The epidemiological evidence for the viral etiology of cancer is strongest for a relationship between hepatitis B virus (HBV) and hepatocellular carcinoma and between human T-cell leukemia virus type 1 (HTLV-1) and T-cell lymphoma.

6.10   **The answer is d.** It is believed that dietary factors affect the exposure of the GI tract to promoters of carcinogenesis. Fats increase the production, and change the composition, of bile salts. These altered bile salts are converted into potential carcinogens. Fiber decreases the effects of fatty acids and may actually protect against the disease, even in the presence of a high-fat diet. Fiber may limit the time the colon is exposed to cancer promoters by speeding intestinal transit time.

6.11   **The answer is b.** The cornerstone of induction therapy in AML is the cell-cycle–specific antimetabolite cytosine arabinoside, plus an anthracycline such as daunorubicin.

6.12   **The answer is b.** Lymphomas are preeminently a malignancy of the lymphocyte. However, there seems to be a separate malignancy for each sequential stage in the developmental sequence from primitive to mature lymphocyte. At each stage of development, the potential exists for the normal maturing lymphocyte to be transformed into a cancer cell. Once transformed, the new clone of malignant cells follows the behavioral pattern of the stage of the lymphocyte at which the transformation occurred. For example, if the function of the maturing cell at the time it is transformed is secretion of an antibody, the tumor cells continue to secrete that normal protein in abnormal quantities. HD and NHL are distinguished on the basis of the Reed-Sternberg giant cells in NHL. The information in choice **d** is reversed.

6.13   **The answer is a.** BCC is the most common form of skin cancer in whites and outnumbers SCC by a ratio of 3:1. Nonmelanoma skin cancers, including BCC, have a higher incidence but a lower metastatic potential and mortality rate than malignant melanoma. Malignant melanoma has a much lower incidence but a mortality rate that is triple that of the nonmelanoma cancers. Increased mortality is directly related to its high potential for metastasis.

6.14   **The answer is a.** The purpose of postremission therapies is to prevent leukemic recurrence related to minimal residual disease. The three types of post-remission therapies are consolidation therapy, intensification therapy, maintenance therapy, and bone marrow transplant (BMT). Consolidation therapy consists of one or two courses of very high doses of the same drugs used for induction (up to 30 times the induction doses of cytosine arabinoside for AML). Intensification regimens use different drugs in the hope that they will not be cross-resistant. Maintenance therapies use lower doses for a prolonged period of time. Maintenance therapy is not currently recommended the treatment of AML.

6.15   **The answer is d.** Approximately 90% of patients with CML have the diagnostic marker Philadelphia chromosome Ph^1.

6.16   **The answer is d.** Although some bone tumors metastasize to the lymph nodes (e.g., Ewing's sarcoma), few, if any, seem to metastasize to the CNS or liver. Most of the more common bone tumors metastasize to the lungs. Whether or not these metastases develop, and when, depends on the stage and aggressiveness of the disease process.

6.17   **The answer is d.** Breast cancer primarily metastasizes to the bone, liver, lungs, nodes, and brain—but not the gastrointestinal tract.

6.18   **The answer is c.** The glioblastoma multiforme (GBM) is the most common adult primary brain tumor. It is most common in individuals who are 50 or older. It shares all the characteristics of anaplastic astrocytoma plus necrosis.

6.19   **The answer is d.** A number of predisposing conditions have been associated with an increased risk of colorectal cancer. These include chronic ulcerative colitis, Crohn's disease, familial polyposis, and a strong family history of predisposition to colon cancer and familial adenomatous polyposis.

6.20   **The answer is c.** A complaint of low back pain frequently indicates that the cancer has spread into the retroperitoneal lymph nodes.

6.21   **The answer is d.** In multiple myeloma, the malignant cell is the plasma cell, the functional mature cell that differentiates and develops from the B lymphocytes.

6.22   **The answer is d.** The major goals of the diagnostic evaluation for a suspected cancer are to determine the tissue type of the malignancy, the primary site of the malignancy, the extent of disease within the body, and also the tumor's potential to recur in the future.

6.23   **The answer is b.** In the case of liver cancer, CT has been preferred for imaging, but MRI with contrast may be equivalent. Ultrasound is preferred for differentiating biliary obstruction from hepatic parenchymal disease.

6.24   **The answer is c.** Ultrasonography (US) can be used to discriminate masses. A *limitation* of the exam is its *inability* to visualize through bone or air. US is most applicable in detecting tumors within the pelvis, the retroperitoneum, and the peritoneum of patients with cancer.

6.25   **The answer is a.** MRI is most applicable in the detection, localization, and staging of malignant disease in the CNS, spine, head and neck, and musculoskeletal system. This imaging method creates sectional images of the body but does not expose the patient to ionizing radiation. It is nuclear imaging, and not MRI, that uses radio-labeled monoclonal antibodies to visualize microscopic sites of metastasis or suspected malignancy. MRI can be enhanced with IV contrast agents.

6.26 **The answer is d.** Since Mrs. Ellis displays no symptoms of bone involvement, a bone scan would not be appropriate. CA-15-3 is used to monitor metastatic disease, not as an early detection test.

6.27 **The answer is d.** Sputum cytology has a diagnostic yield of up to 80% for central tumors, but less than 20% for small peripheral tumors. It is the chest radiograph, however, that is probably the most helpful diagnostic study for lung cancer, and CT can be particularly helpful in evaluating mediastinal lymph nodes.

6.28 **The answer is c.** The diagnosis of lymphoma can be established only by a biopsy of involved tissue, usually a lymph node. Because there are many causes of lymphadenopathy, however—including upper respiratory infection; infectious mononucleosis; allergic reactions; and, in older people, cancer of the head and neck—a careful history and physical examination must first determine whether an enlarged lymph node should be biopsied. For persistent lymphadenopathy or when etiology is not known, a biopsy is usually indicated.

6.29 **The answer is a.** Biopsy is the initial surgical procedure for suspected CM. Because it provides a definitive diagnosis along with microstaging information, an excisional biopsy that entails removal of a few millimeters of normal tissue surrounding the lesion is preferable. An incisional biopsy can be used for lesions in cosmetically sensitive areas or for large lesions. Electrocoagulation, curettage, shaving, and burning are never used to remove a suspicious mole.

6.30 **The answer is d.** Inguinal orchiectomy remains the standard approach for definitive pathological diagnosis. A biopsy or transcrotal approach orchiectomy can cause possible spread of tumor. Both a fine-needle biopsy and a transcrotal approach are contraindicated.

6.31 **The answer is d.** The Pap smear is an effective technique for detecting cervical cancer. When the Pap report shows SIL, biopsy, colposcopy and/or treatment is indicated.

6.32 **The answer is c.** Adenocarcinomas are the most common lung cancer in males, in females, and in nonsmokers, accounting for 40% of all tumors. The squamous cell carcinomas constitute 30% of all lung cancers and are more common in males than in females. They are also the ones that arise from the basal cells of the bronchial epithelium and usually present as masses in large bronchi. Finally, the large cell carcinomas, and not the adenocarcinomas, are the least common type of lung cancer, representing approximately 10–15%.

6.33 **The answer is a.** Carcinoma specifies a malignant tumor arising from epithelial tissues. Epithelium covers or lines surfaces within the body and arises from the ectodermal, mesodermal, or endodermal embryonic layer.

6.34 **The answer is d.** The histological classification most frequently will be adenocarcinoma, but the site of origin may never be determined, even on autopsy.

6.35 **The answer is d.** There are multiple objectives of solid-tumor staging, but the most important is to provide the necessary information for individual treatment planning. Other reasons for using a uniform staging system are to give prognostic information, to assist in treatment evaluation, to facilitate the exchange of information and comparative statistics among the treatment centers, and to stratify individuals who may be eligible for clinical trials.

6.36 **The answer is d.** A stage grouping of Stage III, T4, N2, MO is consistent with a clinical exam that reveals evidence of an extensive primary tumor with fixation to a deeper structure, bone invasion, and lymph nodes of a similar nature. Typically, in such a stage, the lesion may be operable but not resectable, and gross disease is left behind.

6.37 **The answer is a.** A benign tumor is well circumscribed or encapsulated; microscopically, it appears orderly and comprises cells similar to those of its parent tissue. A malignant tumor invades both the organs from which it originated and eventually the surrounding tissues, and it is made up of cells that vary greatly in size and shape.

6.38 **The answer is d.** Malignant tumors arising in glandular epithelial tissues are known as adenocarcinomas.

6.39 **The answer is b.** The term *carcinoma in situ* describes a lesion characterized by full-thickness neoplastic change with no evidence of stromal invasion or metastases.

6.40 **The answer is a.** Bronchogenic cancers are grouped into small cell lung cancer (SCLC) and the non–small cell lung cancers (NSCLC), which include squamous cell carcinoma, adenocarcinoma, and large cell carcinoma. Many tumors are heterogeneous, containing cells from more than one histological type. In both types of cancer, both hyperplasia and carcinoma in situ occur.

6.41 **The answer is a.** In the TNM system, the extent of the primary tumor (T) is evaluated on the basis of depth of invasion, surface spread, and tumor size. The absence or presence and extent of regional lymph node (N) metastasis are considered and the presence of distant metastasis (M) is assessed. The system is further classified by whether the assessment is obtained clinically (cTNM or TNM), after pathological review (pTNM), at the time of retreatment (rTNM), or on autopsy (aTNM).

6.42 **The answer is a.** Stage groupings involve combining the various classification elements of tumor site, regional lymph node involvement, and the presence or absence of metastasis. It involves two main staging periods: pretreatment and retreatment. The two aspects of pretreatment staging of a previously undiagnosed cancer are clinical diagnostic staging, for patients who have had a biopsy, and *postsurgical resection-pathological* staging, which includes a complete evaluation of the surgical specimen by a pathologist.

6.43 **The answer is b.** Restaging focuses particular attention on the disease parameters that were positive at diagnosis, to signal a search for any remaining evidence that treatment should continue. Restaging does not imply that if a remission is obtained the patient reverts to a lesser disease stage. The stage ascribed at the time of diagnosis is the one referenced throughout the illness.

6.44 **The answer is a.** The overall prognosis for cancer of the renal pelvis is poor, with 5-year survival rates of only approximately 40%. This figure is 60% for low-grade, low-stage cancers and drops to 0–33% for higher grades.

6.45 **The answer is b.** The AJCC staging system for lung cancer uses the TNM letters. *T* designates primary tumor and is divided into categories relative to size, location, and invasion. *N*, with three categories, represents regional lymph node status. *M* designates the absence or presence of distant metastases. Lung cancer is also divided into eight stages, each of which is distinctive relative to treatment and 5-year survival statistics. Small cell lung cancer is usually staged using a simple two-stage system. Because most SCLC patients have metastatic disease at the time of diagnosis, this system describes the extent of disease as either "limited" or "extensive."

6.46   **The answer is b.** Determination of the stage of disease in HD is important because it influences which treatment option (radiation therapy or combination therapy) is used. Radiation is very effective for localized HD and is therefore used in early-stage disease. Chemotherapy is more effective than radiation for late-stage disease, when the number of lymph node groups involved is greater, but it also is as effective as radiation in early-stage disease. NHL, on the other hand, is almost always treated with chemotherapy because it usually presents at an advanced stage. A positive bone marrow biopsy indicates a stage IV tumor. A stage II presentation for HD is more likely to indicate a slow-growing malignancy; it is not at all uncommon.

6.47   **The answer is b.** All the other choices, along with a history and physical examination, are standard procedures used in the staging of lymphoma. Other procedures, including a CT scan of the chest and abdomen, a bone marrow biopsy, a percutaneous liver biopsy, a lower limb lymphangiogram (LAG), and an exploratory laparotomy may be done if there is evidence of lymph node involvement below the diaphragm, hepatomegaly or abnormal liver function, extension of the lymphoma to mediastinal lymph nodes, or splenomegaly. Positive results on these tests often indicate a stage IV disease.

6.48   **The answer is b.** Melanoma has been classified into several types, including lentigo maligna (LMM), superficial spreading (SSM), nodular, and acral lentiginous. Each type is characterized by a radial and/or vertical growth phase. In the radial phase, tumor growth is parallel to the skin surface, risk of metastasis is slight, and surgical excision is usually curative. The vertical growth phase is marked by focal deep penetration of atypical melanocytes into the dermis and subcutaneous tissue. Penetration occurs rapidly, increasing the risk of metastasis.

6.49   **The answer is c.** Whereas intermediate-grade tumors can be treated with either chemotherapy or radiation therapy, depending on the stage at presentation, advanced intermediate/high-grade lymphoma is treated with combination chemotherapy. Cyclophosphamide, the most active and effective agent, commonly is used in combination with other agents. Initial responses are usually dramatic but are not long-lived; relapse typically occurs in 4–6 weeks following discontinuation of chemotherapy. In addition, treatment-related neutropenia is severe and sometimes precipitates an opportunistic infection.

6.50   **The answer is c.** Alpha-fetoprotein is a tumor marker that is elevated in the serum of 70–90% of individuals with primary hepatocellular carcinoma, but because levels of alpha-fetoprotein are not specific for liver cancer, histologic diagnosis is required.

6.51   **The answer is c.** A secondary, or metastatic tumor resembles the primary tumor histologically. A second primary lesion refers to an additional, histologically separate malignant neoplasm in the same patient.

6.52   **The answer is b.** For selected tumors, the grade is considered more significant than anatomic staging in terms of prognostic value and treatment. In soft tissue sarcomas, the grade is the primary determinant of stage of disease and of prognosis. In other tumors, such as melanoma, testicular cancer, and thyroid cancer, histological grading has no useful application.

6.53   **The answer is d.** A G2 rating means the tumor is moderately well differentiated. The AJCC recommends the following grading classification:
GX = grade cannot be assessed
G1 = well differentiated
G2 = moderately well differentiated
G3 = poorly differentiated
G4 = undifferentiated

6.54   **The answer is c.** Histopathological type is a qualitative assessment whereby a neoplasm is categorized in terms of the tissue or cell type from which it has originated. Histopathological *grade* is a quantitative assessment of the extent to which the tumor resembles the tissue of origin. A lesion with the same cell type but at a site other than the original site indicates a metastatic tumor; a different cell type originating from another lesion anywhere in the body indicates a second primary cancer.

6.55   **The answer is d.** Clinically important cancers include features such as large tumor volume; Gleason grade 3–5; an invasive, proliferative pattern of growth; elevated PSA; and origination in the peripheral zone. These cancers threaten the patient's life because they progress to fatal metastatic cancers. The vast majority of prostate cancers do not threaten the patient's life and are termed *indolent*.

6.56   **The answer is d.** The primary application of flow cytometry analysis in solid tumors has been to determine DNA content and the percentage of cells synthesizing DNA. Normal DNA is characterized as diploid and contrasts with abnormal, disorganized DNA that is aneuploid.

6.57   **The answer is c.** Although gross hematuria, bladder neck obstruction, and pain in the suprapubic region can all be clinical manifestations of bladder cancer, the most important indicator of disease progression is the depth of tumor penetration into the bladder wall.

6.58   **The answer is d.** The larger the tumor and the more positive nodes involved, the worse the prognosis is.

6.59   **The answer is d.** For HD, prognosis is most closely related to stage. Age and the total number of lymph node groups involved (independent of stage) are other prognostic factors, whereas for NHL prognosis is most closely related to histologic type.

6.60   **The answer is b.** For patients over 70, watchful waiting may be an appropriate option. Research has yet to demonstrate that, for those with stage A or B cancer, treatment is more beneficial than watchful waiting. For men under 70, a physician may often be reluctant to offer watchful waiting, and there is evidence that for younger men with moderately or poorly differentiated localized prostate cancer, treatment may offer a survival advantage.

6.61   **The answer is d.** Microstaging describes the level of invasion of the CM and maximum tumor thickness. The two parameters that are used in assessing the depth of invasion are the anatomic level of invasion or the Clark level and the thickness of tumor tissue or the Breslow level. The prognosis for patients with metastatic disease at the time of diagnosis is poor, with most dying within 5 years. As CM thickness increases, survival rates decrease. Thus, the Breslow level has consistently proved to be a significant prognostic variable in stage I CM.

6.62   **The answer is d.** Chest x-rays and chest scans, together with serum tumor markers consisting of the beta subunit of human chorionic gonadotropin (BHCG) and alpha-fetoprotein (AFP), can be useful in staging testicular cancer and in documenting disease recurrence, as well as in monitoring response to treatment.

6.63 **The answer is d.** A high tumor cell doubling time means he has a favorable prognosis.

6.64 **The answer is a.** In oncology, "cure" is a statistical term that applies to groups of cancer patients rather than to individuals. An individual's normal recovery—with the return to health, weight gain, and the resumption of normal activity—is not conclusive evidence that a cure has been achieved. The nature of cancer is such that even after a long interval of apparent health, the disease may reappear and the person may die. If at autopsy there is no evidence of tumor, a cancer can be said to have been cured, but this is of little practical value.

6.65 **The answer is a.** Poor prognosis has been associated with obstructing or perforating carcinomas, occurrence in young people, location of the tumor below the peritoneal reflection, lymph node involvement, venous invasion, hepatic metastasis, and invasion of the bowel wall.

6.66 **The answer is b.** Radiation is usually indicated if the tumor is found to be invading nearby tissues that cannot be surgically resected. Chemotherapy is used to eliminate micrometastasis.

6.67 **The answer is d.** Situations lending themselves best to surgical treatment include such factors as slow-growing tumors that consist of cells with prolonged cell cycles. A surgical procedure intended to be curative must involve resection of the entire tumor mass as well as a margin of safety of normal, healthy tissue surrounding the tumor. Superficial and encapsulated tumors are more easily resected than those that are embedded in inaccessible or delicate tissues.

6.68 **The answer is c.** Superficial and encapsulated tumors are more easily resected than those that are embedded in inaccessible or delicate tissues or those that have invaded tissues and organs in multiple directions.

6.69 **The answer is b.** Breast reconstruction, although not curative, is considered a reconstructive rather than a palliative procedure. The goal of palliative surgery is to relieve suffering and minimize the symptoms of the disease—for example, amputation of a nonfunctional, painful limb with sarcoma or procedures such as fulguration, electrocoagulation, photodynamic therapy, and bond stabilization.

6.70 **The answer is c.** Because the esophagus is thin-walled and draws upward with each swallow, an anastomosis involving the esophagus has more of a tendency to leak than any other area of the gastrointestinal tract. For this reason, contrast studies are performed 4–6 days after surgery to check for patency of the anastomosis. Small leaks usually close spontaneously; larger leaks often require surgical approximation.

6.71 **The answer is c.** Possible contraindications to major hepatic resection for liver cancer include the following: (1) severe cirrhosis; (2) distant metastases in the lung, bone, or lymph nodes; (3) jaundice, which is often indicative of obstruction of the common bile duct; (4) ascites, which is usually indicative of liver failure and an inability to tolerate a surgical procedure; (5) poor visualization on angiographic studies, which may jeopardize the certainty with which the surgeon resects the tumor; (6) certain biochemical changes that indicate poor liver function and lower the probability of survival; and (7) involvement of the inferior vena cava or portal vein, which would make surgical intervention hazardous.

6.72 **The answer is a.** In women, a radical cystectomy includes the removal of the bladder, urethra, uterus, ovaries, fallopian tubes, and anterior wall of the vagina. In men, the term is synonymous with prostatectomy and includes excision of the bladder with pericystic sac, the attached perineum, the prostate, and the seminal vesicles.

6

6.73 **The answer is a.** Surgical resection is considered standard treatment for stage I (like Mr. Keller's) and stage II (like Ms. Harris's) NSCLC and is performed with the intent to cure the patient. Controversy exists regarding the appropriate treatment for stage IIIA patients, particularly those who have ipsilateral mediastinal lymph node involvement. Most surgeons consider stage IIIB and stage IV lung cancer to be inoperable.

6.74 **The answer is c.** Pneumonectomy is performed only if a tumor cannot be completely excised by lobectomy. It is chosen when the tumor involves the proximal bronchus, is widespread throughout the lung, or is fixed to the hilum. Sleeve resection with bronchoplastic reconstruction is used when the tumor is confined to the bronchus or pulmonary artery and there is no evidence of metastasis. Finally, lobectomy is the most common surgical procedure performed for primary lung cancer that is confined to a single lobe of the lung.

6.75 **The answer is d.** Prostate cancer is not cured by TURP. Rather, TURP is used to treat symptoms of bladder outlet obstruction and, in some patients, provides pathological evidence that a cancer, previously unsuspected, is present.

6.76 **The answer is b.** Megavoltage equipment operates at 2–40 million electron volts (MeV), compared to orthovoltage equipment's 40,000–400,000 electron volts (Kv). It has the advantages of deeper beam penetration, more homogeneous absorption of radiation (minimizing bone absorption), and greater skin sparing. Megavoltage equipment includes cobalt and cesium units, the linear accelerator, the betatron, and such experimental units as those producing neutron beams, heavy ions, and negative pi-mesons.

6.77 **The answer is d.** The presence of these toxins may account for the nausea and anorexia, whereas the increased metabolic rate required to dispose of the waste products might be partially responsible for the frequent complaint of fatigue. The extent of these effects depends on the volume of the irradiated area, the anatomic site, and the dose.

6.78 **The answer is b.** In addition to radioactive implantation, some radioactive isotopes are administered orally or intravenously or by instillation. Liquid sources administered as colloids or solutions are adsorbed or metabolized and present a possibility of contamination of equipment, dressings, and linens, depending on the mode of administration and metabolism.

6.79 **The answer is b.** Efforts to improve the therapeutic ratio have resulted in the development of certain compounds that act to increase the radiosensitivity of tumor cells or to protect normal cells from radiation effect. Radiosensitizers are compounds that apparently promote fixation of the free radicals produced by radiation damage at the molecular level.

6.80 **The answer is d.** During a course of radiotherapy, certain treatment-related side effects can be expected to develop, most of which are site specific as well as dependent on volume, dose fractionation, total dose, and individual differences. Many symptoms do not develop until approximately 10–14 days into treatment, and some do not subside until 2 or more weeks after treatments have ended.

6.81 **The answer is a.** Simulator machinery may involve the use of diagnostic x-rays, fluoroscopic examination, transverse axial tomography, CT scans, and ultrasound, with the goal of localizing a tumor and defining the volume to be treated with radiotherapy. Other aspects of treatment planning include the tattooing of the treatment area, installing various restraining and positioning devices to immobilize the person, shaping the field, and determining what structures are to be blocked and protected from radiation.

6.82   **The answer is a.** The biologic effects of radiation on humans are the result of a sequence of events that follows the absorption of energy from ionizing radiation and the body's attempt to compensate for this assault. Radiation effect takes place at the cellular level, with consequences in tissues, organs, and the entire body.

6.83   **The answer is c.** All of the other choices are opposites of the actual goals of fractionation. Fractionation redistributes cell age within the cell cycle, making tumor cells more radiosensitive. It allows normal cells to repopulate, sparing them from some of the late consequences that occur if new growth is inhibited. It also provides time between treatments for tumor cells to reoxygenate, thus making them more radiosensitive.

6.84   **The answer is c.** Effects of radiation may be acute and immediate (seen within the first 6 months) or may be late (seen after 6 months). Acute effects are due to cell damage in which mitotic activity is altered. If early effects are not reversible, late or permanent tissue changes occur. These late effects are due to the organism's attempt to heal or repair the damage inflicted by ionizing radiation.

6.85   **The answer is b.** Gastric adenocarcinomas are generally radiosensitive; however, the close proximity to dose-limiting organs in the abdomen (i.e., the liver, kidney, and spinal cord) restricts the use of radiotherapy as a treatment modality.

6.86   **The answer is a.** After insertion of the source, hospitalization lasts until decay of the source is reduced to 30 millicuries or less. A condom should be worn during intercourse for 2 months after implantation, but the patient poses no danger as a radioactive source.

6.87   **The answer is c.** Cytokines (which include lymphokines) are substances released from activated immune system cells that affect the behavior of other cells. They may alter the growth and metastasis of cancer cells by augmenting the responsiveness of T cells to tumor-associated antigens, enhancing the effectiveness of B cell activity, or decreasing suppressive functions of the immune system, thereby enhancing immune responsiveness. Included among the cytokines are the interferons and interleukins, tumor necrosis factor (TNF), and colony-stimulating factors (CSFs).

6.88   **The answer is c.** Daily schedules of interferon at doses of 20 million units or greater can result in profound toxicity, including fatigue. Fatigue is a common side effect with nearly all interleukins, particularly in long-term outpatient regimens. Fatigue is not a common side effect of either Mabs or CSFs.

6.89   **The answer is a.** Anaphylactoid reactions have most commonly occurred with Mab therapy. Although anaphylaxis is not described with interferons and most interleukins, high-dose IL-2 administration has been associated with the development of increased sensitivity to other agents.

6.90   **The answer is d.** Biologic response modifiers can be classified as agents that restore, augment, or modulate host antitumor immune mechanisms; cells or cellular products that have direct antitumor effects; and biological agents that have other biological antitumor effects.

6.91   **The answer is d.** The IFNs are a family of naturally occurring complex proteins that belong to the cytokine family. Each of the three major types in humans—α-IFN, β-IFN, and γ-IFN—originates from a different cell and has distinct biologic and chemical properties. All three types of IFNs exhibit the cellular effects listed in choices **a–c**.

6.92   **The answer is c.** Hematologic diseases have responded best to IFN therapy, with measurable responses occurring in the lymphoproliferative malignancies (such as hairy cell leukemia, non-Hodgkin's lymphoma, and multiple myeloma) and in chronic myelogenous and AIDS-associated Kaposi's sarcoma.

6.93   **The answer is a.** It appears that most IFN toxicities, as well as toxicities from most other BRMs, are dose related. Low doses of IFN are well tolerated, whereas high doses often require cessation of therapy. A common reaction to any type of IFN is the occurrence of fever, chills, fatigue, and malaise, referred to collectively as flu-like syndrome.

6.94   **The answer is c.** If possible, following instillation the patient is encouraged to retain the drug for 2 hours in the bladder. A cough can indicate a BCG infection. For home administration, the toilet is disinfected with bleach after every voiding for the first 6 hours.

6.95   **The answer is a.** The metabolic activation and inactivation or catabolism of drugs is carried out primarily by the liver.

6.96   **The answer is d.** Cancer cells can overcome the effects of cytotoxic drugs either by increasing the number of target enzymes or by modifying the enzyme so as to interfere with binding to antagonistic drugs. The ability of cells to repair DNA lesions is an important resistance mechanism seen with alkylating agents and cisplatin.

6.97   **The answer is d.** With therapy such as leucovorin following methotrexate, noncompliance could be fatal. Therefore, give the patient a written schedule to follow, and avoid overdose by giving only one course of oral drug at a time.

6.98   **The answer is b.** It is faulty reasoning to assume that if a vein takes a nonvesicant without any problem, the vesicant will infuse without difficulty. The risk of infiltration of *any* IV increases over time. Other drugs often can cause venous irritation and even spasm that can result in a loss of blood return, a major assessment criteria for safe administration of chemotherapy.

6.99   **The answer is c.** Docetaxel is metabolized by the liver, and elevated liver functions can interfere with metabolism, causing enhanced toxicity of docetaxel. The dose needs to be reduced.

6.100   **The answer is c.** Chemotherapy currently is given preoperatively. The rationale for preoperative chemotherapy is to treat micrometastasis, to decrease the size of the primary tumor (thereby increasing the likelihood of limb-salvage surgery), and to assess the effectiveness of the chemotherapeutic agents for 2–3 months. The route of the chemotherapy is either intravenous or intra-arterial.

6.101   **The answer is b.** Side effects associated with CMF include myelosuppression, hair loss, and hemorrhagic cystitis.

6.102   **The answer is b.** Chemotherapy is the mainstay of treatment in men with advanced or bulky disease. Following orchiectomy, initial cisplatin-based chemotherapy is recommended for cytoreduction and potential cure. The most widely used front-line regimen is BEP.

6.103   **The answer is c.** Although 5-fluorouracil is the cytotoxic agent of choice for colorectal cancer, it is most commonly administered in combination with leucovorin. Floxuridine (FUDR) is used in intraportal chemotherapy through the portal vein or hepatic artery into the liver in individuals with metastasis to the liver.

6.104   **The answer is c.** Patients are monitored closely for signs of renal impairment (increased BUN and creatinine, proteinuria), and the dose of melphalan may need to be reduced based on the severity of renal toxicity. It is also important to closely monitor serial blood counts because the bone marrow–suppressive effects of melphalan may be cumulative in older patients. Hypercalcemia and bone pain are symptoms of the disorder itself, rather than adverse effects.

6.105   **The answer is a.** The use of blood cells, rather than marrow, for allogeneic transplantation is becoming an important area of study. Blood cell transplantation may replace marrow transplantation in the next millennium. The availability of bone marrow makes possible the administration of chemoradiotherapy in supralethal doses—so it is unlikely that chemotherapy or irradiation will replace BMT. Syngeneic transplants do not indicate an alternative treatment, but rather represent a specific source—that of a twin.

6.106   **The answer is d.** Immunosuppressive therapy is aimed at removing or inactivating T-lymphocytes that attack target organs. Cyclosporine and methotrexate inhibit T-lymphocytes that are believed to be responsible for acute GVHD and are the first-line therapy. Used in combination, they are more effective than either agent alone. Several studies demonstrate encouraging results for patients with acute GVHD using psoralen and ultraviolet A irradiation (PUVA).

6.107   **The answer is b.** Veno-occlusive disease is almost exclusive to BMT and is the most common nonrelapse life-threatening complication of preparative-regimen–related toxicity for bone marrow transplantation.

6.108   **The answer is a.** Risk factors for late chronic GVHD include, among others, mismatched donor and recipient, female-to-male transplants, positive herpes simplex and CMV virus, patient age over 18 years, prior grade 2–3 acute GVHD, and CML recipients who received methotrexate and cyclosporine as chronic GVHD prophylaxis.

6.109   **The answer is c.** Marrow transplantation currently is a treatment choice only in the presence of an HLA-matched sibling. BMT for sickle cell anemia is under investigation; however, considerable controversy still exists, and the risks must be balanced against expected morbidity and mortality.

6.110   **The answer is b.** TBI is given before marrow infusion to prevent graft rejection by the patient's immune system. It offers optimal tumor cell kill because it penetrates the CNS and other privileged sites. It is usually given in fractionated doses to reduce toxicities, and it can be given as a booster to patients with bulky disease.

6.111   **The answer is d.** Peripheral blood stem cell transplant (PBSCT) or peripheral progenitor cell transplant (PBPCT) involves obtaining and infusing an unspecified number of true PPSCs with or without committed progenitor and precursor cells. The current terminology for this process is *blood cell transplant* (BCT).

6.112   **The answer is b.** One advantage to using peripheral PPSCs and progenitor cells obtained from peripheral blood is the more rapid recovery of neutrophils and platelets when progenitor cells are used. This is because the committed progenitors collected for BCT are farther along the differentiation pathway than are the PPSCs harvested from the bone marrow. Another advantage is that no anesthesia is required for BCT, so there is less risk of complications and fewer medical contraindications than with bone marrow harvest.

6.113   **The answer is a.** The advantages of ABMT over allogeneic BMT are the absence of GVHD and fewer toxicities. ABMT is less toxic because there is no veno-occlusive disease or GVHD. However, there is a potential risk of tumor contamination in the autologous marrow, and there is no benefit of the GVL effect, which can reduce the risk of relapse.

6.114   **The answer is c.** The macrophage is a primary initiator to an inflammatory immune response. It originates in the bone marrow, circulates as a monocyte, and becomes a macrophage when it enters a tissue at a site of infection. The macrophage is also a secretory cell manufacturing key pyrogenic cytokines such as interleukin-1, tumor necrosis factor, and interleukin-6.

6.115   **The answer is b.** A BRM is any soluble substance that is capable of altering (modifying) the immune system with either a stimulatory or a suppressive effect. It may act by restoring, augmenting, or modulating the host's immunologic mechanisms; by having direct antitumor activity; or by having some other biologic effects, including interfering with tumor cells' ability to survive or metastasize.

6.116   **The answer is c.** AIDS-related diseases such as Kaposi's sarcoma, non-Hodgkin's lymphoma (NHL), and primary CNS lymphoma are referred to as *opportunistic* because they occur in patients with preexisting immunodeficiency. This immunodeficiency can be the result of HIV infection (which destroys the immune system), therapeutic immunosuppression (e.g., chemotherapeutic agents used in organ transplantation), or primary immunodeficiency (e.g., as the result of a genetic defect). These malignancies normally occur at a low incidence and in a more benign form. An AIDS-related opportunistic disease that is not a malignancy is *Pneumocystis carinii* pneumonia.

6.117   **The answer is a.** Cytokines are glycoprotein products of immune cells. They bind to surface receptors of target cells and act as regulators of cell growth or as mediators of defense functions. Natural killer cells are capable of killing transformed cells. Lymphokine-activated killer (LAK) cells are a special population of cytotoxic cells used in cancer therapy that comprise primarily NK cells, which are capable of nonspecific tumor cell killing. B lymphocytes are sedentary cells located in lymph nodes and spleen.

6.118   **The answer is b.** Levamisole is a stimulant of host defense to augment or restore deficient immune function through stimulation of T cells and macrophages after immunosuppression. Side effects of levamisole therapy include mild nausea, liver dysfunction, leukopenia, skin rash, flu-like symptoms, and, rarely, neurological effects such as cerebellar dysfunction and mental confusion. Patients who consume alcohol during levamisole treatment may experience increased side effects, including flushing, throbbing headaches, and respiratory distress.

6.119   **The answer is c.** Immunotherapy is a recent form of melanoma treatment. The rationale for its use parallels the natural history of CM, indicating that immunologic intervention by the host may alter the growth pattern of CM. This immunologic interaction is demonstrated by the occurrence of more spontaneous remission in CM than in other adult tumors. Patients with lymphocytic infiltrates at the tumor site have a more favorable prognosis.

6.120   **The answer is d.** The classic function of the immune system is that cited in choice **a**, distinguishing self from nonself and destroying foreign substances. Homeostasis and surveillance are other important functions.

6.121 **The answer is b.** B memory cells (memory B lymphocytes), along with T memory cells (memory T lymphocytes), make up the recall component of the immune system. They have memory of antigens previously recognized by the body and deal with a particular antigen each time it is encountered.

6.122 **The answer is a.** B lymphocytes form plasma cells, that produce specific immunoglobulins, when stimulated by helper T lymphocytes and an encounter with a foreign antigen. Antibody is an antigen-specific immunoglobulin that is synthesized and secreted by a mature plasma cell, the final cell of B lymphocyte differentiation. Each plasma cell produces only one type of antibody, and each antibody is specific for only one type of antigen.

6.123 **The answer is d.** Data from a number of sources, including familial patterns, have been studied in an attempt to elicit features of genetic predisposition to cancer.

6.124 **The answer is b.** Inheritance of the *BRCA1* susceptibility gene is associated with a strong likelihood that the effect of the mutation will result in the disease for families with multiple breast and ovarian cancers (90%) as well as for those with breast cancers diagnosed before the age of 45 (70%).

6.125 **The answer is a.** Breast cancer, for example, is estimated to have a familial component in about 13% of cases.

6.126 **The answer is c.** The genes are estimated to be involved in 5% of breast cancer cases.

6.127 **The answer is a.** Individuals who have a first-degree relative with colorectal cancer have double the risk for developing adenomatous polyps, which are considered to be precursors of colorectal carcinoma.

6.128 **The answer is b.** The inherited form of retinoblastoma, characterized by multiple primary tumors, originates when both copies of the retinoblastoma antioncogene are absent or damaged. Without the protection of this gene, all retinal cells are predisposed to malignant growth.

6.129 **The answer is d.** Data regarding the genetic basis of cancer have been derived from a number of sources, including familial patterns, which have been studied in an attempt to elicit features of the transmission of neoplastic tendencies.

6.130 **The answer is b.** Germ cell mutations are transmitted to the next generation at birth and are responsible for hereditary (familial) cancer. Most human cancers result from a combination of acquired and inherited mutations with alterations of both oncogenes and antioncogenes.

STUDY NOTES

STUDY NOTES

HEALTH
PROMOTION

PREVENTION

Risk Factors

Lifestyle

7.1 Liver cancer is often associated with:
   a. a long smoking history
   b. obesity
   c. cirrhosis
   d. a bacterial infection

7.2 As long as he is making lifestyle changes, Mr. Jantzen's wife wants him to eat more fiber because his brother had colon cancer. Which of the following sources of fiber has been shown to provide the *most* protection against colon cancer?
   a. cereals
   b. vegetables
   c. fruits
   d. bread

7.3 Mr. Jantzen says, "I heard that beer causes cancer in some people. Is that true?" You answer:
   a. Yes, a variety of beers and whiskeys have been linked to oropharyngeal cancer.
   b. Yes, beer and vodka have definitely been linked to liver cancer.
   c. Yes, beer is associated with esophageal cancer.
   d. Yes, beer is specifically associated with rectal cancer.

7.4 Mr. Jantzen says he just cannot believe that the number of cigarettes he smokes "makes any difference. Either you're a smoker or you're not," he says. You explain that the risk of developing _____ is directly correlated with the number of cigarettes smoked.
   a. bladder cancer
   b. pancreatic cancer
   c. oropharyngeal cancer
   d. kidney cancer

7.5 Your brother-in-law tells you that he is tired of "all the negative talk about smoking. There's more prejudice against it than there is real danger." What percentage of lung cancer deaths are caused by cigarette smoking?
a. 45–50%
b. 50–60%
c. 75–85%
d. 80–90%

7.6 Individuals with esophageal cancer typically have a history of:
a. occupational exposure to radiation
b. obesity
c. oral contraceptive use
d. heavy alcohol intake

7.7 Which of the following are risk factors for cervical carcinoma?
a. herpes simplex virus 2
b. human papillomavirus
c. women exposed to diethylstilbestrol (DES) in utero
d. all of the above

7.8 Which of the following factors may increase a woman's risk of cervical carcinoma?
a. barrier-type contraception
b. limiting the number of sexual partners
c. vitamin A, beta carotene, vitamin C
d. none of the above

Environmental

7.9 Ms. Ellis tells you that her adult daughter is pressuring her to give up suntanning. "I've had a good tan for over 20 years," she says. "I like it. Is my daughter being a little hysterical?" You explain that long-term exposure to the sun has been associated with skin cancer and also with:
a. colorectal cancer
b. breast cancer
c. cancer of the lip
d. uterine cancer

7.10 Although the exact etiology of multiple myeloma is not known, certain factors increase the risk. Which of the following has been associated with an increased incidence of multiple myeloma?
a. chronic low-level exposure to radiation
b. chronic antigenic stimulation
c. chronic high-dose vitamin intake
d. a and b

7.11 Which of the following has been associated with an increased incidence of breast cancer in women?
a. living near high-energy electromagnetic wires
b. mantle radiation for Hodgkin's disease
c. exposure to chemicals used in hair dye
d. all of the above

7.12   Which of the following risk factors is associated with an increased incidence of thyroid cancer?
a. exposure to a nuclear plant disaster
b. iodine insufficiency
c. endemic goiter
d. all of the above

7.13   Esophageal cancer is associated with which of the following risk factors?
a. dietary deficiencies of selenium
b. nitrosamines in food
c. hiatal hernia
d. all of the above

7.14   Gastric cancer is associated with which of the following risk factors?
a. tobacco use
b. alcohol consumption
c. high intake of smoked or salted meats and fish
d. vitamin B_{12} deficiency

7.15   Which of the following environmental factors are associated with a higher incidence of ovarian cancer?
a. industrialized nations
b. higher education and socioeconomic levels
c. lower education and socioeconomic levels
d. a and b

7.16   Which of the following are risk factors for vulvar carcinoma?
a. herpes simplex virus type 2, human papillomavirus, and condylomata
b. herpes simplex virus type 1 and HIV
c. cervical carcinoma in situ, HIV, and human papillomavirus
d. number of sex partners, herpes simplex virus type 2, and condylomata

Occupational

7.17   Mr. Buck's cancer is reportedly related to his years of exposure to asbestos when he was working in construction. Mr. Buck is 67, worked in construction for 50 years, drinks beer occasionally, and smoked "off and on over the years." From this you can infer that Mr. Buck *most likely* has:
a. mesothelioma
b. bronchogenic cancer
c. gastrointestinal cancer
d. lung cancer

7.18   In addition to cigarette smoking and occupational exposure, heavy use of which category of drugs has been shown to increase the risk of cancer of the renal pelvis?
a. antipsychotics
b. non-narcotic analgesics
c. narcotics
d. hypnotics

7.19   During his physical examination, Mr. Pederson, a coal miner, asks you about his relative risk of developing lung cancer. The best response to his question would be to:

    a.   tell him that his risk is due to his exposure to coal

    b.   ask him about his family history of lung cancer, and explain that multiple factors cause the disease

    c.   get his demographic information, and ask him about his exposure to tobacco smoke

    d.   ask him about his diet and his smoking history

7.20   Mr. Frank's cancer has been associated with occupational exposure to a carcinogen. He works as a chemical dye manufacturer. Of the following choices, which type is he most likely to have based on this small clue?

    a.   bladder cancer

    b.   colorectal cancer

    c.   testicular cancer

    d.   esophageal cancer

7.21   Exposure to cytotoxic agents occurs primarily through which of the following routes?

    a.   inhalation

    b.   ingestion

    c.   absorption

    d.   all of the above

7.22   The etiology of bladder cancer can be attributed to four risk factors. Which of the following risk factors has been associated with an increased incidence of bladder cancer?

    a.   cigarette smoking

    b.   occupational exposure to chemicals used in textile dye industry

    c.   exposure to *S. haemotobium*

    d.   all of the above

7.23   Although the cause has not been established, certain occupations increase an individual's risk of developing a glioma or a meningioma, including:

    a.   exposure to wood dust

    b.   exposure to aniline dyes

    c.   exposure to chemicals in pesticides, herbicides, and fertilizers

    d.   exposure to nickel

7.24   Mr. Allen has been exposed to asbestos in the workplace for most of his adult life (he is now 75); Mr. Eliot, 64, has smoked since he was 17; Ms. Frank, 43, calls herself "a dedicated suntanner." Which patient is probably at greatest risk for cancer mortality?

    a.   Mr. Allen

    b.   Mr. Eliot

    c.   Ms. Frank

    d.   the two men

Health Beliefs

7.25   Factors that influence health behaviors include knowledge and education level, socioeconomic status, race, and:

    a.   residential location

    b.   marital status

    c.   age

    d.   employment status

7.26   The *majority* of health behavior is motivated or maintained by:
a. immediate consequences
b. delayed consequences
c. anticipated consequences
d. outcome consequences

7.27   Karen knows that cessation of smoking will decrease her cancer risks, but she doubts that she can do it. This demonstrates that the *most* important prerequisite for behavior change that involves an individual's beliefs is:
a. reactions of others
b. verbal persuasion
c. outcome expectation
d. efficacy expectation

7.28   The Health Belief Model attempts to explain health behavior and is guided by:
a. the assumption that an individual's subjective perception of the environment determines behavior
b. the assumption that people expect treatment and care
c. the assumption that people change their behaviors in response to familial pressures and familial patterns of disease
d. the assumption that people will behave in a specific way in response to intense education and peer pressure

7.29   Predictors of behaviors are determined by three variables. They are:
a. belief in self, perceived susceptibility, and support systems
b. support systems, perceived barriers, and perceived benefits
c. perceived barriers, perceived benefits, and belief in self
d. perceived barriers, perceived susceptibility, and perceived benefits

7.30   The Health Belief Model is based on the principle that:
a. the individual must perceive a threat
b. one can accomplish the behavior change or action required
c. benefits of the behavior change outweigh barriers or negative outcomes
d. all of the above

Prevention Strategies

7.31   One of the early signs of ovarian cancer is:
a. frequent urinary tract infections
b. thin, bloody vaginal discharge
c. heavy and painful menstruation
d. none of the above; there are usually no early signs of ovarian cancer

7.32   Physical recognition of cutaneous melanoma (CM) by practitioners and those at risk can be initiated by using the ABCDE rule. In this rule, *C* stands for:
a. change in symmetry
b. crusting or bleeding
c. color variation or dark black color
d. cause

7.33   A Baltimore study group focuses on smoking cessation among a specific target population. This group's research is focusing on ____ prevention.
a.   primary
b.   secondary
c.   tertiary
d.   integrated

7.34   The Baltimore research team wants to correlate the group's findings with related objectives from the Division of Cancer Protection and Control's (DCPC's) *Cancer Control Objectives for the Nation: 1985–2000*. Which is *not* a target area of prevention addressed by the DCPC?
a.   smoking
b.   exercise
c.   counseling
d.   sun exposure

7.35   The best treatment for cancer is:
a.   prevention
b.   early detection
c.   radiation and excision
d.   new developments in chemotherapy

7.36   Erika is concerned about the number of years she used birth control pills. Although they are associated with some degree of cancer risk, you are able to tell her that the long-term use of oral contraceptives containing both estrogen and progesterone in each pill has been found to offer protection against
a.   vaginal cancer
b.   colorectal cancer
c.   breast cancer
d.   endometrial cancer

7.37   After her father's death from colon cancer, Ellen takes the initiative in preventing colon cancer for herself by eating less fat and more fruits and vegetables and by taking up running. She is engaged in:
a.   illness behavior
b.   sick role behavior
c.   health protective behavior
d.   information-seeking behavior

7.38   Which of the following statements about primary prevention of skin cancers is *false*?
a.   UV radiation is strongest during the midpart of the day.
b.   For most people, sunscreen is not required on overcast days.
c.   Certain medications (e.g., oral contraceptives) can make individuals photosensitive.
d.   Surfaces such as sand and water can reflect more than one-half of the UV radiation onto the skin.

7.39   Which of the following are effective primary preventive strategies for smoking and head and neck carcinoma?
a.   Increase public awareness of the dangers of smoking.
b.   Promote the negative image of smoking in the media.
c.   Promote the "Through With Chew" program.
d.   all of the above

EARLY DETECTION

Epidemiology

Incidence

7.40   Incidence of bone cancer is most common in people with:
   a.   a family tendency for bone cancer
   b.   prior high-dose radiation cancer therapy
   c.   preexisting bone conditions
   d.   all of the above

7.41   Which of the following statements regarding the incidence of breast cancer is true?
   a.   70% of breast cancer occurs in women who are 50 years of age or older.
   b.   The incidence of breast cancer has increased, but the mortality rate—especially among African Americans and Hispanics—has decreased.
   c.   The incidence of breast cancer is approximately 1 of every 4 women.
   d.   The incidence of breast cancer has increased to epidemic proportions among premenopausal women.

7.42   The highest overall incidence of cancer occurs among:
   a.   young adult Asian/Pacific Islanders (APIs)
   b.   native Americans on reservations in the northwest
   c.   African American men
   d.   none of the above

7.43   For breast cancer, the average annual rate per 100,000 individuals has been highest among which females?
   a.   Japanese
   b.   white
   c.   Hawaiian
   d.   black

7.44   In the United States, the highest incidence of esophageal cancer is found among:
   a.   women aged 29–39 years
   b.   African American men
   c.   perimenopausal women
   d.   men aged 30–40 years

7.45   Incidence of cervical cancer is highest in women who are:
   a.   nulliparous
   b.   lifetime celibate
   c.   lifetime monogamous
   d.   multiparous

7.46   Which of the following has *not* been found to be associated with an increased incidence of primary brain tumors?
   a.   inhaled steroids
   b.   AIDS
   c.   genetic disorders
   d.   radiation to the head and neck area

Prevalence

7.47 Jana's research team has identified the relative risk and the frequency of a suspected etiologic factor in an entire defined population. A case-control study is conducted. What is the study *most* likely to be seeking to establish?
   a. causation
   b. attributable risk
   c. a survival risk
   d. prevalence

7.48 Jana's research project is an epidemiologic study of workers in asbestos mines who are free of any cancer. Subjects are to be followed over a 10-year period, and the incidence rates of certain types of cancers are to be determined. This design is an example of a:
   a. prospective study
   b. retrospective study
   c. historical prospective study
   d. historical retrospective study

7.49 Eric is a member of a research team that conducts an epidemiologic study. They determine that in a given year approximately 1 of every 12,000 American men has prostate cancer. This figure represents:
   a. an incidence rate
   b. a mortality rate
   c. a prevalence rate
   d. a survival rate

7.50 The country with the highest incidence of gastric cancer is:
   a. Japan
   b. China
   c. England
   d. the United States

7.51 A fellow nurse remarks that there seems to be an epidemic of breast cancer among young women. Which of the following would be an accurate response to this nurse?
   a. It is true, the prevalence of breast cancer is increased in this population.
   b. It seems that breast cancer is occurring more in younger women only because early detection measures such as mammography are detecting breast cancer sooner.
   c. Breast cancer is being detected earlier when the tumors are smaller because women are more aware of the need to practice early detection measures.
   d. b or c

7.52 Which of the following statements regarding genetic predisposition to cancer is *not* correct?
   a. The *BRCA1* gene is associated with increased susceptibility to both breast and ovarian cancer.
   b. The *BRCA2* gene is associated only with an increase in breast cancer.
   c. The genes are involved in 25% of breast cancer cases.
   d. The genes appear to be more strongly associated with breast cancer diagnosed at an early age.

7.53 The overall smoking prevalence is decreasing in the United States. However, the decrease in smoking prevalence is not uniform among all groups. Which of the following statements regarding the prevalence patterns for smoking is false?
   a. Overall smoking prevalence in women has declined more slowly than in men.
   b. Smoking prevalence has declined more in black than in white adolescents.
   c. The lung cancer mortality rate for white men in the United States has peaked, but the projected peak for mortality rates in women will not occur until the year 2010.
   d. With the predicted declines in mortality rates, the absolute number of lung cancer deaths will also decline.

Health History

Family

7.54 Which of the following statements about dysplastic nevi (DN) is *not* correct?
   a. DN may be familial or nonfamilial.
   b. Most persons affected by DN have about 25–75 abnormal nevi.
   c. DN develop from precursor lesions of cutaneous melanoma (CM) known as congenital nevi.
   d. A distinctive feature of DN is a "fried egg" appearance with a deeply pigmented papular area surrounded by an area of lighter pigmentation.

7.55 Primary risk factors for breast cancer include:
   a. being in the 30- to 45-year age group
   b. family history of breast cancer
   c. two or more heterosexual relationships
   d. lower socioeconomic status

7.56 Which of the following statements regarding the *BRCA2* gene is true?
   a. This gene mutation is associated with postmenopausal breast cancer.
   b. This gene is related to breast cancer in men.
   c. This gene is associated with early-onset female breast cancer.
   d. b and c

7.57 Four patients arrive at a clinic for cancer risk assessment. The most significant risk factor for each patient is listed below. Based on this information, you determine that one risk factor is both specific to the individual and yet outside the individual's control. This patient's risk factor is:
   a. cigarette smoking
   b. exposure to asbestos
   c. air pollution
   d. familial polyposis

7.58 One of the factors that seems to place a woman at higher risk for the development of ovarian cancer is:
   a. occupational exposure
   b. many sexual partners
   c. DES use by the mother
   d. a history of breast cancer

7.59 Which of the following statements regarding involuntary inhalation of tobacco smoke is *not* accurate?
a. There is an increased risk of lung cancer and heart disease among individuals who have never smoked but are living with a spouse who smokes cigarettes.
b. There is no evidence to support the idea that involuntary inhalation of tobacco smoke increases the risk of lung cancer in nonsmokers.
c. Approximately 17% of lung cancers among nonsmokers can be attributed to high levels of exposure to cigarette smoke during childhood and adolescence.
d. Long-term exposure to environmental tobacco smoke increases the risk of lung cancer in women who have never smoked.

7.60 Which of the following statements regarding ovarian cancer risk in families is *not* correct?
a. Women who have two or more first-degree relatives with a history of ovarian cancer have a significantly increased risk for ovarian cancer.
b. Ovarian cancer is an autosomal dominant mode of inheritance with variable penetrance.
c. A woman who has one first-degree relative with ovarian cancer has an overall risk that is two to four times the average risk of having ovarian cancer.
d. Ovarian cancer tends to be common among lower income groups, especially African American, Hispanic, and Native American women.

7.61 Which of the following statements regarding breast cancer risk is *not* accurate?
a. Only 5–10% of all breast cancers are due to tumor suppressor genes *BRCA1* and *BRCA2*.
b. As many as 30% of women diagnosed with breast cancer under the age of 35 have inherited susceptibility.
c. Approximately 1% of women diagnosed after age 75 have breast cancer associated with a dominant susceptibility gene.
d. A woman with a strong family history of breast cancer has a 70% chance that her cancer is caused by an inherited mutation in the *BRCA1* gene.

Previous Malignancies

7.62 Your patient has prostate cancer and is undergoing Lupron therapy. He recently began to complain of pain in his hip. He underwent a bone scan and was found to have an isolated lesion that was thought to be malignant. Biopsy was done and a sarcoma was confirmed. This finding represents which of the following?
a. This is most likely a metassis from his prostate cancer.
b. This is histologically dissimilar from a prostate cancer and is therefore considered to be a second primary cancer and potentially curable.
c. This is most likely a benign condition because he is receiving treatment for cancer.
d. This finding represents a guarded prognosis because his immune system obviously is failing.

7.63 Mr. Svensen has had treatment for a primary tumor, which was completely eradicated. Now, however, the surgeon discovers a metastatic lesion. The metastatic site seems to be solitary, and Mr. Svensen seems very healthy otherwise. Given these limited clues, what method of treatment would you predict will be used for Mr. Svensen's metastatic lesion?
a. chemotherapy to provide systemic control of metastasis
b. cytoreductive surgery to reduce the mass so combination therapy will be effective
c. combination radiation and chemotherapy
d. surgical resection

7.64 The most common second malignant neoplasms following radiation therapy are:
 a. breast carcinomas and gynecologic tumors
 b. cancers of the gastrointestinal tract
 c. sarcomas of the bone and soft tissue
 d. tumors of the bladder and lung

7.65 Your patient is a 5-year survivor of Hodgkin's disease. Your annual workup is conducted with the knowledge that she is most at risk for developing which of the following second primary cancers?
 a. breast cancer
 b. leukemia
 c. lung cancer
 d. non-Hodgkin's lymphoma

7.66 Mr. Allen has lung cancer and has completed his radiation and chemotherapy. He is instructed to return for checkups frequently because he is also at risk for which cancer?
 a. bladder cancer
 b. nasopharyngeal cancer
 c. sarcoma
 d. leukemia

7.67 Tony was treated for bilateral retinoblastoma as a child. His mother comments that he has recently complained of joint pain. You are concerned and order an x-ray of the joint. Your concern is based on which of the following?
 a. Patients with retinoblastoma have a high incidence of metastatic disease to the bone.
 b. Long-term effects of chemotherapy cause joint degeneration.
 c. Radiation causes osteomalagia.
 d. Children with a genetic form of retinoblastoma have a higher incidence of sarcoma.

7.68 Judith had Hodgkin's disease as a child and received mantle radiation therapy. It has been more than 20 years since her treatment. Which of the following statements is *not* correct concerning her follow-up care?
 a. She needs to continue her annual physical exams and mammograms because she is most at risk for second malignancies at this time.
 b. She can relax more because her risk for second malignances decreases every year.
 c. Her highest risk for second malignancies is breast cancer and lung cancer.
 d. Second malignancies are most likely to occur in the field of radiation.

Previous Cancer Treatment

7.69 Late effects involving the central nervous system (CNS) are most likely to occur in which of the following individuals?
 a. a child treated for Hodgkin's disease
 b. a child treated for bone sarcoma
 c. an adult treated for small cell carcinoma of the lung
 d. an adult treated for primary hypothyroidism

7.70   Which of the following statements about the late effects of cancer treatment is *incorrect*?
   a.   Late effects are believed to progress over time.
   b.   Late effects are believed to involve different mechanisms from those of the acute side effects of chemotherapy and radiation.
   c.   Late effects are severe and clinically subtle.
   d.   Late effects are the consequence of biologic cure.

7.71   Scoliosis and kyphosis are most likely to develop as late effects of the treatment of intra-abdominal tumors with:
   a.   combination MOPP therapy
   b.   radiation to one side of the body
   c.   pelvic irradiation combined with alkylating agents
   d.   prolonged used of corticosteroids

7.72   The risk of developing a second malignant neoplasm after treatment for a primary malignancy depends on several factors, including all of the following *except*:
   a.   the type and dose of treatment received (e.g., radiation and alkylating agents)
   b.   a common underlying etiologic factor (e.g., smoking)
   c.   genetic susceptibility (e.g., genetic retinoblastoma)
   d.   the timing of withdrawal of chemotherapeutic agents (e.g., MOPP latency)

7.73   Four years ago, Ms. Jantzen successfully completed treatment for breast cancer. Now she is diagnosed with acute myelogenous leukemia (AML). Which is most likely to have contributed to Ms. Jantzen's AML?
   a.   alkylating agents
   b.   anthracyclines
   c.   vinca alkaloids
   d.   antimetabolites

7.74   Mantle radiation for Hodgkin's disease is associated with an increased risk of which of the following cancers?
   a.   breast cancer, especially in those irradiated prior to the age of 30
   b.   lung cancer
   c.   liver cancer
   d.   none of the above

7.75   Mrs. Ana has breast cancer and has been taking tamoxifen for 4 years. She complains of intermittent vaginal bleeding and thinks she might be menopausal, but is concerned. Your most appropriate advice and rationale would include which of the following?
   a.   She should not be concerned; she is probably experiencing menopause due to the tamoxifen and the bleeding should improve over time.
   b.   Her bleeding is probably due to the hormonal changes caused by the tamoxifen and she should have FSH and LH testing to determine if she is menopausal.
   c.   Tamoxifen can cause endometrial changes and even cancer. She needs to see her gynecologist for an exam and possibly an endometrial biopsy.
   d.   Ovarian cancer is common in women who have breast cancer and she should be examined by her gynecologist.

Assessment of Risk Factors

7.76   Four patients have recently been assessed for possible cancers. Which patient's symptom seems *least likely* to be a warning signal of cancer?
a.   Mr. Jennings reports that he "goes to the bathroom more" and says that the color and consistency of stools have changed.
b.   Ms. Harris has a painful lump in her breast; it is tender on palpation, especially a week before her menstrual cycle.
c.   Twelve-year-old Jill has developed a new mole on her shoulder that is large and has an unusual shape or pattern to it. Her mother thinks it's getting larger.
d.   Mr. Traynor has a sore on his forehead that "just won't clear up."

7.77   In general, health risk assessment models are *most* effective in estimating what type of risk?
a.   relative risk
b.   quantitative risk
c.   empirical risk
d.   absolute risk

7.78   Ms. Ellis asks, "What is the purpose of a cancer risk assessment?" You explain that the following are the purpose of a cancer risk assessment *except*:
a.   identifying the distribution and determinants of diseases and health problems in human populations
b.   providing individuals with information about their health-related behaviors that may increase cancer risk
c.   educating patients about the relationship between risk factors and the likelihood of cancer
d.   stimulating individuals to participate in activities aimed at changing lifestyle and improving health

7.79   Which of the following individuals is probably at greatest risk for developing Kaposi's sarcoma?
a.   a woman who is bisexual, sexually active, and HIV-positive
b.   an intravenous drug user with AIDS
c.   a bisexual man with AIDS
d.   a and c

7.80   One of the primary risk factors associated with the development of endometrial cancer is:
a.   late menopause
b.   oral contraceptive use
c.   radiation exposure
d.   sexual activity at an early age

7.81   One of the factors that seems to put a woman at higher risk for developing cervical dysplasia is:
a.   diethylstilbesterol (DES) exposure
b.   hypertension
c.   diabetes
d.   human papillomavirus

7.82   Which of the following patients is considered at greater risk for developing testicular cancer?
a.   18-year-old Todd, who is very athletic
b.   Todd's great-grandfather
c.   26-year-old Eric, who is an accountant
d.   Frank, who just had his 50th birthday

Physical Exam

7.83 One way that basal cell carcinoma (BCC) is distinguished from squamous cell carcinoma (SCC) is by its:
   a. common occurrence on the head and hands
   b. lower incidence
   c. slower growth rate
   d. less well-demarcated margins

7.84 Which of the following is the *most likely* presenting symptom in a patient with lymphoma?
   a. edema in the upper part of the body
   b. enlarged cervical lymph nodes
   c. a palpable mass in the axillary or inguinal lymph nodes
   d. an upper respiratory infection

7.85 Ms. Allison notices a "funny discoloration" on her arm and comes in for an examination. She tells you that her brother died at age 38 from a common skin cancer. Ms. Allison's brother most likely had, and you should be suspicious for:
   a. squamous cell carcinoma
   b. basal cell carcinoma
   c. melanoma
   d. leukoplakia

7.86 Mr. Eliot, 64 and a smoker for 17 years, has an undifferentiated neoplasm arising in the proximal right bronchus. Which symptom most typically reflects this?
   a. barrel chest
   b. bulges on the thorax
   c. breathlessness
   d. superior vena cava obstruction

7.87 The only early physical finding that is usually suggestive of lung cancer is:
   a. whispered pectoriloquy
   b. egophony
   c. wheezing localized to a single lobe
   d. bagpipe sign

7.88 Mrs. Johns is pregnant and discovers a mass in the upper, outer quadrant of her left breast. Following her physical exam, the physician is most likely to order which of the following tests?
   a. ultrasound
   b. fine-needle aspiration
   c. mammogram (diagnostic)
   d. a or b

7.89   Mrs. Blase has carcinoma of the oral cavity. Although her main complaint initially concerned a painless lesion that she believed she had had for some time, she has recently begun to report a referred pain in her jaw and increased difficulty chewing and swallowing. This kind of referred pain can indicate:
    a. induration
    b. ulceration
    c. pressure affecting adjacent nerves
    d. any of the above

7.90   The most common presenting symptom of testicular cancer is:
    a. a small, hard mass in the scrotum
    b. a dragging sensation
    c. swelling
    d. dull aching or pain in the scrotal area

Recommendations for Screening

7.91   Mr. Vincinnes, 40, is being screened for possible colon cancer. He is asymptomatic. What tests are most important for this patient?
    a. Shifting dullness and fluid wave tests are used first on asymptomatic patients.
    b. Fecal occult blood test and digital rectal exam are the two most important tests for asymptomatic patients.
    c. Hemoccult test and urinalysis are the two standard tests for screening asymptomatic individuals.
    d. None of these answers is completely correct.

7.92   Which of the following women should have an annual Pap smear and pelvic examination?
    a. Lisa, 15, who is sexually active
    b. Marilyn, 55, a widow who has not been sexually active
    c. Glynnis, 17, who is not yet sexually active
    d. Both Lisa and Marilyn

7.93   Which of the following statements is *not true* regarding prostate-specific antigen?
    a. PSA is elevated only in men who have prostate cancer.
    b. When tumor destroys the natural tissue barrier, PSA enters the blood stream.
    c. PSA levels are used as a screening test for prostate cancer.
    d. Procedures such as biopsies can cause false PSA levels.

7.94   Which of the following tests is recommended by the American Cancer Society and the National Cancer Institute to screen for colorectal cancer?
    a. flexible sigmoidoscopy
    b. digital rectal examination
    c. Hemoccult test
    d. all of the above

7.95   Early detection of gastric cancer is unlikely because:
    a. the cancer metastasizes readily
    b. people tend to self-medicate themselves for gastrointestinal distress
    c. risk factors for the disease have not yet been identified
    d. none of the diagnostic tests or procedures currently available accurately detect gastric cancer in its early stages

7.96 The American Cancer Society recommends that all women who are sexually active or who are 18 years of age or older have a Pap smear performed:
    a. every 3 years
    b. every 2 years
    c. annually
    d. biannually

ANSWER EXPLANATIONS

7.1 **The answer is c.** Hepatocellular carcinomas are associated with environmental and hereditary factors, hepatitis B and hepatitis C viruses, and cirrhosis. Alcoholic cirrhosis is a common risk factor for liver cancer in the United States. Ingestion of estrogens, androgens, and oral contraceptives has been reported to be associated with liver tumors.

7.2 **The answer is b.** A majority of studies of differing epidemiologic designs support the hypothesis that high fiber intake is protective against colon cancer, although not all studies are supportive. In studies in which the source of fiber has been examined, fiber from vegetables appears protective against colon cancer, whereas the data for cereal fibers are less supportive of a protective effect.

7.3 **The answer is d.** Alcohol has been causally linked to cancers of the oral cavity, pharynx, larynx, esophagus, and liver, and it may be linked to cancers of the breast and rectum. It is estimated that 3% of cancer deaths are attributable to alcohol. For most cancer sites, alcohol appears to act synergistically with smoking. Although cancers at most sites do not appear to be associated with any particular type of alcohol, rectal cancer appears to be associated specifically with beer consumption.

7.4 **The answer is c.** Active tobacco use has been linked to many cancer types (lung, oropharyngeal, bladder, pancreatic, cervical, and kidney), and a clear linear relationship exists between the number of cigarettes smoked and the risk of lung and oropharyngeal cancers.

7.5 **The answer is d.** Eighty to ninety percent of lung cancer deaths are estimated to be caused by cigarette smoking.

7.6 **The answer is d.** Esophageal cancer appears to be associated with heavy alcohol intake, heavy tobacco use, and poor nutrition; cirrhosis, vitamin deficiency, anemia, and poor oral hygiene may be contributing factors.

7.7 **The answer is d.** Females exposed to DES in utero have a higher incidence of clear cell adenocarcinoma of the cervix and vagina. Human papillomaviruses (HPV) are members of the family of DNA tumor viruses that can cause cellular hyperproliferation and a variety of warty infections. HPV 18 is the most common papillomavirus found in women with adenocarcinoma of the cervix, and HPV 16 is more commonly associated with squamous carcinoma. Herpes simplex virus type 2 has been shown to be carcinogenic in animals. Women with cervical cancer usually have higher HSV2 specific antibody titers than do controls.

7

7.8 **The answer is d.** Several factors may lower a woman's risk of developing preinvasive lesions as precursors to invasive cervical cancer. These include barrier-type contraception; vasectomy; recommended daily allowances of vitamin A, beta carotene, and vitamin C; limiting the number of sexual partners; and initiating sexual activity at a later age.

7.9 **The answer is c.** Long-term exposure to the sun has been associated with cancer of the lip and oral cancer.

7.10 **The answer is d.** Chronic low-level exposure to radiation and chronic antigenic stimulation are associated with an increased incidence of multiple myeloma.

7.11 **The answer is b.** A risk of breast cancer has been associated with radiation therapy for a broad spectrum of health problems, including chronic mastitis, tuberculosis, and thymus disorders. Survivors of the atomic bombs exhibited an increase in breast as well as other cancers. Mantle radiation for Hodgkin's disease is associated with an increased risk relative to age during treatment.

7.12 **The answer is d.** Thyroid cancer has increased dramatically in children exposed to high levels of radioactive fallout from the Chernobyl nuclear plant disaster. High rates of follicular and papillary tumors are noted in areas of endemic goiter. Iodine insufficiency, especially in women, adolescents, and young adults, is a causative factor for thyroid malignancy.

7.13 **The answer is d.** Medical conditions of chronic irritation such as hiatal hernia, reflux esophagitis, and diverticula have been cited as possible etiologic factors. Dietary deficiencies of selenium are considered risk factors.

7.14 **The answer is c.** Both a high intake of smoked or salted meats and fish and nitrates and a low consumption of fresh vegetables and fruits are correlated with increased gastric cancer risk in populations. Neither smoking tobacco nor drinking alcohol has been demonstrated to increase the risk of gastric carcinoma.

7.15 **The answer is d.** With the exception of Japan, industrialized nations have the highest incidence of ovarian cancer. Women with higher educational and socioeconomic levels tend to delay childbearing, have fewer children, and have a higher incidence of ovarian cancer.

7.16 **The answer is a.**

7.17 **The answer is b.** Asbestos, the major carcinogenic fiber, is believed to be related to about 2000 cases of mesothelioma annually in the United States. However, asbestos causes more bronchogenic cancers than mesotheliomas, perhaps 6000, because of its synergism with tobacco smoke. Lung cancer is rare in asbestos workers who do not smoke. Data do not support an association between gastrointestinal cancer and asbestos.

7.18 **The answer is b.** Heavy use of the non-narcotic analgesics aspirin and/or acetaminophen has been shown to increase the risk of cancer of the renal pelvis. Similarly, an association has been made between analgesics and renal cell cancer, but this association has not as yet been substantiated.

7.19 **The answer is c.** It is misleading to suggest that coal poses the most obvious risk. By asking Mr. Pederson for demographic information, the nurse would be able to assess his exposure to air pollution and possibly his exposure to radon (certain areas have been identified as higher in radon activity than others). Since tobacco has an interactive and synergistic effect on the development of lung cancer when combined with other carcinogens, this would also be a good factor to explore. Genetics and diet have not been shown to have a significant effect on the development of lung cancer.

7.20 **The answer is a.** One of the strongest risk factors for bladder cancer involves occupational exposure to 2-naphthylamine, benzidine, and aniline dyes. Workers exposed to aromatic amines have a fourfold greater risk of bladder cancer.

7.21 **The answer is d.** Direct exposure to cytotoxic agents can occur during admixture, administration, or handling. Exposure occurs through inhalation, ingestion, or absorption.

7.22 **The answer is d.** The four etiologic hypotheses related to bladder cancer are cigarette smoking, occupational exposure to industrial chemicals, ingestion of other physical agents, and exposure to *S. haemotobium.*

7.23 **The answer is c.** Agricultural workers exposed to multiple chemicals in pesticides, herbicides, and fertilizers have had a higher than expected incidence of gliomas.

7.24 **The answer is b.** Mr. Eliot is at greatest risk. Cigarette smoking is the largest single preventable cause of premature death and disability and the major single cause of cancer mortality. Individuals like Mr. Allen who are exposed to high levels of asbestos and other respiratory carcinogens in the workplace also have an increased risk, but it is not the single major cause of cancer mortality. Cancers of the skin—most often caused by excessive sun exposure—are the most common cancers in humans, but they too are not the major single cause of cancer mortality.

7.25 **The answer is c.** Age has an influence on health behaviors.

7.26 **The answer is c.** Anticipated consequences, rather than immediate consequences, determine most health behaviors.

7.27 **The answer is d.** Efficacy expectations are the most important prerequisite for behavior change, because stronger efficacy expectations produce more active and sustained efforts in the face of adverse conditions.

7.28 **The answer is a.** The Health Belief Model attempts to explain health behavior and is guided by the assumption that an individual's subjective perception of the environment determines behavior.

7.29 **The answer is d.** Perceived barriers, perceived susceptibility, and perceived benefits are strong predictors of behavior; perceived barriers are the most powerful single predictor. Perceived susceptibility is the weakest predictor but appears to be strongly related to sick role behaviors.

7.30 **The answer is d.** The Health Belief Model is based on the principles that the individual must perceive a threat and believes that something can be done about it. This second expectation has three components: that a behavior change or action will reduce either the severity of or the susceptibility to the threat; that one can accomplish the behavior change or action required; and that benefits of the behavior change outweigh barriers or negative outcomes.

7.31 **The answer is d.** Ovarian cancer is typically asymptomatic in its early stages. As the disease progresses, women may experience vague abdominal discomfort, leading to loss of appetite, flatulence, or urinary frequency; more often than not, these symptoms are no more than annoying and are not taken seriously by the patient and her physician. By the time a diagnosis of ovarian cancer is made, the cancer has spread beyond the ovary in 75% of cases.

7.32 **The answer is c.** Physical recognition of CM by practitioners and those at risk can be initiated by using the "ABCDE" rule. In this rule, *A* = asymmetry, *B* = border irregularity, *C* = color variation or dark black color, *D* = diameter greater than 0.6 cm, and *E* = elevation.

7.33   **The answer is b.** Primary prevention is the avoidance of exposure to carcinogens; secondary prevention is the prevention of promotion by smoking cessation, changes in diet, and administration of chemopreventive agents presumed to act on promotion. Tertiary prevention consists of arresting, removing, or reversing a premalignant lesion to prevent recurrence or progression to cancer.

7.34   **The answer is b.** The four areas of prevention targeted by the DCPC's *Cancer Control Objectives for the Nation: 1985–2000* include smoking, diet, sun exposure, and counseling.

7.35   **The answer is a.** The best treatment for cancer is its prevention. About 90% of the skin cancers could be prevented by protection from the sun. Most cancers caused by cigarette smoking and heavy use of alcohol could be prevented.

7.36   **The answer is d.** The long-term use of combination oral contraceptives has been found to offer some protection against both ovarian and endometrial cancer. Long-term use of conjugated estrogens, on the other hand, is an iatrogenic risk factor for endometrial cancer.

7.37   **The answer is c.** Health protective behavior consists of actions taken by people to protect, promote, or maintain their health.

7.38   **The answer is b.** Sunscreen should always be applied on overcast days because 70–80% of UV radiation can penetrate cloud cover.

7.39   **The answer is d.** Avoiding the use of tobacco and alcohol is key to the prevention of head and neck cancer. As public awareness of the dangers of tobacco use grows and a negative image of smoking is portrayed in the media, it is anticipated that the incidence of head and neck cancer will decrease. The campaign of "Through With Chew" is primarily directed toward boys aged 11–17 who might use smokeless tobacco.

7.40   **The answer is d.** All three factors play some role in the development of bone cancer: familial tendency; prior cancer therapy in the form of high-dose irradiation; and some preexisting bone conditions such as Paget's disease.

7.41   **The answer is a.** 70% of breast cancer occurs in women who are 50 years of age or older.

7.42   **The answer is c.** The highest overall cancer incidence rates occur among African American men.

7.43   **The answer is b.** For breast cancer, the average annual rate per 100,000 individuals has been highest among white females.

7.44   **The answer is b.** In the United States, African American men have a significantly higher incidence of esophageal cancer than white men; similarly, African American women have a higher incidence of the disease than white women. This type of cancer also seems to develop at a younger age in African Americans than it does in whites.

7.45   **The answer is d.** Cervical carcinoma is infrequent in women who are nulliparous and those who are celibate or monogamous throughout their lives. Multiparity is a risk factor.

7.46   **The answer is a.** Increased incidence of primary brain tumors is associated with all these choices *except* inhaled steroids.

7.47   **The answer is b.** Attributable risk is the difference in the incidence or death rates between the group exposed to some factor and unexposed groups. It is used to evaluate the magnitude of change in an outcome (e.g., respiratory cancer) with the removal of the suspect antecedent factor (e.g., smoking). Provided that the relative risk and the frequency of the suspect factor in the entire defined population are known, attributable risk can be estimated from a case-control study. Otherwise, it must be calculated directly from a prospective study.

7.48   **The answer is a.** In this prospective study, subjects (miners) are being selected with varying degrees of exposure to the suspected factor (asbestos). They have not experienced the outcome thought to be associated with the factor (lung cancer or some other cancer). They are then being followed over time to see whether the outcome (e.g., a type of cancer) occurs.

7.49   **The answer is c.** The prevalence rate is the total number of cases—new and existing—in a given population during a specific time period, in this case 1 year. It is a function of both incidence and duration. In other words, the higher the survival rate (duration) for a type of cancer, the higher its prevalence rate will be.

7.50   **The answer is a.** Japan has the highest incidence of gastric cancer in the world, and stomach cancer is the major cause of death in that country. The incidence of gastric cancer is low in the United States. The dramatic differences in geographic distribution of the disease remain an enigma to epidemiologists.

7.51   **The answer is d.** Because women are now more aware of breast cancer and early detection methods, cancer of the breast is being found when tumors are small and the woman is younger. So it is not that breast cancer is occurring more in younger women, it is that it is being discovered before the tumor is large and the woman is older.

7.52   **The answer is c.** The genes are involved in only 5% of breast cancer cases.

7.53   **The answer is d.** Even with the predicted declines in mortality rates, the absolute number of lung cancer deaths will continue to rise because of the increasing size of the population.

7.54   **The answer is c.** DN are precursor lesions of cutaneous melanoma (CM) that develop from normal nevi, usually after puberty. It has been reported that 50% of CM evolves from some form of DN. They may be familial or nonfamilial, with the risk of CM in a family member with DN approaching 100% in melanoma-prone families. DN are often larger than 5 mm and can number from 1–100, with most affected persons having 25–75 abnormal nevi. They appear typically on sun-exposed areas, especially on the back, but also may be seen on the scalp, breasts, and buttocks. Pigmentation is irregular, with mixtures of tan, brown, and black or red and pink. A distinctive feature is a "fried egg" appearance.

7.55   **The answer is b.** The primary risk factors for breast cancer are increasing age, family history of breast cancer, history of benign breast disease, late age at first live birth, nulliparity, early age at menarche, late age at menopause, higher socioeconomic status, being Jewish, estrogen replacement therapy, exposure of the female breast to ionizing radiation in infancy, mammographic parenchymal patterns that are dense, having complex fibroadenomas, and being single.

7.56   **The answer is d.** *BRCA2* has been identified on the long arm of chromosome 13 (13q12-13). This mutation seems to be associated with male breast cancer and early-onset female breast cancer.

7.57   **The answer is d.** Choice **a** is individual but under the person's control; choice **b** is typically a group risk factor shared by persons from the same occupation; choice **c** is typically a group risk factor shared by persons from the same geographic residence. Only choice **d**, an inherited condition, is both specific to the individual and, at the same time, outside the person's control.

7.58   **The answer is d.** Hormonal factors such as nulliparity, infertility, and estrogen therapy have been connected to the development of ovarian cancer. A family history of breast cancer or colon cancer doubles the risk of ovarian cancer.

7.59   **The answer is b.**

7.60   **The answer is d.** Ovarian cancer tends to be more common among white upper-income groups in highly industrialized countries. Jewish women experience a 40% higher incidence rate than do African American, Hispanic, and Native American women.

7.61   **The answer is d.** A woman with a strong family history of breast cancer is generally defined as having four or more genetically related women affected with the disease; about 40% of their cancers are caused by an inherited mutation in the gene *BRCA1* and another 40% by *BRCA2*.

7.62   **The answer is b.** A second primary lesion refers to an additional, histologically separate malignant neoplasm in the same patient. A general rule is always to biopsy the first recurrence, because it may represent a new, curable or treatable malignancy.

7.63   **The answer is d.** Surgery may be used to resect a metastatic lesion if the primary tumor is believed to be eradicated, if the metastatic site is solitary, and if the patient can undergo surgery without significant morbidity.

7.64   **The answer is c.** Sarcomas of the bone and soft tissue are the most common second malignant neoplasms after radiation therapy, with the incidence peaking at 15–20 years following radiation. In a large study of survivors of childhood cancer, the risk of bone cancer was highest among children treated for retinoblastoma and Ewing's sarcoma but also increased significantly in patients treated for rhabdomyosarcoma, Wilms' tumor, and Hodgkin's disease. In addition to sarcomas and leukemia, a variety of solid tumors have been linked to treatment with radiation, including carcinomas of the breast and tumors of the bladder, rectum, and uterus.

7.65   **The answer is b.** In patients with Hodgkin's disease, there is a 77-fold increased risk of the development of leukemia within 4 years of initial treatment.

7.66   **The answer is a.** Patients with lung cancer are at greater risk for the development of bladder cancer because both tumors are associated with smoking.

7.67   **The answer is d.** Genetic susceptibility is an important factor in case finding. Children with the genetic form of retinoblastoma, which is usually bilateral, have a much higher incidence of sarcoma compared with those with the nongenetic form of the disease.

7.68   **The answer is b.** In a study of survivors of Hodgkin's disease, a 17% cumulative risk of second cancers was noted 20 years post-treatment. The most common tumors were lung and breast cancers, with 77% of the tumors occurring in or adjoining the field of radiation.

7.69   **The answer is c.** The late effects of CNS treatment, including neuropsychologic, neuroanatomic, and neurophysiologic changes, have been observed most commonly in children with acute lymphoblastic leukemia (ALL) and brain tumors and in adult small cell carcinoma of the lung (SCCL) patients, all of whom received CNS treatment for the primary tumor or as prophylaxis against meningeal disease.

7.70   **The answer is c.** The late effects of biologic cure result from physiologic changes related to particular treatments or to the interactions among the treatment, the individual, and the disease. Unlike the acute side effects of chemotherapy and radiation, however, late effects are believed to progress over time and by different mechanisms. They can appear months to years after treatment; can be mild, severe, or life-threatening; and can be clinically obvious, clinically subtle, or subclinical. Their impact appears to depend on the age and development stage of the patient.

7.71   **The answer is b.** Uneven radiation to vertebrae, soft tissue, and muscles for the treatment of intra-abdominal tumors frequently results in scoliosis or kyphosis, or both. Although recent therapies have been modified to minimize this problem, it may still occur in some children and tends to become most apparent during periods of rapid growth, such as the adolescent growth spurt.

7.72   **The answer is d.** Adults and children who have received chemotherapy or radiation therapy, or both, for a primary malignancy are at increased risk for the development of a second malignant neoplasm. Alkylating agents and ionizing radiation are the treatments most closely linked to a second malignant neoplasm. In addition to the type and dose of treatment received, the risk of the development of a secondary cancer depends on several predisposing factors, including choices **b** and **c**.

7.73   **The answer is a.** Alkylating agents have a demonstrated causative relationship to acute myelogenous leukemia. AML is the most frequently reported second cancer following aggressive chemotherapy for Hodgkin's disease, non-Hodgkin's lymphoma, multiple myeloma, ovarian cancer, and breast cancer.

7.74   **The answer is a.** The risk of breast cancer correlates with increased radiation dosage, especially if a woman is exposed to radiation in the period of young adulthood.

7.75   **The answer is c.** Tamoxifen acts as an antiestrogen on breast tissue but has a weak estrogenic effect on endometrial tissue and has been associated with thickening of the endometrium and changes from polyps to hyperplasia and cancer. Ovarian cancer does occur in women with breast cancer, but it is not common.

7.76   **The answer is b.** Breast lumps commonly seen in cancer tend to be painless; this is not to say that it is impossible for Ms. Harris to have cancer, but that her sign is less definitive than the others. The seven classic warning signals of cancer include: changes in bowel or bladder habits; unusual bleeding or discharge; a sore that does not heal; obvious changes in warts or moles; painless thickening or lump in the breast or elsewhere; nagging cough or hoarseness; and indigestion or difficulty swallowing.

7.77   **The answer is a.** Risk models have been successful in distinguishing low-, medium-, and high-risk persons and in estimating relative risk but are much less successful in estimating absolute risk in individuals or across populations. Despite the value of a health risk assessment (HRA) in "prospective health assessment," a major concern with HRA is the value of quantitative estimates of absolute risk. The text suggests that more qualitative measures may have more valuable purposes in risk assessment.

7.78   **The answer is a.** Choice **a** is the definition of epidemiology, a study related to but distinct from cancer risk assessment. Categorizing risk factors is an important preliminary step in risk assessment. From this database of risk factors, an individual's cancer risk profile can be developed and specific interventions for risk reduction can be planned. Choices **b** through **d**, however, are the primary objectives of cancer risk assessment.

7.79   **The answer is c.** KS seems to be a disease found predominantly in homosexual and bisexual men with AIDS.

7.80   **The answer is a.** The risk factors associated with the development of endometrial cancer are obesity, nulliparity, late menopause, irregular menses, failure to ovulate, infertility, diabetes, hypertension, history of breast or ovarian cancer, adenomatous hyperplasia, and prolonged use of exogenous estrogen therapy. The more of these factors that apply, the greater the risk of developing endometrial cancer.

7.81   **The answer is d.** Human papillomaviruses have been implicated in an increased risk for both precancerous cervical lesions and invasive cervical carcinoma. The virus is sexually transmitted and can cause a variety of warty infections.

7.82   **The answer is c.** Testicular cancer most commonly affects those in the 20- to 30-year-old age group. It occurs less frequently in adolescents and in men over 40 years of age.

7.83   **The answer is c.** BCC is the least aggressive type of skin cancer and has its origins in either the basal layer of the epidermis or in the surrounding dermal structures. It is most commonly found on the nose, eyelids, cheeks, neck, trunk, and extremities. It grows slowly by direct extension and has the capacity to cause major local destruction. Metastasis is rare and most often occurs in the regional lymph nodes. SCC, on the other hand, may arise in any epithelium. It is most commonly found on the head and hands. It is more aggressive than BCC: it has a faster growth rate, less well-demarcated margins, and a greater metastatic potential. Metastatic disease is usually first noted in the regional lymph nodes.

7.84   **The answer is b.** Three-fourths of lymphoma patients present with enlargement of cervical or supraclavicular lymph nodes, but enlarged axillary or inguinal nodes may be the presenting symptoms. Such nodes are characteristically painless, firm, rubbery in consistency, freely movable, and of variable size. Weakness, fatigue, and general malaise may be a part of the presenting picture.

7.85   **The answer is c.** There are three types of skin cancer: basal cell carcinoma, squamous cell carcinoma, and melanoma. However, melanoma is the most common skin cancer to result in death.

7.86   **The answer is d.** Superior vena cava obstruction is a common complication of lung cancer; approximately 80% of these cases are caused by undifferentiated neoplasms arising in proximal right bronchi. Barrel chest is associated with pulmonary emphysema or normal aging. Bulges on the thorax are often a manifestation of a neoplasm on the ribs. Breathlessness is a more generalized indication of obstruction of the lungs.

7.87   **The answer is c.** The only early physical finding that most strongly suggests lung cancer is wheezing localized in a single lobe of the lung in an elderly person with a long history of smoking.

7.88   **The answer is d.** Sonography is the imaging modality of choice in a young woman, a pregnant woman, or a lactating woman who has not discovered any lumps or other signs of cancer. FNA would also be appropriate.

7.89   **The answer is d.** Referred pain is an important sign that can indicate induration, ulceration, or pressure affecting adjacent nerves. As the lesion increases in size, the individual may experience difficulty chewing foods and swallowing.

7.90   **The answer is a.** The most common sign of testicular cancer is a small, hard mass in the scrotum. However, a dragging sensation, swelling, dull aching, or pain in the scrotal area also may be a presenting symptom.

7.91   **The answer is b.** The two most important screening tests for asymptomatic individuals are examination of the feces for occult blood and the digital rectal examination. The American Cancer Society advocates an annual digital rectal exam beginning at age 40. The ACS, the National Cancer Institute, and the American College of Surgeons recommend that asymptomatic individuals have a sigmoidoscopic exam every 3–5 years beginning at age 50 in conjunction with an annual fecal occult blood test.

7.92   **The answer is d.** The American Cancer Society recommends that all women who are, or who have been, sexually active or who have reached 18 years of age have an annual Pap smear and pelvic examination.

7.93   **The answer is a.** Conditions other than prostate cancer can give rise to elevated PSA levels.

7.94   **The answer is d.** All of these tests are recommended in screening for colorectal cancer.

7.95   **The answer is b.** The earliest symptoms of gastric cancer, such as a sense of fullness or heaviness and moderate distention after meals, are usually vague. Home remedies and self-medications are often employed successfully for a while until other symptoms appear. Because of the elusive nature of gastric disorders, this type of cancer is usually quite advanced by the time medical attention is sought.

7.96   **The answer is c.** The American Cancer Society currently recommends that all women who are or have been sexually active or who are 18 years of age or older should have annual Pap smears. After a woman has had three negative annual Pap smears, the test may be performed less frequently at the discretion of her physician.

STUDY NOTES

STUDY NOTES

PROFESSIONAL PERFORMANCE

APPLICATION OF NURSING STANDARDS

Statement on the Scope and Standards of Oncology Nursing Practice

8.1   As a nurse, you know that which of the following is part of your caregiving role?
    a.   determining the meaning of your patient's pain
    b.   deriving nursing diagnoses
    c.   assisting in selecting interventions
    d.   all of the above

8.2   The Oncology Nursing Society (ONS) endorses the title advanced practice nurse (APN) to designate:
    a.   clinical nurse specialist (CNS) and nurse practitioner (NP) roles in oncology nursing
    b.   the merger of the CNS and NP roles
    c.   exclusion of other master's-prepared nurses in education, administration, or research roles
    d.   all of the above

8.3   Which group has been the *most* active over the years in establishing standards of cancer nursing practice as well as guidelines for cancer nursing education?
    a.   the Oncology Nursing Society (ONS)
    b.   the American Cancer Society (ACS)
    c.   the National Cancer Institute (NCI)
    d.   the American Nurses Association (ANA)

8.4   Within the conceptual framework for cancer nursing education developed in accordance with the Outcome Standards for Cancer Nursing Practice, which of the following concepts is central to oncology nursing practice?
    a.   community-environment
    b.   health care system
    c.   individual and family
    d.   health-illness

8.5 Which of the following generally applies only to the advanced level of nursing education and not to the generalist level?
  a. a baccalaureate degree
  b. a broader scope of practice
  c. clinical experience
  d. conceptual knowledge and skills

Standards of Oncology Education: Patient, Family, and Public

8.6 The purpose of the Standards of Oncology Nursing Education is to provide guidelines for *all but* which of the following?
  a. plan and evaluate generalist education
  b. plan and evaluate continuing education programs
  c. provide certification for advanced education programs
  d. plan and evaluate advanced education

8.7 The mission of the Oncology Nursing Certification Corporation (ONCC) is to advance oncology nursing through the certification process. To be eligible for the certification examination, a nurse must have accomplished *all but* which of the following?
  a. a current RN license
  b. a minimum of 50 CEUs in the area of Oncology Nursing Practice
  c. 1 year of experience as a registered nurse over the 3-year period prior to application
  d. at least 1000 hours of oncology nursing practice within $2^{1}/2$ years of application for a current license

8.8 To be eligible for the Advanced Oncology Nursing Certification examination, the nurse must have accomplished *all but* which of the following?
  a. certification in Oncology Nursing at the basic level
  b. a master's degree or higher
  c. experience in administration, education, practice, or research
  d. a current RN license

8.9 As part of a community-based nursing program, you are assigned to work in a neighborhood health clinic. You notice that women tend to seek little information from the program about early detection measures for breast cancer. Utilizing the Health Belief Model, which of the following strategies would *most likely* increase the women's use of early detection methods for breast cancer?
  a. Inform the women that the physical exam to detect breast cancer is free.
  b. Inform the women that the clinic is extending its hours into the evening to be more convenient.
  c. Teach the women that the earlier the cancer is detected, the better the outcome.
  d. Assure the women that the mammogram does not hurt.

8.10 Mr. Nerry complains that his medication is inadequate to manage his pain. On questioning him, you discover he is not taking the medication on schedule as he has been instructed. According to the Health Belief Model, which of the following nursing actions is most likely to increase your patient's compliance with his medication schedule?
  a. Write down the schedule and have a family member call and remind him.
  b. Explain that the schedule is important and is based on research.
  c. The patient knows what he needs and should take more medicine when he needs it.
  d. Teach him that the benefits of taking the medication on a schedule are worth it because it is the best way to ensure that he will have less pain.

RESEARCH

Clinical Trials

8.11　A phase IV clinical trial is designed:
　　　a.　to address the use of drugs, usually in combination, with cure as the goal of therapy
　　　b.　to answer questions regarding various doses and schedules
　　　c.　to offer new information regarding risks and toxicities
　　　d.　all of the above

8.12　The Breast Cancer Prevention Trial (BCPT) tested the ability of which of the following to prevent breast cancer in healthy women at high risk for the disease?
　　　a.　sulindac
　　　b.　retinoic acid
　　　c.　tamoxifen
　　　d.　beta-carotene

8.13　Ms. Trent's physician is in the process of selecting her treatment plan. His order of preference for protocol, from *most* desirable to *least* desirable choice, is probably:
　　　a.　conventional or standard treatment, a unique individualized treatment plan, a clinical trial, or (last choice) protocol from an abstract or journal article
　　　b.　clinical trial, conventional treatment, unique individualized treatment plan, or (last choice) protocol from an abstract or a journal article
　　　c.　unique individualized treatment plan, clinical trial, conventional treatment, or (last choice) protocol from journal article or abstract
　　　d.　clinical trial, conventional treatment plan, protocol from a journal article or abstract, and (last choice) a unique individualized treatment plan

8.14　A major barrier for both patients and institutions to participation in national studies is that:
　　　a.　trials sponsored by drug companies pose a financial burden for most oncology programs
　　　b.　the NCI rarely is committed to research to prevent cancer since success is fairly limited; thus, it only consistently supports research to improve the quality of life for those who develop cancer
　　　c.　third-party payers often do not cover experimental treatment, which includes all research trials
　　　d.　b and c

8.15　Vanessa works in a lab conducting preclinical toxicology studies to determine safe starting doses for potential anticancer agents for use in humans. She has begun phase I trials for drug E to determine a maximum tolerated dose. Vanessa's study is using patients with advanced cancer as subjects. Dosing starts at 10% of the LD_{10}. This:
　　　a.　will be escalated until significant toxicity is seen in 10% or more of the patients treated
　　　b.　will help in determining the MTD when the dose is raised high enough to produce toxicity in at least 50% of the patients treated
　　　c.　is one step below the MTD
　　　d.　is used for phase II testing

8.16   Historically, there has been underrepresentation of minorities in clinical trials. Which of the following best explains why minorities are less likely to participate in clinical trials?
   a.   unwillingness of researchers to pay for the participants' time
   b.   general distrust of outsiders doing research in their communities
   c.   lack of individuals' ability to pay for tests involved in a study
   d.   religious teachings discouraging research involvement for any reason

Nursing Research Utilization

8.17   The reliability of a measure can be said to depend on:
   a.   the homogeneity or consistency of the items on the measurement scale
   b.   the extent to which the measure produces the same score when applied at to two different times or in two different ways
   c.   test-retest or alternative form and inter-rater repeatability
   d.   all of the above

8.18   Content validity:
   a.   need not depend on the degree to which the scale superficially appears to measure the construct
   b.   includes the degree to which the items represent the range of significant attributes
   c.   includes statistical evidence to support inferences
   d.   must include the physical and psychological domains, but not the social one (which is covered under construct validity)

8.19   The Quality of Life Index (QLI):
   a.   was originally a patient-rated scale of five areas of functioning (activity, daily living, health, support, and outlook)
   b.   can distinguish cancer patients with terminal illness from those with recent disease or active treatment
   c.   is probably the best example of a "cancer-specific" scale that in reality measures generic health concepts
   d.   all of the above

8.20   Evelyn uses the Functional Living Index—Cancer (FLIC) scale to assess a group of patients to determine the impact of cancer on daily issues. The degree to which this scale superficially appears to measure the construct in question is referred to as:
   a.   face validity
   b.   true content validity
   c.   construct validity
   d.   criterion validity

8.21   Pilot studies are useful to:
   a.   assess the feasibility of a research design
   b.   pretest an instrument
   c.   evaluate the risk, side effects, and compliance with a new nursing management approach
   d.   all of the above

EDUCATION PROCESS

Patient

8.22   In the development of patient education materials and resources, pretesting is used primarily during which phase(s)?
   a.   planning and strategy selection
   b.   implementation
   c.   evaluation
   d.   all of the above

8.23   It is important to evaluate the reading grade level of educational materials before giving them to a patient, because it has been shown that over 20% of Americans read at or below which grade level?
   a.   third grade
   b.   fifth grade
   c.   seventh grade
   d.   eighth grade

8.24   To evaluate the reading grade level of a patient education pamphlet or brochure, the nurse would do *all but* which of the following?
   a.   Select approximately 30 sentences at the beginning, the middle, and near the end of the teaching text. Quiz a representative group of patients to determine their level of understanding.
   b.   Select approximately 30 sentences at the beginning, the middle, and near the end of the teaching text. Circle all the words containing three or more syllables and total the number of words circled and divide by 3. More than 12 polysyllabic words is unacceptable.
   c.   Select approximately 30 sentences at the beginning, the middle, and near the end of the teaching text. Circle all the words containing three or more syllables, and total the number of words circled. Estimate the square root of the total number of polysyllabic words counted and add 3. This gives the reading level the person must have to fully understand the text being assessed.
   d.   Find the average number of polysyllabic words per sentence and divide by the total number of sentences. The resulting number is the reading level.

8.25   You are asked to set up a program to teach self-care to patients in follow-up care after major cancer treatments, such as bone marrow or peripheral stem cell transplant patients. Which of the following will you include?
   a.   care of venous access lines
   b.   administration of parenteral fluids
   c.   symptom management
   d.   all of the above

Family

8.26   During a family assessment, the home health care nurse identifies conflict among the family members caring for the patient. The nurse learns that the conflict is "not new" and has existed "for years." The home health care nurse establishes a plan of care for family education that:
a.   attempts to change the behavior among the family members because the patient is upset by the conflict
b.   involves having psychological services counsel the "conflicting members"
c.   schedules family meetings to discuss how the conflict is affecting the patient and what can be done to resolve it
d.   is sensitive to the feelings of the members in conflict but does not attempt educational measures to treat the causes of the conflict

8.27   The husband of a woman with end-stage breast cancer is concerned that his wife is sleeping more and is not even waking to eat or drink. The hospice nurse would explain to the husband that:
a.   these are signs of approaching death
b.   the pain medication has reached a high blood level and needs to be reduced
c.   there is no reason to be concerned
d.   her oncologist should be called to obtain immediate direction for her care

8.28   What is the most appropriate reading level for patient education materials designed to be understood by the majority of readers?
a.   sixth grade
b.   seventh grade
c.   eighth grade
d.   ninth grade

8.29   Which of the following most accurately describes the National Coalition for Cancer Survivorship?
a.   It provides referral to local support services for patients and families.
b.   It addresses barriers to employment and access to health insurance.
c.   It advocates for changes in health care delivery.
d.   all of the above

Community

8.30   During a community education seminar on preventing lung cancer, it is important to note that the use of smokeless tobacco increased significantly in the 1970s because:
a.   it was promoted as a "safe" alternative to smoking
b.   it was cheaper than cigarettes
c.   it became popular among baseball players
d.   it became legal

8.31   In your community seminar, when you explain the proper technique for BSE, you should *not* include which of the following instructions?
a.   For the visual inspection, note symmetry, size, and shape of the breasts.
b.   Examine yourself in front of the mirror with your arms relaxed at your sides.
c.   Examine yourself in front of the mirror with your hands pressed on your hips.
d.   Examine yourself in front of the mirror with your arms folded behind your back.

8.32   The overall goal of home care is:
   a.   to provide holistic and direct care for the patient
   b.   to assist the patient in a peaceful death with dignity
   c.   to provide palliative care
   d.   for patients and families to assume responsibility for the care

8.33   The purpose of the Cancer Patient Education Network is to:
   a.   create a database that is readily accessible to cancer patients through any local or regional ACS office, with the eventual goal of database access from any clinic or physician's office in the United States
   b.   improve communication among health care professionals on cancer education needs and advances
   c.   provide an outreach program from a variety of local or regional offices to serve as a catalyst for cancer education initiatives in these regions and for providing technical assistance for activities related to those initiatives
   d.   a and c

Staff

8.34   A student nurse you know is about to perform her first breast exam on a patient. You know she is using proper technique when she tells you:
   a.   "I should palpate the normal breast first."
   b.   "It is important to press firmly to detect subtle differences beneath the cutaneous layers."
   c.   "After the patient is supine, I will start at the armpit and palpate in increasingly small circles, slowly moving in toward the center and finishing at the nipple area."
   d.   "The patient can have the examination in an upright position if she is more comfortable."

8.35   In planning a staff education program, which of the following would *least likely* be considered critical to the principles of adult learning?
   a.   Adults are independent learners.
   b.   An adult's past experiences may be a hindrance to learning.
   c.   An adult's readiness to learn comes from life's developmental stages.
   d.   Adult learning is task- or problem-oriented.

8.36   *Homebound* is defined as:
   a.   being able to leave one's home only with great difficulty
   b.   being confined to a wheelchair
   c.   requiring home care for over 35 hours per week
   d.   requiring intermittent care

8.37   The *best* teaching approach to enable the cancer nurse to keep up with the changing health care environment, treatment modalities, and the nurse's numerous roles and responsibilities is:
   a.   didactic lecture
   b.   hospital training with minimal lecture
   c.   self-directed learning
   d.   structured, inflexible coursework

LEGAL ISSUES

8.38 What responsibilities should be carried out only by oncology nurses as opposed to assistive personnel?
   a. measuring intake and output
   b. measuring vital signs
   c. extravasation assessment and management
   d. a and c

8.39 If Ann is guilty of misappropriation in the course of conducting her research, she has most likely:
   a. misused the research funds entrusted to her through a grant
   b. committed plagiarism
   c. tagged her study onto an existing protocol, rather than initiating a new project
   d. deliberately omitted facts or fabricated data and findings

8.40 Following World War II, the Nuremberg Code was established to delineate legal responsibility for patient education in the area of informed consent. Content central to this code includes *all but* which of the following?
   a. the use of voluntary consent to protect human subjects in experimentation
   b. the use of coercion as deemed necessary to provide quality care
   c. the individual is capable of providing consent
   d. an understanding of the risks and benefits

8.41 Which of the following organizations have developed specific requirements for cancer patient education, with responsibilities assigned to nurses and other health professionals?
   a. the Joint Commission for the Accreditation of Healthcare Organizations
   b. the Health Care Financing Administration (HCFA)
   c. the Association of Community Cancer Centers
   d. all of the above

ETHICAL ISSUES

8.42 Which of the following have been identified by the Oncology Nursing Society Ethics Advisory Council as the two most important ethical issues to be addressed?
   a. advanced directives and end-of-life care
   b. assisted suicide and end-of-life decisions
   c. assisted suicide and pain management
   d. pain management and end-of-life care

8.43 The Ethical Workup Guide states that health caregivers should:
   a. construct an exhaustive list of possibilities and relevant ethical issues
   b. take a position on ethical theory
   c. decide on an ethically based course of action for a patient
   d. make decisions based on more than one ethical value

8.44 Euthanasia involves one individual making judgments about the value of another person's life. Which of the following should a responsible individual *not* consider?
  a. the objective evaluation of interventions
  b. the outcomes on the well-being of the patient
  c. the economic consequences of prolonging the patient's life
  d. the subjective quality-of-life judgments

8.45 The Ethics Advisory Council of the Oncology Nursing Society has identified five core values for applying the ANA's Code for Nurses. Which of the following is *not* among the ONS's five core values for nurses?
  a. respectful care
  b. quality of care
  c. end-of-life issues
  d. fairness

PATIENT ADVOCACY

8.46 The Patient Self-Determination Act (PSDA) was passed by the United States Congress in 1990. This act requires that all health care institutions do which of the following?
  a. ensure health care to all regardless of ability to pay
  b. provide all patients with written information regarding informed consent
  c. provide written information regarding financial obligations
  d. provide written information about advanced directives

8.47 Which of the following statements concerning advanced directives (AD) is *false*?
  a. An AD is a statement made by a competent person that directs their medical care in the event that they become incompetent.
  b. ADs do not address all possible medical situations, only terminal conditions due to illness or injury.
  c. An AD is a legally binding contract.
  d. A directive may not always be honored due to the inability of medicine to determine the terminality of the patient's condition.

8.48 The primary goal of the Patient Self-Determination Act is to:
  a. facilitate a systematic process of eliciting and honoring patient wishes
  b. control health care costs in the last 6 months of life
  c. require health care institutions to notify patients on admission of their rights under the law to execute an advance directive
  d. facilitate a responsible use of technological intervention

8.49 A patient makes some comments about a living will that lead you to conclude that the patient needs more information. You know that he understands what a living will is when he says it:
  a. specifies disbursement of assets
  b. addresses all possible medical situations
  c. may not always be honored and implemented
  d. all of the above

QUALITY ASSURANCE

8.50   As we increase the quality of any service while maintaining costs, we:
   a.   decrease its value
   b.   lose profitability
   c.   increase the value
   d.   none of the above

8.51   Critical paths consist of:
   a.   emergency oncological care based on triage followed by categorization and individual-
        ized treatment plans
   b.   methods used to resolve oncology care problems through critical thinking
   c.   a series of interventions designed to attain specific patient outcomes for a defined group
        of patients within a specific time frame
   d.   all of the above

8.52   Guidelines for handling antineoplastic agents in the home are in accordance with those
        established by:
   a.   the Food and Drug Administration
   b.   the Occupational Safety and Health Administration
   c.   the American Nurses Association
   d.   the Health Care Financing Administration

8.53   Accurate and timely documentation is crucial to the solvency of a home care agency because
        it is required for:
   a.   reimbursement
   b.   continued referrals
   c.   medical consultations
   d.   access to hospital records

PROFESSIONAL DEVELOPMENT

8.54   Terrence is an oncology advanced practice nurse (OAPN) who chooses to work as a consul-
        tant rather than as a direct care provider. The OAPN in secondary care may be involved in
        any of the following *except:*
   a.   discussing the treatment plan and expected outcomes with the patients and family
   b.   planning and implementing initiatives aimed at patient and family education and
        support
   c.   pain and symptom management
   d.   establishing standards for oncology practice and developing critical pathways

8.55   Primary nursing is a model for:
   a.   promoting health in general or preventing the occurrence of diseases or injuries
   b.   the first level of contact of individuals, the family, and the community with the health
        system
   c.   recognizing patient and family as the unit of care and improving continuity of care
        between settings and specialties
   d.   none of the above

8.56   In the nurse's planning of home care, which of the following measures is most important?
  a.   scheduling extra visits during the working stage
  b.   avoiding upsetting the family by discussing possible emergency situations
  c.   waiting until discharge to order materials and supplies
  d.   being realistic about expected outcomes

8.57   Faculty consultation in clinical settings, faculty-clinical staff research projects, and faculty-clinical staff manuscript preparation are all examples of efforts to:
  a.   identify new research topics
  b.   maintain faculty clinical competence
  c.   increase academic and hospital revenue
  d.   recruit students

8.58   Which of the following is *not* required for use of the designation "oncology certified nurse" (OCN)?
  a.   a minimum of 1 year experience as an RN within the last 3 years
  b.   a baccalaureate degree with credits toward a master's degree
  c.   a minimum of 1000 hours of cancer nursing practice within the last $2^1/2$ years
  d.   a passing score on the ONCC certification examination

MULTIDISCIPLINARY COLLABORATION

8.59   Ambulatory oncology services have increased over the past few years for all of the following reasons *except:*
  a.   economic pressures
  b.   developments in cancer treatment
  c.   innovation in cancer technology
  d.   decreased patient acuity

8.60   The hospital in your community approaches a number of physicians and meets with them, campaigning to form a contractual relationship to increase the opportunity to obtain managed-care contracts and align the organizational structure with the financial incentives found in capitation. Such an arrangement is referred to as a:
  a.   physician-hospital organization
  b.   preferred provider organization
  c.   health maintenance organization
  d.   none of the above

8.61   A Chicago PHO is organized into an integrated delivery system that uses different sites in the community to provide a wide variety of services. This is referred to as:
  a.   vertical integration
  b.   horizontal integration
  c.   depth of services
  d.   none of the above

8.62   Karen is an NP working in a collaborative practice. In general, in a collaborative practice, which of the following is *not* true?
  a.   NPs function independently in caring for a caseload of patients in the ambulatory setting.
  b.   NPs function independently in caring for a caseload of patients in the acute care setting.
  c.   The skills of the provider are matched with the needs of the patient.
  d.   all of the above

8 PROFESSIONAL PERFORMANCE

8.63   You are working in an oncology center that has just hired unlicensed assistive personnel (UAPs). It is your responsibility to determine the basic guidelines for use of UAPs. You establish that UAPs may provide:
   a. treatment assessment
   b. direct patient care
   c. symptom management planning
   d. all of the above

ANSWER EXPLANATIONS

8.1   **The answer is d.** All of these are part of the nursing role as defined by the ONS, as well as describing pain, identifying aggravating and relieving factors, determining individuals' definitions of optimal pain relief, and evaluating efficacy of interventions.

8.2   **The answer is a.** The Oncology Nursing Society (ONS) endorses the title *advanced practice nurse* (APN) to designate clinical nurse specialist (CNS) and nurse practitioner (NP) roles in oncology nursing. The ONS notes that the term *advanced practice nurse* does not imply the merger of the CNS and NP roles, nor does it exclude other master's-prepared nurses in education, administration, or research roles.

8.3   **The answer is a.** The ONS has been promoting excellence in oncology nursing by setting standards, studying ways to improve oncology nursing, encouraging nurses to specialize in oncology nursing, and fostering the professional development of oncology nurses. In addition, the Education Committee of the ONS has been active over the years in developing standards of education that have had significant impact on cancer nursing education.

8.4   **The answer is c.** Central to cancer nursing practice is the individual-family concept. The health-illness concept is the adaptation of the individual and family along a continuum. The practice of cancer nursing occurs in the health care system. The community-environment concept provides the resources and support necessary for individuals with cancer.

8.5   **The answer is b.** Cancer nursing is practiced by both nursing generalists and nursing specialists. Nursing generalists have conceptual knowledge and skills acquired through basic nursing education, clinical experience, and professional development and updated through continuing education. They meet the concerns of individuals with cancer and provide care in a variety of health care settings. Nursing specialists have substantial theoretical knowledge gained through preparation for a master's degree. They meet diversified concerns of cancer patients and their families and function in a broader scope of practice.

8.6   **The answer is c.** The purpose of the standards is to provide guidelines to plan and evaluate generalist education, advanced education, and continuing education programs at all levels. It is also to assess individual knowledge of oncology nursing care. The purpose is to provide guidelines for evaluation, but not to certify.

8.7   **The answer is b.** Nurses are not required to have CEUs to take the exam.

8.8   **The answer is a.** Nurses do not need to be certified in oncology nursing prior to taking the advanced certification exam.

8.9   **The answer is c.** The Health Belief Model is based on several simple principles. The individ-ual must perceive a threat, and feel susceptible to the threat. The behavior change or an action taken will be beneficial in reducing the severity or the susceptibility to the threat.

8.10   **The answer is d.** To assist patients in making decisions about how to respond to the acknowledged threat, in this case pain control, the patient must come to believe that possi-ble actions are of value. The patient needs to be able to weigh the benefits of the actions compared with the barriers. Are the potential benefits of treatment likely to be of greater value than the disadvantages? Patient education must address the issue of efficacy, that the patient believes he or she can accomplish the actions required to undertake treatment.

8.11   **The answer is d.** Postmarketing or phase IV studies are usually designed to answer questions regarding other uses, doses, and schedules, as well as new information regarding risks and toxicity of a new treatment.

8.12   **The answer is c.** The BCPT tested tamoxifen as a chemopreventive agent in a randomized, double-blind trial.

8.13   **The answer is d.** The optimal treatment plan from the physician's point of view is to enter the patient in an existing clinical trial, if one fits the patient's stage of disease and he or she is eligible and willing. If this is not an option, conventional or standard regimens that have been studied extensively are widely accepted for common cancers. If no conventional pro-gram is appropriate, the physician usually tries to find a study in the literature that docu-ments a successful treatment program. Abstracts (synopses of oral presentations) are less detailed and thus less helpful. If all else fails, the physician develops a protocol specific to the situation.

8.14   **The answer is c.** A major barrier for both patients and institutions to participation in national studies is that third-party payers often do not cover experimental treatment, which includes all research trials. Trials sponsored by drug companies generally do not pose a finan-cial concern for oncology programs. The NCI clearly is committed to research to prevent cancer as well as to improve the quality of life for those who develop cancer.

8.15   **The answer is b.** In phase I trials, dosing starts at 10% of the LD_{10} determined in mice and is escalated until significant toxicity is seen in 50% or more of the patients treated. This dose is the MTD, and one step below the MTD is the dosage used for phase II testing.

8.16   **The answer is b.** Two major barriers that have been identified are ethnic minorities' distrust of outsiders doing research in their communities (often referred to as "white-run research") and the lack of culturally sensitive and specific educational materials.

8.17   **The answer is d.** Two synonyms for reliability are repeatability and consistency. Repeatabil-ity is the extent to which a measure, applied two different times (test-retest) or in two dif-ferent ways (alternative form and inter-rater), produces the same score. Consistency is the the homogeneity of the items of a scale. Reliability is not a fixed property of measure, and it cannot be assumed to be generalizable.

8.18   **The answer is b.** Content validity includes both face validity (the degree to which the scale superficially appears to measure the construct in question) and true content validity (the degree to which the items accurately represent the range of attributes covered by the con-struct). Content validity does not include statistical evidence to support inferences made from tests, but it should cut across at least three broad domains (e.g., the physical, psycho-logical, and social) to be considered valid from the perspective of item content.

8.19   **The answer is c.** The QLI is probably the best example of a "cancer-specific" scale that in reality measures generic health concepts. It was originally a physician-rated scale of five areas of functioning (activity, daily living, health, support, and outlook). It has been shown to distinguish cancer patients with terminal illness from those with recent disease or active treatment, as was once popularly assumed.

8.20   **The answer is a.** The degree to which a scale superficially appears to measure the construct in question is referred to as face validity. The degree to which the items accurately represent the range of attributes covered by the construct is called true content validity. Criterion validity includes both concurrent and predictive validity: data collected simultaneously with the scale data provide evidence of concurrent validity. Data collected after the scale data provide evidence for predictive validity. Construct validity extends criterion validity to test the scale in question against a theoretical model and adjusts it according to results to help refine theory.

8.21   **The answer is d.** Pilot studies are useful to assess the feasibility of a research design; to pretest an instrument; and to evaluate the risk, side effects, and compliance with a new nursing management approach.

8.22   **The answer is a.** In the development of patient education materials and resources, pretesting is used primarily in the following phases: planning and strategy selection; selecting processes and materials; and developing materials and pretests.

8.23   **The answer is b.** One aspect of printed patient educational materials that has received considerable attention in the nursing literature is reading level. It is estimated that 20% of Americans read below the fifth-grade level. A fifth-grade reading level has been identified as the minimum reading level for making good use of basic written material.

8.24   **The answer is c.**

8.25   **The answer is d.** Self-care teaching and written guidelines for patients and families about care of venous access lines, administration of parenteral fluids, and symptom management are critical to effective management of patients in an ambulatory environment.

8.26   **The answer is d.** Family units can be identified as supportive, hostile, or ambivalent and their behavior described in terms of cohesion, adaptability, and communication. When crisis occurs or families face the serious and difficult implications of cancer and its treatment, their behavior usually does not change and in some cases can intensify. Therefore, if a family was dysfunctional, hostile, or in conflict before a cancer diagnosis, it is very likely that the behavior will continue. The home health care nurse's primary concern is to support and care for the patient. The chances are high that the home health care nurse would be unable to change the behavior of the family members in conflict.

8.27   **The answer is a.** The hospice team's goal is to help the family prepare for their loved one's death. Families need to be prepared for the actual time of the patient's death and what universal signs they can anticipate. Increasing sleep, a gradual decrease in need for food and drink, increased confusion or restlessness, decreasing temperature of extremities, and irregular breathing patterns may occur. Calling the oncologist indicates the need for intervention, when in fact the goal of care is purely palliative. The pain-relief regimen should not be altered if the patient is comfortable, even if the patient is sleeping more and death is approaching.

8.28   **The answer is a.** It is estimated that 20% of Americans read below the fifth-grade level and that almost half read at the low literacy level. Sixth-grade readability is the typical standard for public education materials aimed at a broad audience.

8.29   **The answer is d.** The NCCS focuses on a wide range of issues related to quality of life for cancer survivors and their families.

8.30   **The answer is a.** A critical public health message is to note that the use of smokeless tobacco increased significantly during the 1970s because it was promoted as a "safe" alternative to smoking. The group of tobacco users changed from men over 50 years of age and older women living in the South to white, male adolescents and young adults in the age range of 14–29 years.

8.31   **The answer is d.** In a proper BSE, the woman should stand in front of the mirror, noting the size, shape, and symmetry of her breasts. She should examine herself with her arms relaxed at her side, with her hands pressed on her hips, and with her arms overhead, but not with her arms folded behind her.

8.32   **The answer is d.** Although home care does consist of holistic and direct physical care, the ultimate goal is to enable the family and/or patient to provide the care. Choices **b** and **c** apply more to hospice care and not necessarily to home care. The patient and family are encouraged to assume responsibility for the care of the patient.

8.33   **The answer is b.** The purpose of the Cancer Patient Education Network is to improve communication among health care professionals regarding cancer education needs and advances.

8.34   **The answer is a.** The examiner should palpate the normal breast first. It is important to press very lightly (not firmly) and gently to detect subtle differences. When the patient is supine, the examiner starts at the areolar area and palpates in increasingly wider concentric circles. Finally, the patient is to be in a supine position.

8.35   **The answer is b.** Adults' past experiences are resources for learning and should be drawn on to enhance the learning process. Self-images are often defined, at least in part, by adults' past experiences, and they have a deep investment in their value.

8.36   **The answer is a.** The homebound status is necessary for insurance and Medicare coverage, and it has to be established and documented by the health care nurse. Homebound means that leaving the home requires considerable effort.

8.37   **The answer is c.** Adult learning concepts, including problem-centered approaches to teaching, immediate application of knowledge, recognition of individual experience, flexible scheduling, and self-directed learning, must be incorporated into educational offerings.

8.38   **The answer is c.** Although patient care activities, such as taking vital signs and measuring intake and output, may be delegated to assistive personnel when the patient is stable, certain nursing care functions, such as extravasation assessment and management, should be performed by oncology registered nurses and should not be delegated to assistive personnel.

8.39   **The answer is b.** Misappropriation refers to an intentional or reckless act of plagiarism or a violation of the confidentiality associated with the review of scientific manuscripts or grants.

8.40   **The answer is b.** Central to this code is the use of voluntary consent to protect human subjects in experimentation. Such consent assumes not only the ability to consent and freedom from coercion, but also that there is an understanding of the risks and benefits and that the subject is giving an informed consent.

8.41 **The answer is d.** In addition to legal obligations for patient education, a variety of accreditation or other certifying standards address specific requirements for patient education, with responsibilities assigned to nurses and other health professionals. In 1993, the JCAHO reorganized its standards for accreditation to bring stronger focus to the area of patient and family education. Other agencies and organizations have joined this call for patient education as an integral part.

8.42 **The answer is b.** Assisted suicide and end-of-life decisions were identified as the two most important ethical issues by the Oncology Nursing Society Ethics Advisory Council and by 900 nurses surveyed by the ANA.

8.43 **The answer is c.** The Ethical Workup Guide requires caregivers to plan an ethically justifiable course of action for their patient. They can use one or more of the ethical values in their decision.

8.44 **The answer is c.** It is important to distinguish between objective evaluation of interventions and outcomes on the well-being of the patient and subjective quality-of-life judgments in which the physician and other caregivers deem that the life the patient is now living is not worthwhile for that person.

8.45 **The answer is c.** The ONS's five core values of respectful care, quality of life, competence, collegiality, and fairness speak from the shared experience of oncology nurses and provide a context for applying the Code for Nurses in oncology nursing practice.

8.46 **The answer is d.** PSDA requires that all health care institutions receiving Medicare or Medicaid reimbursement ask the patients they admit if they have an advance directive. If patients do not, the institution is obligated to provide written information about such directives.

8.47 **The answer is c.** An AD is a one-person statement, not a legally binding contract.

8.48 **The answer is c.** The Patient Self-Determination Act may also serve to control health care costs in the last 6 months of life and to facilitate a responsible use of technological intervention. However, these are not the primary goals of the act. The act does not necessarily facilitate a systematic process of eliciting and honoring patient wishes.

8.49 **The answer is c.** Patients can become confused about what a living will is. It does not specify disbursement of assets. It does not address all possible medical situations. The words "artificial" and "extraordinary" are often used in an AD; however, these words can be interpreted differently. A directive may not always be honored and implemented. An AD is a one-person statement, and not a legally binding contract.

8.50 **The answer is c.** As we increase the quality of any service while maintaining costs, we increase the value.

8.51 **The answer is c.** Critical paths consist of a series of interventions specific to a group of patients with common attributes that are designed to promote the attainment of specific patient outcomes within a specific time frame.

8.52 **The answer is b.** Potential hazards associated with the administration of antineoplastic agents have prompted the Occupational Safety and Health Administration (OSHA) to set guidelines for compounding, transporting, administering, and disposing of toxic chemotherapy agents.

8.53   **The answer is a.** Accurate, descriptive documentation of home health nursing care is vital to reimbursement and continuation of home health services. It has been postulated that the rise in health care expenditures, including those for home health care, has led the government and fiscal intermediaries to enact regulations requiring specific documentation and has increased focused review in an effort to decrease costs by denial of payment for services designated by the reviewer as "noncovered."

8.54   **The answer is a.** As a consultant, the OAPN in secondary care is involved in planning and implementing initiatives aimed at patient and family education and support. The OAPN's expertise is also utilized in symptom management, and OAPNs are often important members of multidisciplinary pain and symptom management teams. They also may act as consultants to an institution in establishing standards for oncology practice and developing critical pathways.

8.55   **The answer is c.** Primary nursing is a model for nursing care delivery designed to improve quality, recognize patient and family as the unit of care, improve coordination of care between specialties, and ensure continuity of care between settings. Primary prevention includes activities that either promote health in general or prevent the occurrence of diseases or injuries. A primary health care model constitutes the first level of contact of individuals, the family, and the community with the health system.

8.56   **The answer is d.** Evaluation of care is based on patient outcomes. Potential limitations must be considered when outcome measures are used. Expected outcomes should be realistic and achievable so that the patient, caregiver(s), and health care providers feel a sense of satisfaction and accomplishment. The family should know what is realistic and achievable from the start. Choice **b** is a serious problem—families are better off when they know how to deal with emergencies.

8.57   **The answer is b.** Faculty need to be prepared in oncology nursing and need to be both knowledgeable in the latest trends and clinically competent. In addition to joint appointments, new and different ways to ensure competence must be explored.

8.58   **The answer is b.** The Oncology Nursing Certification Corporation (ONCC) administers a certification program for cancer nurses. A certification examination is offered twice yearly. Nurses with an RN license, 1 year experience as a registered nurse within the last 3 years, and a minimum of 1000 hours of cancer nursing practice within the last $2^1/2$ years are eligible to take this examination.

8.59   **The answer is d.** Advances in cancer treatment and technology, the influences of economics, and quality-of-life issues have promoted ambulatory services as a method for providing cancer patient and family care. With shortened hospitalizations driven by reimbursement changes, patients are being discharged quicker and sicker; therefore, the patient acuity is actually higher.

8.60   **The answer is a.** In a PHO, a contractual relationship between physicians and the hospital accomplishes several goals: it increases the opportunity to obtain managed-care contracts, aligns the organizational structure with the financial incentives found in capitation, and measures quality of care through outcomes.

8.61   **The answer is b.** Horizontal integration occurs when a PHO is organized into an integrated delivery system that uses different sites in the community to provide a wide variety of services. With vertical integration, these services are capable of being provided within the same system. Vertical integration is sometimes referred to as depth of services, and horizontal integration, as breadth of services.

8.62   **The answer is d.** In a collaborative practice, NPs function independently in caring for a caseload of patients, whether in the ambulatory or the acute care setting. Care is provided based on competence: the skills of the provider are matched with the needs of the patient.

8.63   **The answer is b.** UAPs may provide direct patient care. They should not be used in those situations in which the patient's disease or response is unpredictable or in which specialized knowledge or skills are needed, such as chemotherapy, pain management, symptom management plans, toxicity grading, and unstable patient assessment.

STUDY NOTES

STUDY NOTES